W0245852

Endocrine Autoimmunity and Associated Conditions

Immunology and Medicine Series

VOLUME 27

Series Editors:

Dr. Graham Bird, *Churchill Hospital, Oxford, UK*
Professor Keith Whaley, *University of Leicester, Leicester, UK*

A list of titles in the series can be found at the end of this volume.

Endocrine Autoimmunity and Associated Conditions

Edited by

A. P. Weetman
Clinical Sciences Centre, University of Sheffield, Sheffield, UK

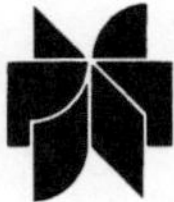

SPRINGER-SCIENCE+BUSINESS MEDIA, B.V.

Library of Congress Cataloging-in-Publication Data is available.

ISBN 978-94-010-6118-6 ISBN 978-94-011-5044-6 (eBook)
DOI 10.1007/978-94-011-5044-6

Printed on acid-free paper

Contents

Preface

Endocrine autoimmunity is the archetype for autoimmune disorders in general. In the four decades since autoimmunity was postulated as the aetiological mechanism in experimental and human autoimmune thyroiditis, there has been a continual development of this idea, not only to encompass conditions affecting other endocrine tissues, but also to identify the exact immunological processes involved. We now know far more about the genetic and environmental susceptibility factors in endocrine autoimmunity and have a detailed molecular knowledge of the interactions occurring within the target organs. As part of the shared immunogenetic predisposition, these disorders occur together more frequently than expected by chance (the autoimmune polyglandular syndromes) and the endocrinopathies in these syndromes are also associated with other autoimmune diseases, in particular pernicious anaemia and vitiligo. While most books on endocrine autoimmunity have tended to ignore these associated disorders, they are so frequent that this book includes a discussion of their pathogenesis. The overall purpose of the book is to present recent advances in our understanding of the immunology of endocrine autoimmunity which will be of interest to immunologists, endocrinologists and general physicians.

The two major autoimmune endocrine disorders are thyroid disease and type 1 diabetes mellitus. Chapter 1 provides an introduction to autoimmune thyroid disease by considering the various animal models of autoimmune thyroiditis and their relation to the human condition. Clearly, such studies have had a fundamental impact on our understanding of disease pathogenesis. Perhaps the major development over the last decade has come from the identification of target autoantigens. In the case of the thyroid these are now well characterized and considered in detail in Chapter 2. The next three chapters concern the three major disorders of thyroid function caused by autoimmunity, namely autoimmune hypothyroidism (Chapter 3), Graves' disease (Chapter 4) and postpartum thyroiditis (Chapter 5). Each of these chapters considers predisposing susceptibility factors, the role of autoantibodies and pathogenic mechanisms. A frequent accompaniment of autoimmune thyroid disease, especially Graves' disease, is thyroid-associated ophthalmopathy. This is perhaps the most difficult management problem for a thyroidologist, and new approaches to treatment will only come from improvements in our understanding of disease mechanisms. These are considered in detail in Chapter 6.

The second major autoimmune endocrinopathy is type 1 diabetes mellitus. Once again there have been major advances in our understanding of the nature of β cell autoantigens and these are detailed in Chapter 7. Chapter 8 contains a comprehensive review of animal and human type 1 diabetes in terms of pathogenesis.

Other endocrine tissues are less frequently the target of autoimmunity and these are considered in the next three chapters. Chapter 9 considers autoimmune Addison's disease and its relation to the polyglandular autoimmunity syndromes. Although rare, Addison's disease is a serious condition where, once again, molecular techniques have had a huge impact in identifying the target autoantigens. Less is known about the role of autoimmunity in premature ovarian failure, a frequent condition likely to be due to a number of different aetiologies, of which autoimmunity is only one. Chapter 10 contains a detailed overview of the clinical background to premature ovarian failure and the evidence that autoimmunity plays a role, in at least some of these cases. Although the pituitary is the master controller of the endocrine system, and therefore of crucial importance to normal endocrine function, autoimmunity seems to affect this gland rarely. A detailed survey of pituitary autoimmunity is provided in Chapter 11.

Finally, as already stated, Chapters 12 and 13 consider pernicious anaemia and vitiligo in detail. Both of these are frequent accompaniments of autoimmune endocrinopathies and recent advances in the understanding of the pathogenesis of these two diseases has matched that of the classical endocrinopathies.

As well as the authors of these chapters, I would also like to thank Mrs Kathryn Watson for her excellent secretarial help in Sheffield and to all at Kluwer for their assistance in producing this book.

Tony Weetman, Sheffield
January 1998

Series Editor's Note

Over the last 30 years there has been a continuing and exponential increase in the understanding of basic immunology mechanisms and their application to the practice of medicine. The aim of this series is to provide a comprehensive and up-to-date review of the scientific basis and clinical relevance of a variety of immunologically-based diseases. The series, producing three new volumes a year, will cover the majority of specialist areas of medicine with diseases of immunological importance and over a four-year cycle will aim continuously to update knowledge and experience in the individual specialist areas. The series is designed for the general or specialist physician or the clinical scientist with an interest in clinical or related problems. We intend to provide in single volumes a synthesis of information which is otherwise difficult to assemble from original papers which are often produced in a variety of specialist medical and immunological journals.

G. Bird and K. Whaley

List of Contributors

J. N. ANASTI
Program Director OB/GYN
St. Lukes Hospital, 801 Ostrum Street
Bethlehem, PA 18015
USA

J. F. BACH
Immunologie Clinique Hôpital Necker
Hôpital Necker
161 rue de Sèvres
75743 Paris Cedex 15
France

R. S. BAHN
Division of Endocrinology
Mayo Clinic
Rochester, MN 55905
USA

J.-P. BANGA
Department of Medicine
King's College School of Medicine and Dentistry
Bessemer Road
London, SE5 9PJ
UK

J. S. BEVAN
Department of Endocrinology
Aberdeen Royal Infirmary
Foresterhill
Aberdeen, AB25 2ZN
UK

P. BURMAN
Department of Medicine
University Hospital
S-751 85 Uppsala
Sweden

R.M. CUDDIHY
Division of Endocrinology
Mayo Clinic
Rochester, MN 55905
USA

D. J. GAWKRODGER
Department of Dermatology
University of Sheffield
Royal Hallamshire Hospital
Sheffield, S10 2JF
UK

F. A. KARLSSON
Department of Medicine
University Hospital
S-751 85 Uppsala
Sweden

Y. M. KONG
Department of Immunology and Microbiology
Wayne State University School of Medicine
Detroit, MI 48201
USA

K. J. E. KROHN
Institute of Medical Technology
University of Tampere
Fin-33101 Tampere
Finland

L. D. K. E. PREMAWARDHANA
Department of Medicine
University of Wales College of Medicine
Heath Park
Cardiff, CF64 2XX
UK

J. H. LAZARUS
Department of Medicine
University of Wales College of Medicine
Heath Park
Cardiff, CF64 2XX
UK

Å. LERNMARK
University of Washington
Department of Medicine
Robert H. Williams Laboratory
1959 Pacific Avenue
Seattle, WA 98195-7710
USA

M. LUDGATE
Department of Medicine
University of Wales College of Medicine
Heath Park
Cardiff, CF64 2XX
UK

J.-Y. MA
Department of Medicine
University Hospital
S-751 85 Uppsala
Sweden

A. M. McGREGOR
Department of Medicine
King's College School of Medicine and Dentistry
Bessemer Road
London, SE5 9PJ
UK

R. S. McINTOSH
Department of Medicine
Clinical Sciences Centre
Northern General Hospital
Sheffield, S5 7AU
UK

A. B. PARKES
Department of Medicine
University of Wales College of Medicine
Heath Park
Cardiff, CF64 2XX
UK

P. PETERSON
Institute of Medical Technology
University of Tampere
Fin-33101 Tampere
Finland

A. PLESNER
University of Washington
Department of Medicine
Robert H. Williams Laboratory
1959 Pacific Avenue
Seattle, WA 98195-7710
USA

H. A. SAWERS
Department of Endocrinology
Aberdeen Royal Infirmary
Foresterhill
Aberdeen, AB25 2ZN
UK

R. UIBO
Institute of General and Molecular Pathology
University of Tartu
Tartu, EE2400
Estonia

P. F. WATSON
Department of Medicine
Clinical Sciences Centre
Northern General Hospital
Sheffield, S5 7AU
UK

A. P. WEETMAN
Department of Medicine
Clinical Sciences Centre
University of Sheffield
Northern General Hospital
Sheffield, S5 7AU
UK

1
Animal models of autoimmune thyroiditis: recent advances

Y. M. KONG

INTRODUCTION

Since the last review in this series in 1986, which focused on the induced model of murine experimental autoimmune thyroiditis (EAT) for Hashimoto's thyroidities (HT) [1], there have been major advances in our understanding of the pathogenic and regulatory mechanisms in autoimmune thyroid disease. These advances have stemmed from new knowledge at the cellular and molecular level of T cell development and interactions with other cell types, and techniques applied to gene cloning and sequencing of thyroid autoantigens. In the interim 10 years, there have been several extensive reviews on EAT induced with thyroid antigens, usually thyroglobulin (TG), and spontaneous autoimmune thyroiditis (SAT), arising from selective breeding in chicken and in rodent colonies exhibiting autoimmune diabetes [2–8]. Some recent papers also correlated findings between both animal and human autoimmune thyroid disease [4–6]. This review will concentrate on studies in the last 6–7 years, primarily in the mouse and rat, where major developments have advanced our understanding of autoimmune diseases.

GENETIC FACTORS CONTROLLING SUSCEPTIBILITY

Major histocompatibility complex (MHC) class II genes

One major advance in immunology has been the increased understanding of the significant role of MHC class II and class I genes in influencing the respective selection and/or deletion of $CD4^+$ and $CD8^+$ T cell subsets during ontogeny,

A.P. Weetman (ed.), Endocrine Autoimmunity and Associated Conditions. 1–23.

thereby shaping the T cell receptor (TCR) repertoire [9]. Thus, the early immunogenetic studies in congenic, recombinant strains within the murine MHC (H2) also correlate with specific selection of the autoreactive TCR repertoire. Genetic susceptibility, as defined by mononuclear cell infiltrates in the thyroid and T cell proliferative response to TG, but not the universal autoantibody production, was mapped to the class II H2A region of $H2^{k,s}$ and not $H2^{b,d,f}$ strains [reviewed in Reference 1]. Susceptibility is unaltered by the mammalian source of TG chosen for immunization, the adjuvant applied or when only mouse (M) TG in multiple doses is used. It should be noted, however, that MTG generally induces more severe thyroid inflammation than heterologous TGs, partly because MTG has unique thyroiditogenic epitope(s) stimulating the autoreactive T cells in mice, in addition to conserved epitopes shared with heterologous TGs. The use of congenic strains in the rat has also shown $RT.1^c$ strain to be susceptible and $RT.1^u$ to be resistant [10]. In SAT, breeding between the BUF ($RT.1^b$) and BB/Wor ($RT.1^u$) rat, a diabetes model, has linked SAT to $RT.1^b$, dissociating it from pancreatic insulitis under $RT.1^u$ influence [11]. The role of H2E, the other murine class II region, is less clear; susceptible k strains express H2E molecules while similarly susceptible s strains do not. H2E molecules are known to participate in shaping the TCR Vβ gene repertoire in conjunction with MMTV (murine mammary tumour virus; also known as mls) superantigen expression [12].

The extent of class II gene regulation is driven home by the selective use of transgenic models provided with murine or human (H) MHC (HLA) class II transgenes. When we introduced H2AaAb transgene from susceptible k haplotype into resistant B10.M ($H2^f$) mice which express only endogenous H2A but not H2E molecules, severe thyroiditis involving up to 80% of the gland was observed in Aa^kAb^{k+} mice, compared with none to moderate inflammation in Aa^kAb^{k-} sibs [13]. Susceptibility was likewise acquired after the introduction of HLA-DRB1*0301 (DR3) transgene into B10.M mice [14]. Similar to EAT-susceptible strains, thyroid inflammation was observed after either MTG or HTG immunization. Since endogenous $H2^f$ molecules were also present, it appears that resistance in B10.M mice is due more to the absence of appropriate class II molecules for clonal selection than to the stimulation of regulatory T cell subset suppressing EAT induction.

To define the precise role of DR3 molecules in the absence of H2 molecules, we introduced the DR3 transgene into class II-negative $H2Ab^0$ mice. Both MTG and HTG immunization induced moderate to severe thyroiditis in $DR3^+$ mice [14]. The responsiveness to MTG was specific for DR3 molecules, since the introduction of HLA-DRB1*1502 (DR2) β-chain transgene, in conjunction with an Ea^k transgene to aid DR2 expression, into Ab^o mice resulted in essentially negative response (Table 1.1); in contrast to $DR3^+$ mice, most $DR2^+$ mice did not exhibit thyroiditis and anti-MTG titres were negligible (at 1:800 dilution). This allelic specificity demonstrates that HLA polymorphism is a determinant in EAT susceptibility to MTG. It should be noted that, in the DR2 β-chain transgenic mice with the HLA-DRa homologue, Ea^k, transgene,

Table 1.1 Induction of EAT with mouse TG after HLA-DRB1*0301 (DR3) but not after HLA-DRB1*1502 (DR2) gene transfer into H2Ab^0 mice

		Thyroiditis[a]					
		No. mice with % thyroid involvement					
Transgene expression	*MTG antibody (O.D. at 1:800)*	*0*	*>0–10*	*>10–20*	*>20–40*	*>40–80*	*Incidence (%)*
$DR3^+ E^+$	0.95±0.20	–	2	2	3	2	100
$DR3^- E^+$	<0.2	6	1	–	–	–	14
$DR3^- E^-$	<0.2	6	–	–	–	–	0
$DR2^+ E^+$	0.29±0.11	7	–	–	–	–	0
$DR2^- E^+$	<0.2	5	1	–	–	–	17
$DR2^- E^-$	<0.2	7	1	–	–	–	13

[a]Mice were immunized with 40 μg MTG and 20 μg LPS i.v. 3 h later on days 0 and 7, and were killed on day 28

H2E ($E\alpha^k E\beta^b$) molecules may also be expressed. Although it is clear that both $DR3^-E^+$ and $DR2^-E^+$ mice responded very poorly to MTG immunization, H2E restriction in normal k strains have been reported in T cells responding to HTG [15] and a 17-mer TG epitope [16]. Thus, it remains to be determined whether the response to HTG is polymorphic in the same degree or if the same thyroiditogenic epitopes in the large TG molecule (660 kDa) are involved.

The DR3 molecules apparently function as regular antigen presenters *in vivo*, since the proliferative responses of T cells from MTG- and HTG-immunized $DR3^+E^-$ mice, respectively, to MTG (Figure 1.1A) and HTG (Figure 1.1B) were blocked by monoclonal antibody (mAb) to the DRβ chain. These findings support HLA-DR3 association with HT reported in some patient studies, but not in others [cited in Reference 14]. The data further implicate TG as a relevant autoantigen in the human, not just a diagnostic tool to be replaced by thyroid peroxidase (TPO). Further studies with TG or other thyroid antigens and their peptides in mice given DR- or DQ-region genes as they become available will help clarify specific MHC control in autoimmune thyroid disease without the complication of linkage disequilibium.

Bearing in mind that humans are polygenic, early studies in F_1 mice have shown that susceptibility is dominant. However, the use of lipopolysaccharide (LPS) as adjuvant rather than the stronger but non-physiological complete Freund's adjuvant (CFA), has revealed that F_1 mice develop less severe thyroiditis [1,5]. In addition to heterozygosity, human class II genes with different specificities generally co-exist. Thus, similar to other autoimmune disease models, we tested an H2Ea transgene in susceptible B10.S mice which do not express H2E molecules; the resultant E^+ B10.S mice displayed reduced thyroiditis, indicating a moderating effect due to H2E expression [13]. Indeed,

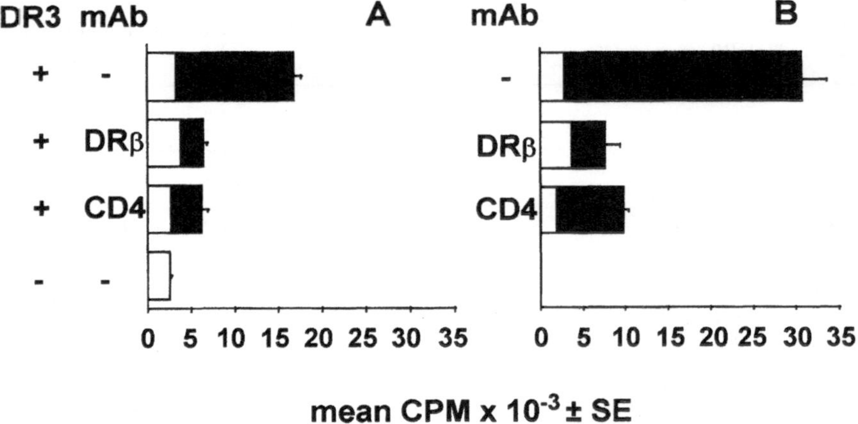

Figure 1.1 TG presentation to spleen cells from MTG-immunized or HTG-immunized mice was blocked by mAb to the HLA-DRβ chain. (**A**) Spleen cells from MTG-immunized $DR3^{+}E^{-}$ mice showing reduced proliferative response to MTG in the presence of mAb to DRβ and to mouse CD4; immunized $DR3^{-}E^{-}$ mice did not respond to MTG stimulation. (**B**) Spleen cells from HTG-immunized mice showing reduced proliferative response to HTG in the presence of mAb to DRβ and to mouse CD4. [^{3}H]Thymidine uptake was measured after 4 days in culture in the presence of mAb only (background c.p.m., open bar) or 40 μg/ml of TG plus mAb (black bar); control spleen cells were cultured without mAb or TG (open bar) or with TG (black bar)

with the availability of DNA typing and transgenic mouse models, interactions of class II genes which may result in an interplay between protective and susceptible traits in autoimmune disease are increasingly receiving investigative attention [17].

MHC class I genes

Class I genes are also involved in clonal selection and/or deletion of autoreactive $CD8^{+}$ TCR repertoire [9]. As reviewed previously [1], the use of H2K- and D-end recombinant strains has shown the D-end to play a definite role in reducing autoantibody production and/or thyroiditis. Whether the D-end is involved depends on the particular H2A/D combination and may include H2E influence in some strains [13,18]. The K-region exerts some effect on autoantibody level and incidence or severity of thyroiditis. Both K and D molecules are involved in thyroid target cell destruction by cytotoxic T cells (Tc) after MTG priming, demonstrating the importance of class I restriction at the effector/target cell level as in natural disease [19,20]. The early suggestion of genetic differences within the murine thyroid affecting susceptibility has not been corroborated by more recent studies in the rat [21].

Autoreactive TCR repertoire

As mentioned above, the autoreactive TCR repertoire is largely shaped by MHC class II and class I molecules since ontogeny, as further evidenced by class II gene transfer of susceptibility traits [13,14]. Since the large and partially sequenced MTG molecule [22] has many unidentified, unique and shared epitopes and no known immunodominant epitopes, the specific TCR gene usage cannot be determined until more thyroiditogenic TG epitopes are identified. Indeed, partly because there are a number of such epitopes on TG, there is increasing evidence that the TCR repertoire is sufficiently diverse and flexible to respond to different autoepitopes under the same MHC umbrella. EAT susceptibility to MTG is unaltered in some k or s strains despite multiple MMTV-influenced deletions (CBA) or 50% genomic deletions (SJL, C57BR) of $V\beta^+$ T cells. The plasticity of the TCR repertoire is apparent when EAT induction is unaffected by 50–70% TCR Vβ genomic deletions in congenic strains of susceptible B10.K mice [23]. Moreover, after the introduction into CBA mice of an irrelevant Vβ8.2 transgene, which represented about 76% and 90% T cells in the $CD4^+$ and $CD8^+$ subsets, respectively, EAT induction with MTG in these CBA-Vβ8.2 k/k mice was unabated [24]. On the other hand, thyroid inflammation in CBA-Vβ8.2 k/q mice was significantly reduced; the q haplotype is intermediate in EAT susceptibility. As discussed above, heterozygosity as found in polygenic man may be protective, diminishing the host's capacity to recognize multiple thyroiditogenic epitopes.

Non-MHC factors

Compared with the major influence of MHC genes, a number of non-MHC genes, many unmapped, contribute in a minor way to antibody levels, thyroiditis incidence or inflammation [1]. The dissociation between autoantibody titres and extent of thyroiditis is well documented [25], even when small (12–18mer) TG peptides are used for immunization [26–28]. Thus, sex hormones [29] and Igh V-gene complex [30] with influence primarily on anti-MTG levels have little bearing on thyroid pathology.

Studies on MTG-induced EAT in aging mice, however, show age of induction to be a crucial factor in the severity and chronicity of thyroiditis. Immunization of 2-month-old mice led to 100% incidence and more severe destruction lasting up to 18 months, compared with incidences of 60% in 6-month-old and 38% in 12-month-old animals [31]. The duration of chronic disease is also dependent upon non-MHC background genes in different strains.

Other genetic and environmental factors may also affect thyroiditis incidence and/or severity in susceptible animals [see Reference 4]. Briefly, in SAT models, the incidence in BUF rat has decreased with time and now thymectomy or immunization with rat TG in CFA is required [32], whereas intentional inbreeding resulted in the extreme manifestations of OS chicken [7,8] and a highly thyroiditis-prone line derived from the diabetic BB/Wor rat [33]. One nonobese diabetic (NOD) mouse colony has a >77% incidence of thyroiditis [34], in contrast to 10–18% in most colonies [35]. The contributing factors are unknown; diabetes in NOD mice is favoured by conditions of low microbial load, but whether this same environment affects thyroiditis in this model is unknown. In thymectomized and irradiated PVG/c rats with an altered T cell compartment, the incidence of thyroiditis is increased by orally introduced microbial flora [36]. Others have studied the effect of increased and prolonged iodine intake which appears to have a greater effect on SAT than EAT models [4,14]; its role is addressed below. Diet may also influence EAT incidence and severity in mice [37], but reduction is associated with a highly caloric breeder chow not generally in use for maintenance.

PATHOGENIC T CELL MECHANISMS

TCR Vβ gene usage

Thyroiditogenic T cells in CBA/J mice infiltrating the thyroid are mostly TCRα/β$^+$ [38]. Because CBA/J mice have about 25% Vβ8$^+$ T cells and these cells have been implicated in several autoimmune diseases, we examined their thyroiditogenicity by *in vivo* depletion or *in vitro* enrichment of Vβ8$^+$ T cells with Vβ8 mAb or the superantigen, staphylococcal enterotoxin B (SEB), prior to adoptive transfer. As shown in Table 1.2, the highly enriched Vβ8$^+$ population did not transfer thyroiditis, indicating that they are not a major player in MTG-induced EAT. These findings have recently been confirmed in the same mouse strain [39].

Examinations of the thyroidal infiltrates from HTG-immunized CBA/J mice [40] or from NOD colony with a high incidence of thyroiditis [41] have suggested biased TCR Vβ gene usage. In CBA/J mice, restricted TCR use is

Table 1.2 Noninvolvement of Vβ8$^+$ T cells in MTG-induced EAT as shown by adoptive transfer

			Thyroiditis[b]: No. mice with % thyroid involvement			
Expt.	*In vitro activator[a]*	*MTG antibody[b] (mean log^2 titre ± SE)*	*0*	*>0–10*	*>10–20*	*>20–40*
1	SEB	1.5 ± 0.3	4	–	–	–
	MTG	6.2 ± 1.8	–	–	2	2
2	F23.1	1.0 ± 0.0	5	–	–	–
	MTG	11.7 ± 0.2	–	–	1	6

Modified from Fuller *et al.* [38].

[a]Spleen cells from MTG-immunized CBA/J mice were cultured for 3 days with SEB (0.5 μg/ml), SEA (0.003 μg/ml), Vβ8 mAb (F23.1, 5 μg/ml) or MTG (20 μg/ml), and 2×10^7 viable cells were injected i.v. into normal recipients on day 0.

[b]Determined on day 14.

reflected by the clonal selection of two CDR3 motifs on thyroidal Vβ13$^+$ T cells after HTG immunization. In a subsequent study, the same motifs are observed in recipient thyroids following adoptive transfer of MTG-primed and -activated T cells [42]. Although the TG epitope driving clonal expansion of these Vβ13$^+$ T cells is unknown, the data suggest that the autoepitope is shared between HTG and MTG. Moreover, unlike SEB (Table 1.2), SEA activates MTG-primed T cells to transfer thyroiditis and the transfer population contains activated Vβ13$^+$ T cells (Qiang Wan *et al.*, unpublished data). Our identification of Vβ13 CDR3 motifs among other Vβ$^+$ T cells by adoptive transfer of MTG-primed cells is in contrast to the multiple Vβ gene usage recently observed in a similar transfer protocol [39]. In addition to our primers being different, another divergence could be our examination of individual recipient thyroids for clonal expansion rather than pooling the thyroids [39].

Composition and kinetics of thyroid-infiltrating cells

The temporal participation of CD4$^+$ and CD8$^+$ T cells at the time of EAT induction in mice and their subsequent infiltration into the thyroid during development has been followed by using two synergistic pairs of rat mAbs, each pair recognizing nonoverlapping epitopes on CD4 or CD8 molecules [43]. The early predominance of CD4$^+$ T cells in the thyroid with a CD4:CD8 ratio of 7, which declines to about 2 by day 17 [44], is corroborated by the finding that treatment with CD4 mAbs up to day 14 post-immunization interferes with EAT induction. Similarly early treatment with CD8 mAbs reduces infiltration slightly without enhancing antibody production, indicating the lack of pre-existing CD8$^+$ suppressor T cells (Ts). *In situ* analysis by immunocytochemical staining for up to 6 weeks reveals the same reduced but shifting CD4:CD8 ratio between 2.4 and 3.0 [45]. This shift in ratio reflects the increase and decline of CD8$^+$ T cells with no significant variations occurring in the CD4$^+$ subset. On day 70, total thyroidal T cells remain at about 30% with a ratio of about 2; throughout this period, macrophages are stable at 30–35%, and B cells at <2–6% [43]. Thyroid inflammation shows little change up to 18 months after immunization [31]. Similarly in rat EAT, there is a high number of CD8$^+$ T cells and few B cells [10]. In BUF SAT brought on by neonatal thymectomy, a CD4:CD8 ratio of 1 is present for several months [46].

In the adoptive transfer protocol in which CD4$^+$ T cells are preferentially expanded with MTG during the 3-day *in vitro* activation period, the total thyroidal T cells could reach 56% [47]. There is also a substantial infiltration of CD8$^+$ T cells possibly due to recruitment, resulting in a CD4:CD8 ratio of about 1.7. Cyclic changes in %CD8$^+$ T cells, similar to the active immunization protocol, are also observed. In contrast to our immunohistochemical studies cited above, a reverse CD4:CD8 ratio determined by flow cytometry of pooled thyroid suspension at a later interval after transfer has been reported [48]. These workers also observed the same reverse ratio in their granulomatous model derived by including mAb to interleukin (IL)-2 receptor or interferon (IFN)-γ during *in vitro* activation [49,50]. The differences in results could be due to different mAbs used and *in situ* analysis versus pooled suspensions at a later time point. It is clear, however, that any shift in subset ratio with time can only be observed by *in situ* analysis of sequential samples after either active immunization or adoptive transfer; the subtle differences are unlikely to be discernible in the peripheral blood leukocytes.

Effector mechanisms

A T cell-mediated disease is likely to evoke a number of mechanisms leading to damage, including the production of inflammatory cytokines [2]; the mechanisms are not mutually exclusive. $CD4^+$ T cells in induced EAT proliferate in response to signals generated by class II molecules presenting TG epitopes on macrophages and/or dendritic cells. B cells are not required for EAT induction [51], although complement-fixing antibodies could participate in damage at late stages. Anti-CD4 treatment up to 14 days after MTG immunization interferes with EAT development [43]. These $CD4^+$ T cells are also the ones responding to TG and initiating SAT after the removal of regulatory T cells. They then aid in recruiting macrophages and $CD8^+$ Tc to the thyroid by producing T_H1-type inflammatory cytokines. While it is difficult to demonstrate directly cytotoxic activity *in situ*, our initial demonstration of Tc differentiating in the presence of $CD4^+$ T cells and destroying thyroid epithelial cells in a class I-restricted manner [19] has been confirmed by a number of laboratories [20,33,52]. Both $CD4^+$ T cell clones and $CD8^+$ Tc clones from the T cell depletion model produce IL-2, IFN-γ and tumour-necrosis factor [52,53]. The reduction in thyroid pathology and a Tc phenotype after anti-IFN-γ treatment throughout EAT development in porcine (P) TG-immunized mice further shows the involvement of IFN-γ in pathogenesis [54]. Another important inflammatory cytokine for T_H1 cell activation is IL-1, which can serve as an adjuvant for EAT induction with MTG, similar to LPS; its early administration can also prevent induction of Ts [55].

Once the $CD4^+$ and $CD8^+$ subsets are established in the thyroids, they appear independent of each other; mAb treatment to one subset essentially leaves the other intact in either the active induction or adoptive transfer regimen [43,56]. The effector function of $CD8^+$ T cells is in contrast to another report [48]. As illustrated above, the TCR repertoire is quite versatile. Indeed, in MTG-immunized, class I-deficient (β2m$^-$/$_-$) B10.K mice, thyroid inflammation is as severe as in B10.K mice [57]. However, the presence of macrophages appears dependent on both subsets, since only combined treatment with anti-CD4 and anti-CD8 can clear the thyroids completely of T cells as well as macrophages [43]. The cyclic changes shown by only the $CD8^+$ subset [45,47] is intriguing. It is unknown at present whether the early cells are MTG-driven Tc and the later arrival represent $CD8^+$ Ts, which have been observed after vaccination with irradiated MTG-activated T cells. In the granulomatous model in which both mononuclear and polymorphonuclear cells are observed and anti-MTG producing B cells may play a role [59], $CD8^+$ T cells have been reported to aid its resolution [60].

Short and long-term effects of immunotherapy

Using synergistic pairs of CD4 and CD8 mAbs highly efficient in depleting T cells *in vivo*, we have examined the immediate and long-term effects of immunotherapy by injecting the mAbs singly or in combination on days 21 and 25 after MTG immunization. On day 28, the thyroids show significant reduction in inflammation after either anti-CD4 or anti-CD8 treatment [43]. The most efficacious regimen is combining the CD4 and CD8 mAb; $>50\%$ of the thyroids are purged of all inflammatory cells, including macrophages. On day 70, control thyroids continue to display a CD4:CD8 ratio of 2, while those from anti-CD4-treated mice show elevated percentages of $CD8^+$ T cells and those from anti-CD8-treated mice contain primarily $CD4^+$ T cells. After combined therapy, the very few lesions that can be found in some mice have a subset ratio of 1. Since T cell subsets have been undergoing recovery from the thymus, the newly emerging T cells apparently do not enter the thyroid, despite continuing antigenic stimulus as reflected by ongoing MTG antibody production. Thus, the short two-dose therapy has a long-lasting effect.

After reimmunization of such treated groups on day 70 and assay for EAT on day 98, only control rat IgG- or anti-CD8-treated groups exhibit the equivalent of a secondary response with high MTG antibody titres and severe inflammation [61]. By contrast, most mice treated with anti-CD4 or combined mAbs show the equivalent of a primary response, apparently following a re-establishment of self tolerance. Thus, efficient clearance of both T cell subsets from the thyroid can eliminate immunological memory of thyroiditogenicity. Although such treatment is usually not required for autoimmune thyroid disease, this approach can serve as a model for other autoimmune diseases.

Other treatments have included recombinant (r) hIL-10 or mAbs to IFN-γ, intercellular adhesion molecule-1 (ICAM-1) and lymphocyte function-associated antigen-1 (LFA-1). Treatment with multiple rhIL-10 doses during MTG immunization moderates thyroid inflammation in association with apoptotic T cell death and reduced cytotoxicity without affecting antibody levels [62], and the same group shows doses of anti-IFN-γ to have similar effects in PTG-immunized mice [54]. Both anti-ICAM-1 and anti-LFA-1 in multiple doses reduce thyroid infiltration in rat EAT [63]. The immunosuppressive agent FK 506, given after the appearance of TG antibodies in thymectomized and irradiated rats, reduces thyroid infiltration and ICAM-1 expression [64]. In murine transfer EAT, anti-ICAM-1 shows no effect, but anti-α4 (VCAM-1) integrin can lower thyroid inflammation [65]. These treatments deal with moderating EAT development and are unlikely to have long-term effects.

T CELL REGULATION IN NATURAL AND ACQUIRED RESISTANCE

Genetic susceptibility and the constant presence of circulating TG in conjunction with periodic, environmental, polyclonal stimuli do not generally result in autoimmune thyroiditis, as discussed elsewhere [1,5]. Only by immunization of susceptible mice with MTG plus adjuvant, including LPS and rIL-1β [55], or with MTG alone in repeated doses can EAT be induced. The use of syngeneic MTG injections without adjuvant [25] has provided us with several clues into self tolerance and autoimmunity.

(i) Autoreactive T cells are not clonally deleted and can respond to self peptides without 'molecular mimicry';

(ii) Natural resistance is normally operating; only 50% of animals develop thyroiditis, whereas 100% produce MTG antibodies, albeit contingent upon continuing MTG administration. In humans, autoantibodies are often found without thyroid dysfunction;

(iii) Clonal anergy is not of major importance in maintaining self tolerance.

Although it could be argued that repeated MTG injections stimulate production of cytokines, especially IL-2, thereby overcoming anergy, this does not explain how self tolerance can be strengthened with MTG to prevent EAT induction with adjuvant or why depletion of certain T cell subset results in low incidence of SAT, as described below.

Induction of resistance (suppression) with mouse thyroglobulin (MTG)

The three protocols we have found efficacious in inducing resistance in susceptible mice to EAT induction are: two 100 μg doses of deaggregated (d) MTG [55,66], LPS 24 hr before two sub-tolerogenic, 20 μg doses of dMTG [67], and thyroid-stimulating hormone (TSH) infusion for 3–4 days [66,67]. All three protocols lead to reduction in or prevention of thyroid inflammation, T cell proliferative response to MTG and autoantibody production. The link among all three is the 3- to 5-fold increase of circulatory MTG level over a period of ⩾2–3 days. Since this can be achieved physiologically by means of TSH infusion, we have hypothesized that one function of circulatory TG is to maintain a low level of Ts, holding autoreactive T cells in abeyance against low levels of periodic stimuli in the environment [1,5]. As mentioned above, normal tolerance can be re-established after EAT induction if the animals are given immunotherapy combining CD4 and CD8 mAbs, a two-dose regimen that purges the thyroid of inflammatory cells [61].

When the circulatory TG level is raised by exogenous or endogenously released MTG, self tolerance is heightened to such a degree that the host is resistant to strong immunogenic challenge with MTG plus adjuvant. This induced resistance is durable, lasting for at least 2–3 months [68]. It is transferable with T cells which require 2–3 days to expand/differentiate, and exerts its effect on the afferent phase to prevent EAT induction [69,70]. Induced resistance is mediated by a cyclophosphamide-insensitive population of $CD4^+$ regulatory T cells: depletion of $CD4^+$, but not $CD8^+$, T cells in the tolerized host abrogates resistance [71]. Moreover, MTG-induced resistance cannot be overcome by the infusion of normal immunocompetent cells [71] or rescued by IL-2 administration [55], arguing against clonal anergy as the major mechanism of resistance.

Others have induced suppression with milligram amounts of orally administered heterologous HTG [72] or PTG [73] and challenged the mice with HTG or MTG, respectively. Since both heterologous TGs contain foreign epitopes, hyporesponsiveness rather than strong suppression to HTG-induced EAT was observed, and T cell proliferation, but not the anti-MTG response, was reduced in PTG-fed mice after challenge with MTG. After inducing tolerance by injecting HTG [74], PTG or HTG + PTG [75] and challenging with MTG, we have also observed suppressed proliferation to the shared epitopes but, with time, thyroiditis was observed, suggesting that MTG has unique, thyroiditogenic epitope(s) not shared with other TGs. The cells mediating oral tolerance have not been defined.

$CD4^+$ regulatory T cells

We [71] and others [76] have confirmed that resistance induced by MTG injection is mediated by $CD4^+$ T cells and the characteristics of suppression have been described above. Although T_H1 and T_H2 cells are involved in the production of certain cytokines which promote and moderate various disease states [77], and although IFN-γ, a T_H1-like cytokine, has been implicated in EAT pathogenesis [54], it is unknown at present whether T_H2-like cells or cytokines mediate the induced resistance. Thus, we have used the term, $CD4^+$ Ts, to distinguish them from TG-reactive inducer T cells (Ti), which may become T_H1-like cells. To understand the requirements for suppressor activation, which takes 2–3 days [66,69] but lasts for >2–3 months [68], we have examined when resistance becomes irreversibly induced. rIL-1β, used as an early inflammatory cytokine produced by antigen-presenting cells, interferes with activation of Ts efficiently when given 3 h after dMTG. It is less efficacious 24 h after dMTG and is ineffective when given 3 h before dMTG [55] (Table 1.3). The short half-life of IL-1 indicates that, in reference to the tolerogenic signal, the timing of this second signal is critical in diverting the commitment of Ts toward Ti.

We next used a non-depleting rat CD4 mAb which modulates surface CD4 for about 3 days without depleting this subset *in vivo*. Reducing the surface CD4 molecules at the time of tolerance induction with dMTG has no effect on the expansion/differentiation of $CD4^+$ Ts, but the presence of low levels of CD4 mAb interferes with their suppressive action on Ti during immunization [78].

Table 1.3 Time-dependency of rIL-1β interference with induction of resistance

Pretreatment										
dMTG[a] *(days −17, −10)*	*rIL-1β*[b] *Dose*	*rIL-1β*[b] *Time ± dMTG*	*MTG Ab (mean* log_2 *titre)*	*T cell prolif-eration (SI)*	*Thyroiditis: no. mice with % thyroid involvement* 0	>0–10	>10–20	>20–40	>40–80
+	–	–	<1.0	<1.0	4	1	1	–	–
+	10 000 U	−3 h	7.6	<1.0	3	4	–	1	–[c]
+	10 000 U	+ 3 h	16.6	4.3	–	2	1	3	1
+	10 000 U	+24 h	9.1	<1.0	1	2	2	2	–
–	–	–	16.3	6.8	–	–	3	3	–[c]

Adapted from Nabozny and Kong [55].

[a]100 μg dMTG before MTG and LPS immunization on days 0 and 7; data from day 28.

[b]rIL-1β was given i.v. before (–) or after (+) dMTG.

[c]$p < 0.01$.

This interference suggests the need for close proximity between Ts and Ti, and may implicate local cytokine involvement. High doses of the same non-depleting CD4 mAb has also been shown to interfere with MTG immunization and induces a suppressor population [79]. One T_H2-like cytokine, rIL-10, but not rIL-4, interferes with the *in vitro* activation of MTG-primed cells for adoptive transfer [80], and moderates EAT development *in vivo* [62]. However, more studies are required to determine whether T_H2-like or other cytokines, such as TGF-β, play any major role in the inhibition by Ts at the critical afferent phase of EAT induction.

The small increase of circulatory TG level, attainable by TSH infusion for 3–4 days, leading to suppression of thyroid infiltration by $CD4^+$ T cells, demonstrates the likelihood of this effect operating periodically *in vivo* [67]. That low levels of Ts exist in nature is supported by two T cell depletion protocols in which a particular T cell subset is removed to enable the remaining Ti to induce SAT. One protocol entails the removal of an Lyt-1^+,2,3^- ($CD4^+$) subset in EAT-resistant mice before transfer into nu/nu mice to permit the subsequent development of SAT [81,82]. EAT resistance may involve a number of different mechanisms; however, since resistance in B10.M mice appears to be due to a lack of appropriate class II molecules rather than the presence of Ts [14]. Another protocol depletes a $CD5^{bright}$ subset from F_1 responder donors before transfer into 'B' mice, resulting in SAT [53,83]. These data help pinpoint the cell types which might have been depleted in the course of thymectomy with or without irradiation in mice [84] and rats [46,85]; the animals subsequently develop SAT.

Induction of resistance with idiotype-bearing T cells

In general, after *in vivo* triggering of autoreactive Ti, a population of idiotype-bearing T cells expand and differentiate, which may or may not lead to frank thyroid dysfunction. To examine if such cells can induce anti-idiotype regulatory T cells, we have used irradiated, MTG-primed and -activated spleen cells [58], and others have employed an MTG-derived thyroiditogenic cell line [86] and a PTG-derived, cytotoxic $CD8^+$ hybridoma [87] to vaccinate mice. In addition to reduced thyroiditis observed by others in the challenged mice, we also found lowered antibody response. While irradiated $CD4^+$ T cells alone are sufficient for vaccination, full protection requires both $CD4^+$ and $CD8^+$ Ts [58]. A synergistic effect is observed between dMTG- and the weaker vaccination-induced resistance, since a regimen of subtolerogenic doses of dMTG preceding one dose of irradiated cells affords stronger protection than either alone [88] (Table 1.4). It is possible that both mechanisms operate *in vivo*, with normally low MTG levels activating $CD4^+$ Ts and idiotype-bearing T cells activating idiotype-specific $CD4^+$ and $CD8^+$ Ts, particularly if autoreactive Ti have been triggered to some extent. Anti-idiotype antibodies are involved in protecting mice vaccinated with PTG-derived hybridoma against PTG-induced EAT [89]. Whereas these antibodies play a role in shared epitope-induced EAT which lasts for only weeks [90], their role in protecting against MTG-induced EAT which lasts for up to 18 months [31] is unknown.

AUTOANTIGENS AND THYROIDITOGENIC PEPTIDES

Since the chemical and physical properties of thyroid autoantigens are discussed in Chapter 2, this section will deal only with autoantigens and their peptides that have been tested in experimental models.

Table 1.4 Synergistic suppression of EAT induction by pretreatment with a single dose of MTG followed by irradiated spleen cells

Pretreatment[a]			*MTG antibody*[b] *(mean* log_2 *titre* ± *SE)*	*Thyroiditis incidence*[b] *(%)*
day −28	*day −21*	*day −7*		
–	–	–	15.00 ± 0.8	100
dMTG	dMTG	–	< 1	50
–	–	γSC	16.0 ± 0.5	100
dMTG	dMTG	γSC	< 1	17
dMTG	dMTG	dMTG	< 1	100

Modified from Nabozny *et al.* [88].

[a]Each mouse was given 20 μg dMTG and/or 2.0×10^7 irradiated MTG-primed and -activated (γSC) at the intervals shown and was challenged i.v. with 20 μg MTG and 20 μg LPS on days 0 and 7.

[b]Determined on day 28.

TGs and TG epitopes

Not only is TG the prototype antigen that has been used to induce EAT for more than 30 years, its importance as a potential initiator of autoimmunity eventuating in thyroid damage in nature has recently been reinforced. In addition to the OS chicken long known for unusual susceptibility and responses to TG [7], TG autoreactivity has been observed in recent SAT models. Manipulation of the T cell subset compartment followed by transfer into 'B' mice results in thyroiditis development and isolation of TG-reactive T cell lines and clones [53]. TG-reactive T cell lines from the thyroiditis-prone subline of BB/Wor rat adoptively transfer thyroiditis and exhibit cytotoxicity [33]. The NOD-H2^{h4} mouse, bearing EAT-susceptible genes from both the k haplotype and the NOD strain which responds to MTG-induced EAT (Kong and David, unpublished data), develops a low incidence of thyroiditis and exhibits autoantibodies to MTG [91]. Neither the BB/Wor- nor NOD-derived strain produces antibodies to TPO. Moreover, our HLA-DR3 transgenic mice respond to either HTG or MTG immunization, supporting TG as an important, and not merely a bystander, autoantigen [14].

It is unknown at present which TG epitopes are thyroiditogenic in DR3^{+} transgenic mice, but they undoubtedly include epitopes shared between MTG and HTG. Early reciprocal stimulation studies of MTG- or HTG-primed cells for adoptive transfer and generation of Tc have revealed the presence of thyroiditogenic, shared epitopes between HTG and MTG [92]. The observations of two identical CDR3 motifs on thyroidal Vβ13^{+} T cells after either HTG [40] or MTG [42] immunization also demonstrate the importance of shared epitopes. That some of the shared epitopes are also conserved in PTG and bovine (B) TG has been inferred by earlier studies [5]. While one should bear in mind in using rodents that there is ample evidence indicating unique thyroiditogenic epitopes on MTG not shared with heterologous TGs [5,74,75], they have not been identified. Thus, studies have focused on peptide derivatives from heterologous TGs [26–28,93,94], of which the complete amino acid sequence of HTG and BTG and partial sequence of PTG and RTG are known. The recent sequencing of 287 amino acids (less than one-ninth) from the C-terminus of MTG [22] confirms the conservation of these small peptides. That no immunodominant epitopes have emerged from these studies of shared/conserved epitopes supports our earlier hypothesis that conserved and MTG-unique T cell epitopes contribute to the total thyroiditogenicity of MTG [74].

Since TG is a prominent antigen in several SAT and certainly in EAT models, it is perhaps not too surprising that excessive intake of dietary iodine, related to iodination of TG and enhanced immunogenicity, increases thyroiditis incidence and/or severity [91,95,96]. However, the TG-reactive lymphocytes from thyroiditis-prone BB/Wor rat recognize TG regardless of iodine content [97]. Furthermore, most iodine residues normally are incorporated into the four primary hormonogenic sites on TG [98], and, as reviewed recently [5], necropsy studies in Caucasians, black Americans and Japanese show that the distinct ethnic/genetic differences in susceptibility are little influenced by environmental factors such as high iodine intake in the USA compared with the UK, and in coastal regions of Japan compared with mountainous regions [99,100]. Whether iodination is really critical for immunogenicity of TG is better addressed using defined peptides to induce EAT, wherein the antigenicity can be clarified by *in vitro* expansion of primed cells, followed by adoptive transfer of thyroiditis to demonstrate thyroiditogenicity. In such studies, both an 18-mer [28] and a 40-mer [93] pathogenic peptide contain one tyrosine which was not iodinated prior to immunization, while a 14-mer closer to the HTG C-terminus and sharing 5 amino acids with human TPO does not contain tyrosine [101]. Another 17-mer has no tyrosine but induces moderate thyroiditis [27] and contains a 9-mer pathogenic peptide which can be presented by either $H2E^k$ and $H2A^s$ molecules in two different haplotypes [102].

Since T cells responding to these peptides are not expanded by culture with intact TG, it was necessary to examine the importance of iodine residues after priming with intact TG or peptide. Testing with a 12-mer peptide from the hormonogenic site at position 2553, it was determined that the peptide was not thyroiditogenic unless the tyrosine had been substituted with thyroxine (T4) [94]. However, since non-iodinated, thyronine (T0)-containing peptide was not compared, we undertook to determine if iodination was indeed required for site 2553 to be an autoepitope and if other primary hormonogenic sites were likewise immunogenic and required iodine residues. By comparing three pairs of 12-mer peptides 1–12, 2549–2560, 2559–2570, containing T0 or T4 at positions 5, 2553, or 2567, respectively, we found that, of the three T4-containing peptides, hT4(5) and hT4(2553), but not hT4(2567), stimulated MTG-primed or HTG-primed T cells *in vitro*, with hT4(2553) being the stronger. However, as shown in Table 1.5, hT0(2553) is also stimulatory. Comparing hT0(2553) and hT4(2553), both activated MTG-primed, or peptide-primed, T cells to transfer thyroiditis [14]. A summary is presented in Table 1.6. hT4(2553) is highly stimulatory *in vitro* for self-primed and hT0(2553)-primed cells, while hT0-(2553) is less stimulatory for hT4(2553)-primed cells. Since hT0(2553)-primed cells have never seen the iodinated peptide, iodination appears to enhance binding affinity *in vitro*. Given the differences in *in vitro* reactivity, it is not surprising that hybridomas can be selected to respond only to T4- but not T0-containing peptide which was not used for priming, as reported recently [103]. The marked immunogenicity of non-iodinated hT0(2553) and the poor antigenicity of hT4(5) and hT4(2567) demonstrate that immunogenicity of a conserved hormonogenic site depends more on its amino acid composition than on T4 substitution [14]. The secondary role of iodine residues in TG is also supported by the findings that none of these peptides are immunodominant and that only by vigorous immunization can T0 or T4 at either position 5 or 2553 lead to mild thyroiditis, but only in $H2^k$ and not in susceptible $H2^s$ strains [104].

Table 1.5 Capacity of T0-containing synthetic peptide derivatives of HTG to induce EAT or prime T cells

Immunizing antigen	*No. mice with thyroid infiltration*[a]	*In vitro activator*[b]	*[^{3}H]Thymidine uptake mean CPM ± SE (stimulation index)*
MTG	4/6	–	2 400 ± 300
		MTG	23 100 ± 1 700 (9.8)
hT0(5)	0/6	–	5 200 ± 300
		MTG	4 600 ± 100 (< 1.0)
		hT0(5)	4 200 ± 600 (< 1.0)
hT0(2553)	0/6	–	3 200 ± 100
		MTG	1 500 ± 200 (< 1.0)
		hT0(2553)	45 800 ± 4 300 (14.4)

[a]Mice were immunized i.v. with 20 μg MTG or 100 μg peptide derived from HTG(1-12) or (2549–2560)+20 μg LPS on days 0 and 7, and their thyroids examined on day 28.

[b]Spleen cells from day 28 were cultured at 9×10^5/well for 4 days with 20 μg/ml MTG or 5 μg/ml peptide.

Table 1.6 Capacity of hT0(2553) and hT4(2553)-containing synthetic peptide derivatives to induce EAT and cross-stimulate each other for adoptive transfer

Immunizing antigen	*No. mice with thyroid infiltration*[a]	*In vitro*		
		Activator[b]	*Stimulation index*	*Adoptive transfer*[c]
MTG	4/4	MTG	9.0	Yes
		hT0(2553)	2.7	Yes
		hT4(2553)	9.5	Yes
hT0(2553)	0/6	MTG	1.3	No
		hT0(2553)	17.0	Yes
		hT4(2553)	23.2	Yes
hT4(2553)	0/6	MTG	<0.1	No
		hT0(2553)	2.1	No
		hT4(2553)	51.9	Yes

Adapted from Kong *et al.* [14].

[a]Mice were immunized i.v. with 50 μg MTG or peptide on day 0 (tail base) and day 7 (hind footpads), and their thyroids examined on day 28.

[b]Lymph node cells were activated for 3 days in the presence of irradiated spleen cells with 20 μg/ml MTG or peptide hT0(2553) or 5 μg/ml peptide hT4(2553), both derived from HTG(2549-2560).

[c]Peptide-activated cells were injected at twice the cell number of MTG-activated cells into normal recipient mice and thyroid inflammation was assessed on day 14.

TPO and TSHR in EAT induction

Porcine TPO induces thyroiditis in $H2^b$ mice, a haplotype resistant to EAT induction with TG [105]. A 15-mer is found to be thyroiditogenic and at a different site from the five amino acids shared with HTG [101]. Limited by quantity, the use of mouse TPO awaits production by recombinant technology. Similarly, the unavailability of mTSHR has led workers to attempt hTSHR immunization as a means of producing a Graves' disease model but with limited success. In a study with congenic strains, repeated immunization with hTSHR or peptides led to antibody production, transient variations of T3 levels and thyroiditis in $H2^q$ and $H2^s$ mice, but not in $H2^d$ mice; there were inconsistent gender variations among the strains [106]. On the other hand, others reported producing thyroiditis in $H2^d$ and NOD mice, which can be transferred, with extracellular domain raised in bacteria as a fusion protein [107]. Using rTSHR extracellular domain produced in insect cells, antibodies blocking TSH binding but not thyroiditis have been reported in a number of strains including $H2^d$ mice [108–110]. With larger quantities available, efforts to produce TSHR antibodies that have stimulatory or inhibitory activity and thyroiditis are continuing. As reviewed elsewhere [6,111], others have examined Graves' disease lymphocytes and thyroid tissues in athymic and SCID mice, which have served primarily as hosts for the study of interactions of transferred cells and not as actual animal models of Graves' disease.

SUMMARY

It is clear in both HT and animal models that the major players are the T cells and their subsets. Thus, the recent major advances have paralleled our understanding of T cell immunobiology and their interactions with MHC class II molecules presenting small T cell epitopes to the appropriate TCR repertoire. There are convincing data from studies on T cell regulation to suggest:

(i) Both $CD4^+$ and $CD8^+$ T cells contribute to pathogenicity by producing inflammatory cytokines, expressing adhesion molecules, and direct cytotoxicity on target cells;

(ii) Immunotherapy with anti-CD4 and anti-CD8 mAbs not only demonstrates each subset's involvement but also their independence within the thyroid, whereas the efficient clearance of both subsets and macrophages by combined immunotherapy reveals the secondary involvement of inflammatory macrophages and the potential of removing memory T cells and re-establishing self-tolerance;

(iii) $CD4^+$ regulatory T cells exist and are maintained by circulatory TG threshold in nature to suppress periodic autoimmune stimuli, with idiotype-specific $CD8^+$ Ts and antibodies as possible back-up;

(iv) The TCR repertoire is highly adaptable and can respond to different, small TG epitopes presented on different MHC molecules.

Two other major advances of note are the complete or partial sequencing of several mammalian TGs including the mouse, and the finding of HLA-DRB1 polymorphism as one determinant in EAT susceptibility in transgenic mice. The potential of TG as an initiator and not a bystander autoantigen is confirmed by data from SAT models showing a primary role for TG. Given the high homology in mammalian TGs, the study of conserved epitopes in rodents, some of which are identical to the human, is justified. Indeed, studies of conserved, primary hormonogenic sites as well as other uniodinated pathogenic peptides have revealed the secondary role of iodine residues in TG immunogenicity. Necropsy studies in several countries also confirm the importance of genetic/ethnic factors over dietary/environmental factors. That HLA (e.g. DR3) association with HT is difficult to affirm appears related to the lack of immunodominant epitopes, plasticity of the TCR repertoire, HLA-DR/DQ linkage disequilibrium as well as possible interactions between these loci. HLA-DR and -DQ transgenic models and the use of defined epitopes may help dissect such influences.

Finally, it is often said that no model represents HT in every aspect but that induced EAT is less representative than any SAT model. Excluding the OS chicken which harbours other abnormal features, the major similarity between HT and other SAT models appears to be the unpredictable time of onset. Given that the appropriate MHC, the autoantigen and the TCR repertoire are already present, it seems likely that, similar to induced EAT, HT is also induced, but the actual second signals or triggering factors, ultimately affecting the T cells, may vary among the polygenic humans. Otherwise, studies in TG-induced EAT would not find such parallels in the human.

Acknowledgements

The author is grateful for the continuing collaborations and stimulatory discussions of Alvaro A. Giraldo and Chella S. David, who have made the ongoing studies possible and enjoyable, and for the assistance of Lesley Lomo in manuscript preparation. This work was supported by the National Institute of Diabetes, and Digestive and Kidney Diseases, DK 45960.

References

1. Kong YM. The mouse model of autoimmune thyroid disease. In: McGregor AM, ed. Immunology of Endocrine Diseases. Lancaster, UK: MTP Press Limited; 1986:1–24.
2. Charreire J. Immune mechanisms in autoimmune thyroiditis. Adv Immunol. 1989;46:263–334.
3. Kong YM, Lewis M. Animal models of autoimmune endocrine diseases: diabetes and thyroiditis. In: Volpé R, ed. Autoimmune Diseases of the Endocrine System. Boca Raton, FL: CRC Press; 1990:23–50.

4. Kong YM, Giraldo AA. Experimental autoimmune thyroiditis in the mouse and rat. In: Cohen IR, Miller A, eds. Autoimmune Disease Models: A Guidebook. San Diego: Academic Press; 1994:123–45.
5. Kong YM. Regulatory mechanisms in autoimmune thyroiditis: recent lessons from a murine model. Fund Clin Immunol. 1994;2:199–213.
6. Weetman AP, McGregor AM. Autoimmune thyroid disease: further developments in our understanding. Endocr Rev 1994;15:788–830.
7. Wick G, Brezinschek HP, Hala K, Dietrich H, Wolf H, Kroemer G. The Obese strain of chickens: an animal model with spontaneous autoimmune thyroiditis. Adv Immunol. 1989; 47:433–500.
8. Wick G, Cole R, Dietrich H, Maczek Ch, Muller P-U, Hala K. The obese strain of chickens with spontaneous autoimmune thyroiditis as a model for Hashimoto disease. In: Cohen IR, Miller A, eds. Autoimmune Disease Models: A Guidebook. San Diego: Academic Press; 1994:107–22.
9. Rothenberg EV. The development of functionally responsive T cells. Adv Immunol. 1992;51: 85–214.
10. De Assis-Paiva HJ, Rayner DC, Roitt IM, Cooke A. Cellular infiltration in induced rat thyroiditis: phenotypic analysis and relationship to genetic restriction. Clin Exp Immunol. 1989;75:106–12.
11. Colle E, Guttmann RD, Seemayer TA. Association of spontaneous thyroiditis with the major histocompatibility complex of the rat. Endocrinology. 1985;116:1243–7.
12. Kotzin BL, Leung DYM, Kappler J, Marrack P. Superantigens and their potential role in human disease. Adv Immunol. 1993;54:99–166.
13. Kong YM, David CS, Lomo, LC et al. Role of mouse and human class II transgenes in susceptibility to and protection against mouse autoimmune thyroiditis. Immunogenetics. 1997;46:312–17.
14. Kong YM, Lomo LC, Motte RW et al. HLA-DRB1 polymorphism determines susceptibility to autoimmune thyroiditis in transgenic mice: definitive association with HLA-DRB1*0301 (DR3) gene. J Exp Med. 1996;184:1167–72.
15. Krco CJ, Gores A, David CS, Kong YM. Immunogenetic aspects of human thyroglobulin-reactive T cell lines and hybridomas. J Immunogenet. 1990;17:361–70.
16. Chronopoulou E, Carayanniotis G. H-2E^k expression influences thyroiditis induction by the thyroglobulin peptide (2495-2511). Immunogenetics. 1993;38:150–3.
17. Zanelli E, Gonzalez-gay MA, David CS. Could HLA-DRB1 be the protective locus in rheumatoid arthritis? Immunol Today. 1995;16:274–8.
18. Kong YM, David CS, Giraldo AA, El Rehewy M, Rose NR. Regulation of autoimmune response to mouse thyroglobulin: influence of H-2D-end genes. J Immunol. 1979;123:15–18.
19. Creemers P, Rose NR, Kong YM. Experimental autoimmune thyroiditis: in vitro cytotoxic effects of T lymphocytes on thyroid monolayers. J Exp Med. 1983;157:559–71.
20. Salamero J, Charreire J. Syngeneic sensitization of mouse lymphocytes on monolayers of thyroid epithelial cells. VII. Generation of thyroid-specific cytotoxic effector cells. Cell Immunol. 1985;91:111–18.
21. Eishi Y, McCullagh P. The relative contributions of immune system and target organ to variation in susceptibility of rats to experimental allergic thyroiditis. Eur J Immunol. 1988; 18:657–60.
22. Kuppers RC, Hu Q, Rose NR. Mouse thyroglobulin: conservation of sequence homology in C-terminal immmunogenic regions of thyroglobulin. Autoimmunity. 1996;23:175–80.
23. Fuller BE, Giraldo AA, Motte RW et al. T cell receptor Vβ gene usage in experimental autoimmune thyroiditis. Ann NY Acad Sci. 1995;756:450–2.
24. Lomo LC, Motte RW, Giraldo AA et al. Vβ8.2 transgene expression interferes with development of experimental autoimmune thyroiditis in CBA k/q but not k/k mice. Cell Immunol. 1996;168:297–301.
25. El Rehewy M, Kong YM, Giraldo AA, Rose NR. Syngeneic thyroglobulin is immunogenic in good responder mice. Eur J Immunol. 1981;11:146–51.
26. Kong YM, McCormick DJ, Wan Q et al. Primary hormonogenic sites as conserved autoepitopes on thyroglobulin in murine autoimmune thyroiditis: secondary role of iodination. J Immunol. 1995;155:5847–54.
27. Chronopoulou E, Carayanniotis G. Identification of a thyroiditogenic sequence within the thyroglobulin molecule. J Immunol. 1992;149:1039–44.

28. Carayanniotis G, Chronopoulou E, Rao VP. Distinct genetic pattern of mouse susceptibility to thyroiditis induced by a novel thyroglobulin peptide. Immunogenetics. 1994;39:21–8.
29. Okayasu I, Kong YM, Rose NR. Effect of castration and sex hormones on experimental autoimmune thyroiditis. Clin Immunol Immunopathol. 1981;20:240–5.
30. Kuppers RC, Neu N, Rose NR. Animal models of autoimmune thyroid disease. In: Farid NR, ed. Immunogenetics of Endocrine Disorders. New York: Alan R. Liss, Inc.; 1988:111–31.
31. Okayasu I, Hatakeyama S, Kong YM. Long-term observation and effect of age on induction of experimental autoimmune thyroiditis in susceptible and resistant mice. Clin Immunol Immunopathol. 1989;53:254–67.
32. Cohen SB, Weetman AP. Characterization of different types of experimental autoimmune thyroiditis in the Buffalo strain rat. Clin Exp Immunol. 1987;69:25–32.
33. Allen EM, Thupari JN. The pathogenicity of spontaneously-occurring thyroglobulin-reactive T lymphocytes from BB/WOR rats. Autoimmunity. 1996;23:35–44.
34. Bernard NF, Ertug F, Margolese H. High incidence of thyroiditis and anti-thyroid autoantibodies in NOD mice. Diabetes. 1992;41:40–6.
35. Asamoto H, Oishi M, Akazawa Y, Tochino Y. Histologic and immunologic changes in the thymus and other organs in NOD mice. In: Tarui S, Tochino Y, Nonaka K, eds. Insulitis and Type I Diabetes: Lessons from the NOD Mouse. Tokyo: Academic Press; 1986:61–71.
36. Penhale WJ, Young PR. The influence of the normal microbial flora on the susceptibility of rats to experimental autoimmune thyroiditis. Clin Exp Immunol. 1988;72:288–92.
37. Bhatia SK, Rose NR, Schofield B, Lafond-Walker A, Kuppers RC. Influence of diet on the induction of experimental autoimmune thyroid disease. Proc Soc Exp Biol Med. 1996;213:294–300.
38. Fuller BE, Giraldo AA, Motte RW, Nabozny GH, David CS, Kong YM. Noninvolvement of $V\beta8^+$ T cells in murine thyroglobulin-induced experimental autoimmune thyroiditis. Cell Immunol. 1994;159:315–22.
39. McMurray RW, Hoffman RW, Tang H, Braley-Mullen H. T cell receptor Vβ usage in murine experimental autoimmune thyroiditis. Cell Immunol. 1996;172:1–9.
40. Matsuoka N, Unger P, Ben-Nun A, Graves P, Davies TF. Thyroglobulin-induced murine thyroiditis assessed by intrathyroidal T cell receptor sequencing. J Immunol. 1994;152:2562–8.
41. Matsuoka N, Bernard N, Concepcion ES, Graves PN, Ben-Nun A, Davies TF. T-cell receptor V region β-chain gene expression in the autoimmune thyroiditis of non-obese diabetic mice. J Immunol. 1993;151:1691–701.
42. Nakashima M, Kong YM, Davies TF. The role of T cells expressing TcR Vβ13 in autoimmune thyroiditis induced by transfer of mouse thyroglobulin-activated lymphocytes: identification of two common CDR3 motifs. Clin Immunol Immunopathol. 1996;80:204–10.
43. Kong YM, Waldmann H, Cobbold S, Giraldo AA, Fuller BE, Simon LL. Pathogenic mechanisms in murine autoimmune thyroiditis: short- and long-term effects of in vivo depletion of $CD4^+$ and $CD8^+$ cells. Clin Exp Immunol. 1989;77:428–33.
44. Creemers P, Giraldo AA, Rose NR, Kong YM. T-cell subsets in the thyroids of mice developing autoimmune thyroiditis. Cell Immunol. 1984;87:692–7.
45. Conaway DH, Giraldo AA, David CS, Kong YM. *In situ* kinetic analysis of thyroid lymphocyte infiltrate in mice developing experimental autoimmune thyroiditis. Clin Immunol Immunopathol. 1989;53:346–53.
46. Cohen SB, Dijkstra CD, Weetman AP. Sequential analysis of experimental autoimmune thyroiditis induced by neonatal thymectomy in the Buffalo strain rat. Cell Immunol. 1988;114:126–36.
47. Conaway DH, Giraldo AA, David CS, Kong YM. In situ analysis of T cell subset composition in experimental autoimmune thyroiditis after adoptive transfer of activated spleen cells. Cell Immunol. 1990;125:247–53.
48. McMurray RW, Sharp GC, Braley-Mullen H. Intrathyroidal cell phenotype in murine lymphocytic and granulomatous experimental autoimmune thyroiditis. Autoimmunity. 1994;18:93–102.
49. Braley-Mullen H, Sharp GC, Bickel JT, Kyriakos M. Induction of severe granulomatous experimental autoimmune thyroiditis in mice by effector cells activated in the presence of anti-interleukin 2 receptor antibody. J Exp Med. 1991;173:899–912.

50. Stull SJ, Sharp GC, Kyriakos M, Bickel JT, Braley-Mullen H. Induction of granulomatous experimental autoimmune thyroiditis in mice with *in vitro* activated effector T cells and anti-IFN-γ antibody. J Immunol. 1992;149:2219–26.
51. Vladutiu AO. Experimental autoimmune thyroiditis in mice chronically treated from birth with anti-IgM antibodies. Cell Immunol. 1989;121:49–59.
52. Sugihara S, Fujiwara H, Niimi H, Shearer GM. Self-thyroid epithelial cell (TEC)-reactive $CD8^+$ T cell lines/clones derived from autoimmune thyroiditis lesions. J Immunol. 1995;155: 1619–28.
53. Sugihara S, Fujiwara H, Shearer GM. Autoimmune thyroiditis induced in mice depleted of particular T cell subsets: characterization of thyroiditis-inducing T cell lines and clones derived from thyroid lesions. J Immunol. 1993;150:683–94.
54. Tang H, Mignon-Godefroy K, Meroni PL, Garotta G, Charreire J, Nicoletti F. The effects of a monoclonal antibody to interferon-gamma on experimental autoimmune thyroiditis (EAT): prevention of disease and decrease of EAT-specific T cells. Eur J Immunol. 1993;23:275–8.
55. Nabozny GH, Kong YM. Circumvention of the induction of resistance in murine experimental autoimmune thyroiditis by recombinant IL-1β. J Immunol. 1992;149:1086–92.
56. Flynn JC, Conaway DH, Cobbold S, Waldmann H, Kong YM. Depletion of $L3T4^+$ and Lyt-2^+ cells by rat monoclonal antibodies alters the development of adoptively transferred experimental autoimmune thyroiditis. Cell Immunol. 1989;122:377–90.
57. Lomo LC, Zhang FS, Giraldo AA, David CS, Kong YM. Flexibility of the thyroiditogenic T cell repertoire for murine autoimmune thyroiditis in $B2m^{-}/-$ and TCR-$V\beta^{c}$ mice. Autoimmunity. 1997; [in press].
58. Flynn JC, Kong YM. In vivo evidence for $CD4^+$ and $CD8^+$ suppressor T cells in vaccination-induced suppression of murine experimental autoimmune thyroiditis. Clin Immunol Immunopathol. 1991;60:484–94.
59. Braley-Mullen H, Sharp GC, Kyriakos M. Differential requirement for autoantibody-producing B cells for induction of lymphocytic versus granulomatous experimental autoimmunue thyroiditis. J Immunol. 1994;152:307–14.
60. Braley-Mullen H, McMurray RW, Sharp GC, Kyriakos M. Regulation of the induction and resolution of granulomatous experimental autoimmune thyroiditis in mice by $CD8^+$ T cells. Cell Immunol. 1994;153:492–504.
61. Fuller BE, Giraldo AA, Waldmann H, Cobbold SP, Kong YM. Depletion of $CD4^+$ and $CD8^+$ cells eliminates immunologic memory of thyroiditogenicity in murine experimental autoimmune thyroiditis. Autoimmunity. 1994;19:161–8.
62. Mignon-Godefroy K, Rott O, Brazillet M-P, Charreire J. Curative and protective effects of IL-10 in experimental autoimmune thyroiditis (EAT): evidence for IL-10-enhanced cell death in EAT. J Immunol. 1995;154:6634–43.
63. Metcalfe RA, Tandon N, Tamatani T, Miyasaka M, Weetman AP. Adhesion molecule monoclonal antibodies inhibit experimental autoimmune thyroiditis. Immunology. 1993;80: 493–7.
64. Tamura K, Woo J, Murase N, Carrieri G, Nalesnik MA, Thomson AW. Suppression of autoimmune thyroid disease by FK 506: influence on thyroid-infiltrating cells, adhesion molecule expression and anti-thyroglobulin antibody production. Clin Exp Immunol. 1993; 91:368–75.
65. McMurray RW, Tang H, Braley-Mullen H. The role of a4 integrin and intercellular adhesion molecule-1 (ICAM-1) in murine experimental autoimmune thyroiditis. Autoimmunity. 1996; 23:9–23.
66. Lewis M, Giraldo AA, Kong YM. Resistance to experimental autoimmune thyroiditis induced by physiologic manipulation of thyroglobulin level. Clin Immunol. Immunopathol. 1987;45:92–104.
67. Lewis M, Fuller BE, Giraldo AA, Kong YM. Resistance to experimental autoimmune thyroiditis is correlated with the duration of raised thyroglobulin levels. Clin Immunol Immunopathol. 1992;64:197–204.
68. Fuller BE, Okayasu I, Simon LL, Giraldo AA, Kong YM. Characterization of resistance to murine experimental autoimmune thyroiditis: duration and afferent action of thyroglobulin- and TSH-induced suppression. Clin Immunol Immunopathol. 1993;69:60–8.
69. Kong YM, Okayasu I, Giraldo AA et al. Tolerance to thyroglobulin by activating suppressor mechanisms. Ann NY Acad Sci. 1982;392:191–209.
70. Parish NM, Rayner D, Cooke A, Roitt IM. An investigation of the nature of induced suppression to experimental autoimmune thyroiditis. Immunology. 1988;63:199–203.

71. Kong YM, Giraldo AA, Waldmann H, Cobbold SP, Fuller BE. Resistance to experimental autoimmune thyroiditis: L3T4+ cells as mediators of both thyroglobulin-activated and TSH-induced suppression. Clin Immunol Immunopathol. 1989;51:38–54.
72. Guimaraes VC, Quintans J, Fisfalen M-E et al. Immunosuppression of thyroiditis. Endocrinology. 1996;137:2199–207.
73. Peterson KE, Braley-Mullen H. Suppression of murine experimental autoimmune thyroiditis by oral administration of porcine thyroglobulin. Cell Immunol. 1995;166:123–30.
74. Nabozny GH, Simon LL, Kong YM. Suppression in experimental autoimmune thyroiditis: the role of unique and shared determinants on mouse thyroglobulin in self-tolerance. Cell Immunol. 1990;131:140–9.
75. Nabozny GH. Functional characteristics and autoantigenic requirements of CD4+ suppressor T cells in murine experimental autoimmune thyroiditis. Ph.D. Dissertation, Wayne State University, 1991.
76. Parish NM, Roitt IM, Cooke A. Phenotypic characteristics of cells involved in induced suppression to murine experimental autoimmune thyroiditis. Eur J Immunol. 1988;18:1463–7.
77. Sad S, Mosmann TR. Single IL-2-secreting precursor CD4 T cell can develop into either Th1 or Th2 cytokine secretion phenotype. J Immunol. 1994;153:3514–22.
78. Nabozny GH, Cobbold SP, Waldmann H, Kong YM. Suppression in murine experimental autoimmune thyroiditis: in vivo inhibition of CD4+ T cell-mediated resistance by a nondepleting rat CD4 monoclonal antibody. Cell Immunol. 1991;138:185–96.
79. Hutchings PR, Cooke A, Dawe K, Waldmann H, Roitt IM. Active suppression induced by anti-CD4. Eur J Immunol. 1993;23:965–8.
80. Mignon-Godefroy K, Brazillet M-P, Rott O, Charreire J. Distinctive modulation by IL-4 and IL-10 of the effector function of murine thyroglobulin-primed cells in 'transfer-experimental autoimmune thyroiditis'. Cell Immunol. 1995;162:171–7.
81. Sakaguchi S, Fukuma K, Kuribayashi K, Masuda T. Organ-specific autoimmune diseases induced in mice by elimination of T cell subset. I. Evidence for the active participation of T cells in natural self-tolerance;deficit of a T cell subset as a possible cause of autoimmune disease. J Exp Med. 1985;161:72–87.
82. Sakaguchi S, Sakaguchi N. Thymus and autoimmunity: capacity of the normal thymus to produce pathogenic self-reactive T cells and conditions required for their induction of autoimmune disease. J Exp Med. 1990;172:537–45.
83. Sugihara S, Izumi Y, Yoshioka T et al. Autoimmune thyroiditis induced in mice depleted of particular T cell subsets. I. Requirement of Lyt-1^{dull} L3T4^{bright} normal T cells for the induction of thyroiditis. J Immunol. 1988;141:105–13.
84. Kojima A, Tanaka-Kojima Y, Sakakura T, Nishizuka Y. Spontaneous development of autoimmune thyroiditis in neonatally thymectomized mice. Lab Invest. 1976;34:550–7.
85. Penhale WJ, Farmer A, Irvine WJ. Thyroiditis in T cell-depleted rats: influence of strain, radiation dose, adjuvants and antilymphocyte serum. Clin Exp Immunol. 1975;21:362–75.
86. Maron R, Zerubavel R, Friedman A, Cohen IR. T lymphocyte line specific for thyroglobulin produces or vaccinates against autoimmune thyroiditis in mice. J Immunol. 1983;131:2316–22.
87. Remy J-J, Texier B, Chiocchia G, Charreire J. Characteristics of cytotoxic thyroglobulin-specific T cell hybridomas. J Immunol. 1989;142:1129–33.
88. Nabozny GH, Flynn JC, Kong YM. Synergism between mouse thyroglobulin- and vaccination-induced suppressor mechanisms in murine experimental autoimmune thyroiditis. Cell Immunol. 1991;136:340–8.
89. Roubaty C, Bedin C, Charreire J. Prevention of experimental autoimmune thyroiditis through the anti-idiotypic network. J Immunol. 1990;144:2167–72.
90. Tang H, Bedin C, Texier B, Charreire J. Autoantibody specific for a thyroglobulin epitope inducing experimental autoimmune thyroiditis or its anti-idiotype correlates with the disease. Eur J Immunol. 1990;20:1535–9.
91. Rasooly L, Burek CL, Rose NR. Iodine-induced autoimmune thyroiditis in NOD-H2h4 mice. Clin Immunol Immunopathol. 1996;81:287–92.
92. Simon LL, Justen JM, Giraldo AA, Krco CJ, Kong YM. Activation of cytotoxic T cells and effector cells in experimental autoimmune thyroiditis by shared determinants of mouse and human thyroglobulins. Clin Immunol Immunopathol. 1986;39:345–56.

93. Texier B, Bédin C, Tang H, Camoin L, Laurent-Winter C, Charreire J. Characterization and sequencing of a 40-amino-acid peptide from human thyroglobulin inducing experimental autoimmune thyroiditis. J Immunol. 1992;148:3405–11.
94. Hutchings PR, Cooke A, Dawe K, et al. A thyroxine-containing peptide can induce murine experimental autoimmune thyroiditis. J Exp Med. 1992;175:869–72.
95. Champion BR, Rayner DC, Byfield PGH, Page KR, Chan CTJ, Roitt IM. Critical role of iodination for T cell recognition of thyroglobulin in experimental murine thyroid autoimmunity. J Immunol. 1987;139:3665–70.
96. Sundick RS, Herdegen DM, Brown TR, Bagchi N. The incorporation of dietary iodine into thyroglobulin increases its immunogenicity. Endocrinology. 1987;120:2078–84.
97. Allen EM, Thupari JN. Thyroglobulin-reactive T lymphocytes in thyroiditis-prone BB/Wor rats. J Endocrinol Invest. 1995;18:45–9.
98. Xiao S, Dorris ML, Rawitch AB, Taurog A. Selectivity in tyrosyl iodination sites in human thyroglobulin. Arch Biochem Biophys. 1996;334:284–94.
99. Okayasu I, Hatakeyama S, Tanaka Y, Sakurai T, Hoshi K, Lewis PD. Is focal chronic autoimmune thyroiditis an age-related disease? Differences in incidence and severity between Japanese and British. J Pathol. 1991;163:257–64.
100. Okayasu I, Hara Y, Nakamura K, Rose NR. Racial and age-related differences in incidence and severity of focal autoimmune thyroiditis. Am J Clin Pathol. 1994;101:698–702.
101. Hoshioka A, Kohno Y, Katsuki T et al. A common T-cell epitope between human thyroglobulin and human thyroid peroxidase is related to murine experimental autoimmune thyroiditis. Immunol Lett. 1993;37:235–9.
102. Rao VP, Balasa B, Carayanniotis G. Mapping of thyroglobulin epitopes: presentation of a 9mer pathogenic peptide by different mouse MHC class II isotypes. Immunogenetics. 1994; 40:352–9.
103. Dawe KI, Hutchings PR, Geysen M, Champion BR, Cooke A, Roitt IM. Unique role of thyroxine in T cell recognition of a pathogenic peptide in experimental autoimmune thyroiditis. Eur J Immunol. 1996;26:768–72.
104. Wan Q, Motte RW, McCormick DJ et al. Primary hormonogenic sites as conserved autoepitopes on thyroglobulin in murine autoimmune thyroiditis: role of MHC class II. Clin Immunol Immunopathol. 1997;85:187–94.
105. Kotani T, Umeki K, Yagihashi S, Hirai K, Ohtaki S. Identification of thyroiditogenic epitope on porcine thyroid peroxidase for C57BL/6 mice. J Immunol. 1992;148:2084–9.
106. Marion S, Braun JM, Ropars A, Kohn LD, Charreire J. Induction of autoimmunity by immunization of mice with human thyrotropin receptor. Cell Immunol. 1994;158:329–41.
107. Costagliola S, Many M-C, Stalmans-Falys M, Vassart G, Ludgate M. Transfer of thyroiditis, with syngeneic spleen cells sensitized with the human thyrotropin receptor, to naive BALB/c and NOD mice. Endocrinology. 1996;137:4637–43.
108. Carayanniotis G, Huang GC, Nicholson LB et al. Unaltered thyroid function in mice responding to highly immunogenic thyrotropin receptor: implications for the development of a mouse model for Graves' disease. Clin Exp Immunol. 1995;99:294–302.
109. Wagle NM, Patibandla, SA, Dallas, JS, Morris, JC, Prabhakar, BS. Thyrotropin receptor-specific antibodies in BALB/cJ mice with experimental hyperthyroxinemia show a restricted binding specificity and belong to the immunoglobulin G1 subclass. Endocrinology. 1995;136: 3461–9.
110. Vlase H, Nakashima M, Graves PN, Tomer Y, Morris JC, Davies TF. Defining the major antibody epitopes on the human thyrotropin receptor in immunized mice: evidence for intramolecular epitope spreading. Endocrinology. 1995;136:4415–23.
111. Volpé R, Kasuga Y, Akasu F et al. The use of the severe combined immunodeficient mouse and the athymic 'nude' mouse as models for the study of human autoimmune thyroid disease. Clin Immunol Immunopathol. 1993;67:93–9.

2
Thyroid autoantigens

M. LUDGATE

INTRODUCTION

The thyroid gland, which has a central role in the control of metabolism via T_3 and T_4 hormones, is the target of the most common autoimmune diseases [1]. The thyroid hormone precursor is thyroglobulin (TG), which is iodinated on tyrosine residues. A fraction of these residues is coupled to form T_4, which is de-iodinated to form T_3. Both the iodination and coupling steps are catalyzed by thyroid peroxidase (TPO). The thyroid is under the control of the hypothalamic/pituitary axis: thyrotropin releasing hormone (TRH) acts on the pituitary resulting in the release of thyrotropin (TSH) which modulates the growth, differentiation and function of the thyroid via the TSH receptor (TSHR). TRH and TSH levels are themselves under the control of T_4 and T_3, in a negative feedback which results in the maintenance of homeostasis [2].

Three of the thyroid-specific proteins, TG, TPO and the TSHR are directly implicated in the production of thyroid hormones and have been identified as major autoantigens in a spectrum of diseases ranging from primary myxoedema (PM) and Hashimoto's thyroiditis (HT), in which the immune-mediated destruction of the gland results in hypothyroidism (Chapter 3), to Graves' disease (GD) in which antibodies to the TSHR act as TSH agonists with consequent hyperthyroidism (Chapter 4).

In recent years considerable progress has been made in defining the transcription factors which are implicated in thyroid-specific expression of TG, TPO and the TSHR. As already mentioned, TSH controls the differentiated function of the thyroid and increases in cAMP levels result in the up-regulation of the transcription of TG and TPO; thyroid stimulating antibodies (TSAb) of GD mediate the same effect. Characterization of the promoter regions of TG and

A.P. Weetman (ed.), Endocrine Autoimmunity and Associated Conditions. 25–38.

TPO have not identified classical cyclic AMP response elements (CREs) and their transcription seems to be controlled by TTF-1 (expressed in the thyroid and the lung) and PAX-8 (expressed in the thyroid and kidney). Regions in the promoters of all three thyroid autoantigens which bind these factors have been identified, although the control of TSHR expression is more complex since, in some circumstances, increased cAMP results in down-regulation of the receptor [3]. A detailed description is beyond the scope of this chapter which will concentrate on the structure/function characteristics of TG, TPO and TSHR, particularly as relates to their role as autoantigens. The possibility that other thyroid proteins may be autoantigens will also be discussed.

THYROGLOBULIN

Gene structure, similarities and variants

TG is a homodimeric (2×330 kDa) glycosylated iodoprotein, with a sedimentation rate of 19 S, which accumulates in the thyroid follicular lumen. Its abundance and degree of iodination vary greatly depending on the activity of the gland. Immunoreactive TG is also found in the plasma where its role, if any, remains unknown.

The TG promoter is translated from an 8.4 kb mRNA encoded by a large (>250 kb) transcription unit on the long arm of chromosome 8, distal to the c-myc locus [4]. Cloning and sequencing of the human [5] and bovine [6] TG cDNAs have provided a detailed picture of the primary structure of the protein. Following a 19 amino acid signal peptide, the polypeptide chain is composed of 2748 residues. Analysis for internal homology led to its subdivision into four regions, A–D from the amino to the carboxyl terminus. Domain A is composed of 10 type I repeats containing about 60 amino acids including 24 highly conserved residues, 6 of which are cysteines. Domain B (1439–1486), contains three type II repeats of a shorter motif. Domain C (14860–2111) is composed of the repetition of a type III motif existing as two subtypes, sharing a similar pattern of cysteine residues and both repeated twice. Domain D is the remaining 600 residues which has no internal homologies.

Structure/function relationships have emerged from the comparison of its primary structure with that of iodothyronine-containing peptides. In the coupling reaction, one iodotyrosine is considered as the electron donor and the other as the acceptor, the latter being the hormonogenic site. Four tryptic peptides containing thyroid hormone have been isolated from TG of various species and sequenced [7]. The corresponding tyrosine residues have been identified in the primary structure. Two of them map at sub-terminal positions (residues 5 and 2746 in the human sequence) and correspond to sites involved preferentially with the synthesis of T_4 and T_3, respectively. The two other sites are at positions 1290 and 2553.

Comparison of the primary structure of TG with available polypeptide sequences revealed a significant similarity between domain D and the whole sequence of acetylcholinesterase (AChE) [8], between domain A and the invariant chain of class II antigens [9] and also GA773, a major gastrointestinal tumour-associated antigen [10]. In all cases the similarity is suggestive of a common ancestor but does not reveal functional relationships.

In terms of its role as an autoantigen, the similarity with AChE has been suggested as a possible link between the thyroid and eye orbit which might explain the eye disease which frequently accompanies autoimmune thyroid disease, thyroid-associated ophthalmopathy (TAO; Chapter 6), which is briefly discussed below. Potentially of more significance is the similarity with the invariant chain of the major histocompatibility complex (MHC) class II antigen. In the absence of endogenous peptide for antigen presentation, a portion of the invariant chain, known as the CLIP peptide, is inserted into the groove of the class II antigen ensuring its correct folding and localization at the cell surface [11]. Thus antigen presenting cells bearing peptides sharing similarities with TG are generated, which in susceptible individuals may be sufficient to trigger normally anergic TG-specific T cell clones. The predisposition to autoimmune thyroid disease is the consequence of multiple genes, including HLA-DR, in particular DR3 and DR5. In elegant transgenic studies, the human DR3 gene has been introduced into mice normally resistant to the induction of thyroiditis using TG as an immunogen, and the animals subsequently developed disease (see Chapter 1).

Apart from the heterogeneity related to glycosylation and hormone content, analysis of TG cDNA has revealed variations in primary structure as the consequence of alternative splicing. Minor transcripts in which one or two exons are missing have been sequenced in bovine and human species, and alternative splicing in all regions of human TG mRNA has been described [12]. A 1.1 rat TG mRNA, which encodes the first five exons followed by a short carboxyl terminal unrelated to TG, seems to be up-regulated by TSH [13]. The function and relationship of these minor transcripts to the role of TG as an autoantigen, or indeed as a hormone precursor are unknown.

TG as an autoantigen

Despite its central role in the function of the thyroid gland and the fact that most progress in animal models of thyroid autoimmunity has been made using TG, this autoantigen is generally regarded as a bystander in human disease since TG antibodies probably have no pathological rule. Despite this, and in an attempt to determine whether TG antibodies in normal individuals and patients vary, several different approaches have been applied to try to define the antibody epitopes of TG. Screening a lambda gt11 human thyroid library with hetero-antibodies (rabbit anti-human TG) revealed 10 epitope-bearing segments and demonstrated that the 22 amino acids at the carboxyl-terminus of the protein contain a highly reactive epitope. When extensive screening was performed using sera having higher titres of TG antibodies predominantly from patients with HT, either individually or pooled, not a single positive plaque was isolated

[14]. An indirect approach was used to identify autoepitopes of TG, based on the sequence similarity between TG and AChE: the same library was screened with a rabbit anti-AChE antibody and two clones encoding virtually identical TG peptides were isolated. Subsequently they were shown to be recognized by patients with autoimmune thyroid disease and thus could be considered as an autoepitope [15].

These results, which demonstrate that the majority of TG autoantibodies are directed against conformational or iodine-containing epitopes and that a major heteroepitope is located at the C-terminus of TG, are at variance with a more recent study which has employed fragments of TG expressed as a bacterial fusion protein [16]. Seven immunoreactive peptides were identified: none of them included a hormonogenic site and five of them were located in the central part of the molecule. Further progress in identifying the predominantly conformational autoepitopes will require site-directed mutagenesis studies of the type already applied to TPO and the TSHR (see below), but the production of monoclonal antibodies which compete with human sera for TG binding should also be informative [17].

THYROID PEROXIDASE

Gene structure, similarities and variants

TPO is a glycosylated haemoprotein bound to the apical plasma membrane of thyroid follicular cells with its catalytic domain facing the colloid space. It seems to exist in two molecular forms of 105 and 110 kDa and was identified as the major antigenic component of the thyroid microsomal antigen [18,19]. This was confirmed by one of the cloning strategies in which a thyroid expression library was screened with microsomal autoantibodies and a polyclonal antibody to porcine TPO, and many of the clones isolated were proved to be identical. The primary structure of human TPO was subsequently elucidated by sequencing its cDNA [20,21]. It contains 933 amino acids, including a putative signal peptide, five potential glycosylation sites and 21 cysteine residues which may be implicated in disulphide bonds: there is evidence for at least one disulphide bond creating a loop in the protein [22]. Analysis of hydropathy profiles indicates that the protein is anchored in the membrane by a 25 amino acid segment located near the C-terminus.

The extracellular domain has similarities with myeloperoxidase, indicative of a common evolutionary origin, and the C-terminus extension has two domains encoded by modules belonging to the epidermal growth factor and complement C4b families. The TPO gene is located on the short arm of chromosome 2 [23]. It comprises 17 exons and 16 introns and extends over 150 kb [24]. Comparisons with other peroxidases has suggested that one of the histidines, at position 407 or 494, is the proximal and that at 414 is the distal haem binding site in TPO [25].

The major transcript of TPO is 3.1 kb (TPO1) but there are a number of splice variants. The most abundant has 171 bp in exon 10 spliced out, resulting in a protein 57 amino acids shorter (TPO2), which was suggested might explain the 105 kDa species. Several lines of evidence argue against this. When full length TPO is transfected into a non-thyroidal cell, the 105/110 doublet is obtained [26]. Furthermore an antibody to the 57 amino acids unique to TPO1 revealed the same 105/110 kDa doublet [27]. In the same study, using antibodies to various regions of TPO, no proteins which could be the product of the other variants described [26,28] were detected, indicating that only the full length transcript is translated and consequently responsible for all enzymatic activity. Variations in glycosylation or other post-translational modification must explain the two molecular forms.

TPO as an autoantigen

Unlike TG, antibodies to the thyroid microsomal antigen have been shown to be capable of fixing complement and participating in antibody-dependent cellular cytotoxicity (ADCC), both mechanisms which would lead to immune destruction of the thyroid gland, autoimmune hypothyroidism (Chapter 3). This condition is associated with high titres of antibodies to the thyroid microsome and, with the demonstration that TPO is the major component of this antigen complex, it seemed logical to assume that the biological activity of microsomal antibodies is directed to TPO. This has been confirmed indirectly in the case of ADCC, since preincubation of sera with TPO dramatically reduced their cytotoxicity for porcine thyroid follicular cells [29]. Results of studies aimed at determining whether TPO autoantibodies are able to fix complement are awaited.

In common with TG autoantibodies, those against TPO are also present in normal individuals, although their reported prevalence varies. Thus it became relevant to characterize the B cell epitopes of the protein to identify putative disease-specific epitopes which might improve diagnostic assays and also to determine whether autoantibodies inhibit the enzymatic activity of TPO. Currently there is a debate between groups finding linear sequential epitopes of TPO and those who consider that, again like TG, the majority of TPO autoantibodies bind conformational 3-dimensional epitopes.

In one of the original studies to clone human TPO, a major epitope, C2, was identified which was recognized by 95% of HT sera and two-thirds of patients with autoimmune thyroid disease [30]. Subsequently C2, and a second fragment C21, were delimited by screening a TPO epitope library using autoimmune thyroiditis sera, as antigenic linear hot spots, C2 (590–622) and C21 (710–722) [31], and these have been confirmed in other studies in which fragments of TPO have been expressed as various bacterial fusion proteins [32,33]. Furthermore it has been shown that autoantibodies affinity purified on the larger (590–675) C2 fragment retain their activity in a radio-immunoassay which employs the intact full length human protein [34].

In more recent studies, the reactivity of TPO antibody-positive sera from normal individuals was not found to be different from patients with autoimmune thyroid disease [35]. The frequency of antibodies to a 513–633 fragment (which contains C2) was greater in HT patients than in GD [36], although both groups of patients had similar frequencies of antibodies to a 633–933 fragment (which contains C21).

The definition of conformational epitopes is less straightforward, as exemplified by the limited progress made with TG autoepitopes. One approach involves the production of monoclonal antibodies which may be capable of competing for TPO binding with autoantibodies and whose reaction with various peptide fragments of TPO can be elucidated to build up a map of the contact residues involved [37]. Chimeric molecules in which portions of myeloperoxidase have been substituted into TPO and expressed in eucaryotic cells have shown that autoantibody recognition does not require the amino terminal 121 amino acids [38].

Of 13 monoclonal antibodies which bind non-denatured TPO and were used to screen a TPO epitope library, only one, mAb 47 [39], was shown to bind a linear sequence which corresponded to the C21 epitope. However the binding of human TPO FAb fragments, generated in combinational libraries, was not found to be diminished by mAb 47 and it was concluded that this epitope is not recognized by autoimmune thyroiditis sera [40]. However, even though the FAbs generated resemble serum autoantibodies in terms of affinity, most evidence suggests that the heavy and light chain pairs formed do not reflect the combinations found *in vivo* [41].

Thus the data from the linear and conformational camps complement rather than contradict each other and we can conclude that TPO autoantibody epitopes bind to the carboxyl end of the extracellular domain of the molecule, with contact residues at 590–622 and 710–722. There is no difference between normal and autoimmune thyroid disease autoepitopes in general, but HT sera seem to recognize preferentially the C2 region. Since the proximal and distal histidine residues, which constitute the active site, are located some 200 residues upstream from the antigenic hot-spot, it seems unlikely that TPO autoantibodies would inhibit enzymatic activity, although allosteric interference might create this effect. Data to investigate this point are contradictory and would be facilitated by the expression of enzymatically active TPO on a non-thyroid background. To date, most systems tried, including baculovirus [42] and yeast [43], generate inactive enzyme, and the fact that most autoantibodies retain their immunoreactivity with these TPO proteins also argues against their being inhibitory.

THYROTROPIN RECEPTOR

Gene structure, similarities and variants

The human TSHR is a member of the G protein-coupled receptor family. It is a glycoprotein of 744 amino acids, with 398 residues comprising the large extracellular domain (ECD), a feature shared with the receptors for the other glycoprotein hormones, luteinizing hormone (LH) and follicle stimulating hormone (FSH), and shown to be involved in hormone binding (see below). The remaining 346 residues are arranged into seven membrane spanning regions, characteristic of the G protein-coupled receptors [44]. There are six potential N-linked glycosylation sites and 11 cysteines in regions predicted to be outside the cells. An odd number of cysteines is a feature of receptors which cross link. Recent studies [45] have confirmed those from the pre-cloning era [46], showing that the receptor undergoes post translational modification into two subunits, A of M_r 55 kDa which is the ECD, and B of M_r 40 kDa, the membrane spanning regions, the two held together by disulphide bonds. Furthermore, quantitative western blot analysis has revealed that the B subunit is more abundant than the A subunit, suggesting that the latter can be shed from the thyrocyte surface and this shedding is increased in the presence of TSH [47]. Whether this is the activation mechanism has yet to be resolved, but the fact that trypsin treatment (see below) increases cAMP levels would tend to support this theory [48]. The ECD of the receptor is comprised of a number of leucine-rich repeats, modules which are found in a number of other proteins particularly those involved in protein–protein interactions such as RNAsin. The crystal structure of this protein has recently been obtained and by analogy a doughnut structure for the ECD of the receptor has been proposed [49].

The TSHR shares similarity with the LHR and FSHR, which is approximately 70% when comparing the membrane spanning regions and 45% in the ECD. The gene for the TSHR is located on the long arm of chromosome 14 [50]. It comprises 10 exons, (1–9 encoding the ECD and 10 the membrane spanning region) and 11 introns, spanning about 100 kb. The major TSHR transcripts are 4.6 and 4.4 kb and are the consequences of differing polyadenylation. In addition a number of alternative transcripts have been described, the most abundant being of 1.3 and 1.8 [51]. They seem to be the product of exons 1–8 or 1–9, followed by a short intronic sequence containing a stop codon. Proteins which could be the translation products of these transcripts have yet to be demonstrated although if expressed they would not be membrane bound (lacking exon 10) and thus could be circulating TSH binding proteins analogous to that for growth hormone. The LHR and FSHR also have a number of alternatively spliced variants but, as in the case of the TSHR, their pathophysiological role remains conjectural.

The TSHR has a central role in the pathogenesis of toxic adenoma and congenital hyperthyroidism, since point mutations leading to single amino acid changes can result in the constitutive activation of the receptor. Similarly, loss of function mutations are associated with congenital hypothyroidism [reviewed in Reference 52]. However in the case of autoimmunity the receptor seems to be a bystander, since a mutation originally thought to be implicated in autoimmunity (Pro52Thr) has been found in 12% of the normal population and when characterized *in vitro* was found to behave like the wild type TSHR in signal transduction and hormone binding studies [53].

The TSHR as an autoantigen

The TSHR is the target of a heterogeneous collection of autoantibodies: TSAb, usually measured by their ability to increase cAMP levels in thyroid cells (very potent TSAb also stimulate phospholipase C); thyroid blocking antibodies (TBAb), which inhibit TSH-mediated cAMP production and thyrotropin binding inhibiting immunoglobulins (TBII) which are routinely assayed using porcine thyroid membranes and I^{125}-labelled bovine TSH [reviewed in Reference 46]. These differing antibodies may co-exist in the same patient and also TSHR antibodies having no agonist or antagonist activity but able to bind directly to a TSHR preparation in a western blot [54].

TSHR autoantibodies are known to be directly involved in pathogenesis, as elegantly demonstrated in nature by their placental transfer and subsequent development of hyper- or hypothyroidism in neonates of mothers having TSAb or TBAb respectively. These conditions are transient, in keeping with the half-life of an immunoglobulin [55]. The recent demonstration of TSHR in the fat of young rats suggests that receptor antibodies may also be implicated in thyroid-associated ophthalmopathy [56] although thyrotropin receptors have yet to be found in adult human fat from any location (see Chapter 6).

Since the cloning of the TSHR it has been possible to develop binding and bioassays using cell lines stably transfected with the human TSHR, which escape many of the practical problems associated with non-recombinant methods yet display a good correlation with them and may even be more sensitive [57,58]. An important point to emerge from the development of these assays is that a single gene product expressed in a non-thyroidal cell is sufficient to couple both to Gs and Gq and is able to account for all TSAb/TBAb/TBII activities detected with thyrocytes, and it is not necessary to invoke the existence of other sub-types or components of the TSHR. Having said that, a minority of untreated Graves' sera are negative for TSAb and TBII, regardless of how they are measured. It is worth noting that most assays for receptor antibodies are performed in the absence of NaCl, sometimes with isotonicity maintained with sucrose, and these conditions are known to increase the natural constitutive activity of the unliganded receptor [59], thereby making it easier to be triggered by an agonist such as TSAb. Stimulation of cAMP production *in vitro* also requires relatively high concentrations of serum or IgG (1 in 10 dilution) indicating that circulating levels of these antibodies and their affinity for the receptor are low, although local effects in the thyroid, a major site of TSHR antibody production, are sufficient to result in clinical hyperthyroidism.

In an attempt to understand why receptor antibodies may be TSH agonists or antagonists, and with the aim of developing improved assays for diagnosis and prediction of clinical outcome, considerable effort has gone into attempting to define the regions of the TSHR involved in the binding and bioactivity of TSH, TSAb and TBAb. The main findings of the two groups who have contributed most to this difficult area are as follows:

(i) Numerous discontinuous residues (of the ECD of the TSHR) comprise the high affinity TSH binding site.

(ii) Binding sites for TSH/TSAb/TBAb are dissimilar in the amino part of the ECD and similar at the carboxyl end of the ECD.

(iii) Residues 1–260 are required for the binding of all three ligands [reviewed in Reference 60]. Some of these findings are in agreement with those reviewed by Kohn *et al.* [61].

(iv) The high affinity TSH binding site is located in the carboxyl terminus of the ECD, implicating in particular Tyr 385, and residues 295–302 and 387–395, especially the cysteine residues.

(v) TSH agonist activity acts through the amino end of the ECD, particularly thr 40 and residues 30–33, 34–37, 42–45, 52–56 and 58–61.

Binding to different regions of the receptor provide some explanation for the existence of antibodies having agonist or antagonist activities, but the fact that TBAb inhibit the activity of both TSH, and TSAb and that TBAb can be transformed into TSAb by the addition of anti-human immunoglobulin [62], imply the existence of other mechanisms, e.g. variation in pI or degree of glycosylation. Progress in this area awaits elucidation of the mode of TSH activation. Studies of the constitutive mutations of the receptor mentioned above indicate that the TSHR is in a constrained conformation in the absence of hormone, which prevents it coupling to the G protein. Point mutations can modify the structure sufficiently to relax that constraint. Recently mild trypsin treatment has been found to do the same; by removing a portion of the receptor, probably located in the 317–366 region, the cAMP response to bovine TSH was slightly decreased [48]. In earlier studies, TSAb were shown to retain their bioactivity, in common with human TSH, whereas bovine TSH activity was reduced on human thyroid cells treated with trypsin [63]. The physiological relevance of these observations and whether TSH itself has proteolytic activity remain to be resolved.

Finally, access to recombinant forms of receptor should enable the establishment of animal models of Graves' disease and PM. Results so far are promising for the latter, since it is possible to induce TBAb and thyroiditis in mice by hyperimmunization with recombinant TSHR [64]. However less progress has been made in Graves' disease, although some studies have produced antibodies which, at high concentrations, have weak stimulatory activity [65] and some animals have transiently reduced or elevated T_4 levels [66]. The less than perfect receptor preparations used may be one reason for the failure to induce TSAb and a second may be the fact that TSAb are predominantly of the kappa light chains, which comprise about one-third of immunoglobulins in man but only 5% in mice. However, if TSAb prove to be unique to the human condition, this would be further evidence that their agonist activity is attributable to more than a mere coincidence of heavy and light chain variable regions.

OTHER THYROID-ASSOCIATED AUTOANTIGENS

The possible involvement of the TSHR in thyroid-associated ophthalmopathy has already been mentioned. Another candidate antigen is a 64 kDa protein, cloned by screening a thyroid expression library with autoimmune thyroid disease sera. It was shown to be expressed in the thyroid and extraocular muscle but not skeletal muscle, by northern blotting; the broader tissue distribution obtained by RT-PCR studies probably reflects illegitimate transcription. The protein shares similarity with tropomodulin, which interacts with tropomyosin, both being components of the cytoskeleton [reviewed in Reference 67].

Prior to its cloning, the Na^+/I^- symporter was described as an autoantigen [68]. Some 150 sera were screened for their ability to inhibit the uptake of iodide but not rubidium and one positive was found from a 55-year-old female having HT and autoimmune gastritis. The rat symporter has recently been cloned [69]. It has 12 membrane spanning segments, a molecular weight of 80 kDa and is expressed predominantly in the thyroid and, to a lesser extent, in the stomach and salivary gland. The protein has been expressed in a prokaryotic system as a fusion protein and almost 90% of GD patients were shown to have antibodies to it [70]. The real prevalence is probably between these two extremes, as in the first study detection depended on the antibody inhibiting the symporter rather than just binding to it and previous extensive western blotting studies with thyroid antigens have not identified an 80 kDa band with the majority of GD sera, which would be predicted from the second study if it were accurate.

FUTURE PROSPECTIVES

A variety of techniques has been used to identify and characterize thyroid autoantigens: screening expression libraries, generation of combinatorial libraries, site directed mutagenesis, chimera studies, production of monoclonal antibodies, prokaryotic and eukaryotic expression, etc. A current goal is the ability to perform X-ray diffraction to analyse antigen/antibody and receptor/ligand interactions, which would require crystals of TPO and the TSHR. Several eukaryotic expression systems have already been tried but despite generating the quantity required, the proteins are inactive either as enzymes (TPO) or in TSH binding.

More progress is being made in the T cell cloning area as both TPO and the TSHR have been stably transfected into EBV-transformed B cells, which can thus assume the role of antigen presenting cells. There is little doubt that studies of this type, coupled with transgenic mouse experiments permitting the dissection of the human autoimmune response, will yield real insights into the pathogenesis of autoimmune thyroid disease.

References

1. Weetman AP, McGregor AM. Autoimmune thyroid disease: further developments in our understanding. Endocrine Rev. 1994;15:788–830.
2. Taurog A. Hormone synthesis; thyroid iodide metabolism. In: Braverman L, Utiger R, eds. Werner and Ingbar's The Thyroid. Philadelphia: Lippincott Co.; 1996:47–81.
3. DiLauro R, Damante G, Defelice M et al. Molecular events in the differentiation of the thyroid gland. J Endocrinol Invest. 1995;18:117–9.
4. Baas F, Bikker H, Guerts van Kessel A et al. The human thyroglobulin gene: a polymorphic marker localised distal to c-myc on chromosome 8 band g24. Hum Genet. 1985;69:138–42.
5. Malthierry Y, Lissitzky S. Primary structure of human thyroglobulin deduced from the sequence of its 8448 base cDNA. Eur J Biochem. 1987;165:491–8.
6. Mercken L, Simons MJ, Swillens S, Massaer M, Vassart G. Primary structure of bovine thyroglobulin as deduced from the sequencing of its 8431 base cDNA. Nature. 1985;316:647–51.
7. den Hartog M, Sijmons C, Bakker O, Risstalpers C, Devijlder J. Importance of the context and localisation of tyrosine residues for thyroxine formation within the N-terminal part of human thyroglobulin. Eur J Endocrinol. 1995;132:611–17.
8. Swillens S, Ludgate M, Mercken L, Dumont J, Vassart G. Analysis of sequence and structure homologies between thyroglobulin and acetylcholinesterase: possible functional and clinical significance. Biochem Biophys Res Commun. 1986;137:142–8.
9. Koch N, Lauer W, Hibichi J, Dobberstein B. Primary structure of the gene for the murine I-A antigen associated invariant chain. An alternatively spliced exon encodes a cysteine-rich domain homologous to a repetitive sequence of thyroglobulin. EMBO J. 1987;6:1677–83.
10. Linnenbach A, Wojcierowski J, Wu S et al. Sequence investigation of the major gastro-intestinal tumor associated antigen gene family GSA773. Proc Natl Acad Sci USA. 1989;71: 223–6.
11. Wolf P, Hidde L. DM exchange mechanism. Nature. 1995;376:464–5.
12. Targovnik H, Medeiros-Neto G, Varela V, Cochaux P, Wajchenberg B, Vassart G. A nonsense mutation causes human hereditary congenital goitre with preferential production of a 171 nucleotide deleted thyroglobulin ribonucleic acid messenger. J Clin Endocrinol Metab. 1993; 77:210–15.
13. Graves P, Davies T. A second thyroglobulin mRNA species (rTg-2) in rat thyrocytes. Mol Endocrinol. 1990;4:155–61.
14. Dong Q, Ludgate M, Vassart G. Towards an antigenic map of thyroglobulin: identification of ten epitope bearing sequences within the primary structure of thyroglobulin. J Endocrinol. 1989;122:169–76.
15. Ludgate M, Dong Q, Dreyfus P et al. Definition at the molecular level of a thyroglobulin-acetylcholinesterase shared epitope: study of its pathophysiological significance in patients with Graves' ophthalmopathy. Autoimmunity. 1989;3:167–76.
16. Malthierry Y, Henry M, Zanelli E. Epitope mapping of human thyroglobulin reveals a central immunodominant region. FEBS Lett. 1991;279:190–92.
17. Schultz E, Benker G, Bethauser H, Stempka L, Hufner M. An auto-immunodominant thyroglobulin epitope characterised by a monoclonal antibody. J Endocrinol Invest. 1992; 15:25–30.
18. Portmann L, Hamada N, Heinrich G, DeGroot L. Anti-thyroid peroxidase antibody in patients with autoimmune thyroid disease: possible identity with anti-microsomal antibody. J Clin Endocrinol Metab. 1985;61:1001–3.
19. Czarnocka B, Ruf J, Fernand M, Carayon P, Lissitzky S. Purification of human thyroid peroxidase and its identification as the microsomal antigen involved in autoimmune thyroid disease. FEBS Lett. 1985;190:147–52.
20. Kimura S, Kotani T, Bride O et al. Human thyroid peroxidase: complete cDNA and protein sequence, chromosome mapping and identification of two alternatively spliced mRNAs. Proc Natl Acad Sci USA. 1987;86:394–403.
21. Libert F, Ruel J, Ludgate M et al. Thyroperoxidase, an autoantigen with a mosaic structure made of nuclear and mitochondrial gene modules. EMBO J. 1987;6:4193–6.
22. Taurog A, Dorris M, Yokoyama N, Slaughter C. Purification and characterisation of a large, tryptic fragment of human thyroid peroxidase with enzymatic activity. Arch Biochem Biophys. 1990;278:333–41.

23. Endo Y, Onogi S, Umeki K et al. Regional localisation of the gene for thyroid peroxidase to human chromosome 2p25 and mouse chromosome 12c. Genomics. 1995;25:760–1.
24. Kimura S, Hong Y-S, Kotani T, Ohtaki S, Kikkawa F. Structure of the human peroxidase gene; comparison and relationship to the human myeloperoxidase gene. Biochemistry. 1989; 28:4481–9.
25. Taurog A, Dorris M, Yokoyama N, Slaughter C. Purification and characterisation of a large tryptic fragment of human thyroid peroxidase with high catalytic activity. Arch Biochem Biophys. 1990;287:333–41.
26. McLachlan S, Rapoport B. The molecular biology of thyroid peroxidase: cloning, expression and role as autoantigen in autoimmune thyroid disease. Endocrine Rev. 1992;13:192–206.
27. Cetani F, Costagliola S, Tonacchera M, Panneels V, Vassart G, Ludgate M. The thyroperoxidase doublet is not produced by alternative splicing. Mol Cell Endocrinol. 1995;15:125–32.
28. Zanelli E, Henry M, Charvet B, Malthierry Y. Evidence for an alternate splicing in the thyroperoxidase messenger from patients with Graves' disease. Biochem Biophys Res Commun. 1990;170:735–41.
29. Rodien P, Madec A-M, Ruf J et al. Antibody dependent cell mediated cytotoxicity in autoimmune thyroid disease – relationship to anti-thyroperoxidase antibodies. J Clin Endocrinol Metab. 1996;81:2595–600.
30. Ludgate M, Mariotti S, Libert F et al. Antibodies to human thyroid peroxidase in autoimmune thyroid disease; study with a cloned recombinant cDNA epitope. J Clin Endocrinol Metab. 1989;68:1091–6.
31. Libert F, Ludgate M, Dinsart C, Vassart G. Thyroperoxidase, but not the thyrotropin receptor, contains sequential epitopes recognised by autoantibodies in recombinant peptides expressed in the pUEX vector. J Clin Endocrinol Metab. 1991;73:857–60.
32. Banga JP, Barnett P, Ewins D, Page M, McGregor A. Mapping of autoantigenic epitopes on recombinant thyroid peroxidase fragments using the polymerase chain reaction. Autoimmunity. 1990;6:257–68.
33. Zanelli E, Henry M, Malthierry Y. Epitope mapping of human thyroid peroxidase defined 7 epitopes recognised by sera from patients with thyroid pathologies. Cell Mol Biol. 1993;39: 491–501.
34. Elisei R, Mariotti S, Swillens S, Vassart G, Ludgate M. Studies with recombinant autoepitopes of thyroid peroxidase: evidence suggesting an epitope shared between the thyroid and the gastric parietal cell. Autoimmunity. 1990;8:65–70.
35. Tonacchera M, Cetani F, Costagliola S et al. Mapping thyroid peroxidase epitopes using recombinant protein fragments. Eur J Endocrinol. 1995;132:53–61.
36. Bermann M, Magee M, Koenig R et al. Differential autoantibody responses to thyroid peroxidase in patients with Graves' disease and Hashimoto's thyroiditis. J Clin Endocrinol Metab. 1993;77:1098–101.
37. Czarnucka B, Pastuszko D, Carayon P, Ruf J, Gardas A. Majority of thyroid peroxidase autoantibodies in patients with autoimmune thyroid disease are directed to a single TPO domain. Autoimmunity. 1996;23:145–54.
38. Nishikawa T, Rapoport B, McLachlan S. Exclusion of two major areas on human thyroid peroxidase from the immunodominant region containing the conformational epitopes recognised by human autoantibodies. J Clin Endocrinol Metab. 1994;79:1648–54.
39. Finke R, Seto P, Ruf J, Carayon P, Rapoport B. Determination at the molecular level of a B cell epitope likely to be associated with autoimmune thyroid disease. J Clin Endocrinol Metab. 1991;73:919–21.
40. Chazenbalk G, Costante G, Portolano S, McLachlan S, Rapoport B. The immunodominant region on human thyroid peroxidase recognised by autoantibodies does not contain the monoclonal antibody 47/C21 linear epitope. J Clin Endocrinol Metab. 1993;77:1715–18.
41. Rapoport B, Portalano S, McLachlan S. Combinational libraries – new insights into human organ specific autoantibodies. Immunol Today. 1995;16:43–9.
42. Wedlock N, Furmaniak J, Fowler S et al. Expression of human thyroid peroxidase in the yeast *Saccharomyces cerevisiae* and *Hansenula polymorpha*. J Mol Endocrinol. 1993;10:325–36.
43. Haubruck H, Mauch L, Cook N et al. Expression of recombinant human thyroid peroxidase by the baculovirus system and its use in ELISA screeningn for diagnosis of autoimmune thyroid disease. Autoimmunity. 1993;15:275–84.

44. Libert F, Lefort A, Gerard C et al. Cloning, sequencing and expression of the human thyrotropin (TSH) receptor: evidence for binding of autoantibodies. Biochem Biophys Res Commun. 1989;165:1250–5.
45. Nagayama Y, Kaufman K, Seto P, Rapoport B. Molecular cloning, sequence and functional expression of the cDNA for the human thyrotropin receptor. Biochem Biophys Res Commun. 1989;165:1187–90.
46. Rees Smith B, McLachlan S, Furmaniak J. Autoantibodies to the thyrotropin receptor. Endocrine Rev. 1988;9:106–21.
47. Loosfelt H, Pichon C, Jolivet A et al. 2 subunit structure of human thyrotropin receptor. Proc Natl Acad Sci USA. 1992;89:3765–9.
48. Van Sande J, Massart C, Costagliola S et al. Specific activation of the thyrotropin receptor by trypsin. Mol Cell Endocrinol. 1996'119:161–8.
49. Kajava A, Vassart G, Wodak S. Modeling of the 3 dimensional structure of proteins with the typical leucine rich repeats structure. Structure. 1995;3:867–77.
50. Gross B, Misrahi M, Sar S, Milgrom E. Composite structure of the human thyrotropin receptor gene. Biochem Biophys Res Commun. 1991;177:679–87.
51. Graves P, Tomer Y, Davies T. Cloning and sequencing of a 1.3 kb variant of human thyrotropin receptor mRNA lacking the transmembrane domain. Biochem Biophys Res Commun. 1992;187:1135–43.
52. Van Sande J, Parma J, Tonacchera M, Swillens S, Dumont J, Vassart G. Somatic and germ-line mutations of the TSH receptor gene in thyroid disease. J Clin Endocrinol Metab. 1995; 80:2577–85.
53. Tonacchera M, Cetani F, Costagliola S, Van Sande J, Refetoff S, Vassart G. Functional characteristics of a variant thyrotropin receptor. Eur J Biochem. 1996;238:490–4.
54. Tonacchera M, Costagliola S, Cetani F et al. Patient with monoclonal gammopathy, thyrotoxicosis, pretibial myxedema and thyroid associated ophthalmopathy; demonstration of direct binding of autoantibodies to the thyrotropin receptor. Eur J Endocrinol. 1995;134: 97–103.
55. McKenzie J, Zakarija M. The clinical use of thyrotropin receptor antibody measurements. J Clin Endocrinol Metab. 1989;69:1093–6.
56. Endo T, Ohta K, Haraguchi K, Onaya T. Cloning and functional expression of a thyrotropin receptor cDNA from rat fat cells. J Biol Chem. 1995;270:10833–7.
57. Costagliola S, Swillens S, Niccoli P, Ruf J, Vassart G, Ludgate M. Binding assay for thyrotropin receptor antibodies using recombinant protein. J Clin Endocrinol Metab. 1992; 75:1540–4.
58. Vitti P, Elisei R, Tonacchera M et al. Detection of thyroid stimulating antibody using Chinese hamster ovary cells transfected with cloned recombinant human thyrotropin receptor. J Clin Endocrinol Metab. 1993;76:499–503.
59. Cetani F, Tonacchera M, Vassart G. Differential effects of NaCl concentration on the constitutive activity of the thyrotropin and the luteinizing hormone chorionic gonadotropin receptors. FEBS Lett. 1996;378:27–31.
60. McLachlan S, Rapoport B. Autoimmune endocrinopathies. 2. Recombinant thyroid auto-antigens – the keys to pathogenesis of autoimmune thyroid disease. J Int Med. 1993;234:347–59.
61. Kohn L, Shimura H, Shimura Y et al. The thyrotropin receptor. Vitam Horm. 1995;50:287–384.
62. Taniguchi S, Yoshida A, Shigemasa S. The mechanism involved in the conversion of thyrotropin receptor bound blocking type immunoglobulin G to the stimulating type by anti-human IgG antibodies. Endocrinology. 1990;126:796–803.
63. Foti D, Russo D, Costante G, Filetti S. The biological activity of bovine and human thyrotropin is differently affected by trypsin treatment of human thyroid cells; thyroid stimulating antibody is related to human thyrotropin. J Clin Endocrinol Metab. 1991;73: 710–16.
64. Costagliola S, Many M-C, Stalmans-Falys M, Tonacchera M, Vassart G, Ludgate M. Recombinant thyrotropin receptor and the induction of autoimmune thyroid disease: a new animal model. Endocrinology. 1994;135:2150–9.
65. Hidaka Y, Guimaraes V, Soliman M et al. Production of thyroid stimulating antibodies in mice by immunisation with T cell epitopes of human thyrotropin receptor. Endocrinology. 1995;136:1642–7.

66. Wagle N, Patibandla S, Dallas J, Morris J, Prabhakar B. Thyrotropin receptor specific antibodies in BALBc mice with experimental hyperthyroxinemia show a restricted binding specificity and belong to the immunoglobulin G1 subclass. Endocrinology. 1995;136:3461–9.
67. Ludgate M. Back to the drawing board for antigens in thyroid associated ophthalmopathy? In: Wall J, Kahaly G, eds. Developments in Ophthalmopathy, Vol. 25. Basel: Karger; 1993:36–43.
68. Raspe E, Costagliola S, Ruf J, Mariotti S, Dumont J, Ludgate M. Identification of the Na^+/I^- cotransporter as a potential autoantigen in thyroid autoimmune disease. Eur J Endocrinol. 1995;132:399–407.
69. Dia G, Levy O, Carrasco N. Cloning and characterisation of the thyroid iodide transporter. Nature. 1996;379:456–60.
70. Endo T, Kogai T, Nakazoto M, Saito T, Kaneshige M, Onaya T. Autoantibody against $Na^+/^-$ symporter in the sera of patients with autoimmune thyroid disease. Biochem Biophys Res Commun. 1996;224:92–5

3
Autoimmune hypothyroidism

A. P. WEETMAN, R. S. McINTOSH and P. F. WATSON

Autoimmune hypothyroidism is the prototype for autoimmune diseases, and is one of the most common, with a prevalence of around 1% in Caucasian women and 0.5% in men. The chronicity of the disease, the characterization of autoantigens (Chapter 2) and the availability of several animal models (see Chapter 1) have all helped in its study. This chapter provides an overview of the main features of autoimmune hypothyroidism and summarizes recent research on its pathogenesis.

CLINICAL FEATURES

Epidemiology

Autoimmunity is by far the most common cause of spontaneous (non-iatrogenic) hypothyroidism in iodine-sufficient areas, accounting for over 90% of cases. Hypothyroidism develops gradually, and clinically apparent disease represents the culmination of ongoing thyroid damage over many months or years. This is evident from the high frequency of focal thyroiditis in the general population: up to 45% of women and 20% of men in the UK and USA have 1–10 foci of thyroiditis/cm^2 at routine autopsy, with more severe thyroiditis (>10 foci/cm^2) occurring in 5–15% of women and 1–5% of men [1,2]. The presence of focal thyroiditis is strongly correlated with circulating thyroglobulin (TG) and/or thyroid peroxidase (TPO) antibodies, discussed further below [3].

In the most detailed survey of autoimmune hypothyroidism to date, in which a population from the North East of England was followed for 20 years, the mean incidence of spontaneous hypothyroidism was 3.5/1000 women/year and, for men, 0.6/1000/year [4]. The mean age at diagnosis was 58–59 in both sexes,

A.P. Weetman (ed.), Endocrine Autoimmunity and Associated Conditions. 39–61.

although there was a steady accumulation of cases over time. However, in extreme old age the proportion of the population with autoimmune hypothyroidism falls and this may reflect the fact that healthy centenarians are a self-selected group with a resulting low frequency of autoimmunity [5]. There are also racial variations, thyroiditis being less frequent in black and Japanese Americans than in white Americans [2].

Presentation

The goitrous form of autoimmune thyroiditis (Hashimoto's thyroiditis) often presents with a small to large goitre without overt hypothyroidism; the gland is firm or even hard, and occasionally irregular, giving rise to the suspicion of malignancy. This possibility should be taken seriously, as coincidental thyroid tumours are not diminished (or increased) in frequency in this condition, while the uncommon B cell lymphoma of the thyroid is strongly associated with long-standing Hashimoto's thyroiditis [6]. Pain in an enlarging thyroid suggests the presence of a lymphoma, but can also rarely occur as part of the inflammatory process. Serum thyroid stimulating hormone (TSH) levels are the best initial guide to thyroid status, an elevated value despite normal circulating thyroxine (T_4) levels being termed subclinical hypothyroidism; there is an increased risk of future overt hypothyroidism in such patients [4]. Indeed, T_4 treatment often improves non-specific symptoms such as fatigue in patients with subclinical hypothyroidism.

Patients without an obvious goitre (atrophic thyroiditis or primary myxoedema) generally only come to attention when symptomatic hypothyroidism is apparent, although the widespread use of TSH assays and a low threshold for suspecting the diagnosis mean that the classical features of hypothyroidism are less common nowadays. A number of conditions may be associated with autoimmune hypothyroidism (Table 3.1) including the autoimmune polyglandular syndromes (Chapter 9).

Treatment

It would be difficult to find a more straightforward (or cheap) treatment than T_4 replacement, as doses can now be matched precisely to the patient's requirements using a sensitive TSH assay. In turn this means that immunosuppression is unlikely to be useful in this condition, unless a risk-free and simple one-off treatment could be used which would then only have the advantage over T_4 of not requiring the patient to take tablets each day. Compliance can be a problem with T_4 replacement, and patients should receive an annual check of TSH levels initially, with the interval between testing increasing to every 3 years if the TSH is repeatedly normal.

Goitre size usually decreases over a year or two on T_4 replacement and thyroidectomy is only indicated rarely, when there is a suspicion of tumour or in patients with painful thyroiditis, which responds poorly to steroids [7]. T_4

Table 3.1 Disorders associated with autoimmune hypothyroidism

Autoimmune polyglandular syndromes type 1 (uncommon) and type 2 (common) – see Chapter 9

Individual, non-endocrine components of these syndromes:
- Vitiligo (Chapter 13)
- Pernicious anaemia (Chapter 12)
- Alopecia areata
- Leucotrichia

Other organ-specific disorders:
- Myasthenia gravis
- Coeliac disease
- Dermatitis herpetiformis
- Chronic active hepatitis
- Idiopathic thrombocytopenic purpura

Non-organ-specific disorders
- Rheumatoid arthritis
- Systemic lupus erythematosus
- Systemic sclerosis
- Sjögren's syndrome
- Polymyalgia rheumatica

replacement is life-long, although remissions have been reported in 5–10% patients, particularly in those who have TSH-receptor (TSHR) blocking antibodies, discussed below [8]. The duration of such remissions is unknown and at present it is questionable whether withdrawal of T_4 is warranted; we do not attempt this.

PATHOLOGY

In keeping with the diversity in clinical features, a spectrum of histopathological features occurs in autoimmune thyroiditis [9]. The frequent occurrence of focal thyroiditis has already been noted: thyroid follicles are generally normal in this entity, although there may be destruction of those adjacent to the infiltrate. The factors which determine if and how focal thyroiditis progresses to more serious thyroid damage are unknown.

Diffuse thyroiditis is the key feature of both goitrous and atrophic thyroiditis, although the infiltrate is far more extensive in the former. There is a dense accumulation of lymphocytes, plasma cells and macrophages, with germinal centre formation. Thyroid follicles are destroyed and therefore their number in histological sections is obviously reduced; the remaining follicular cells show evidence of injury, with hyperplasia and oxyphilic metaplasia (Hürthle or Askanazy cells; Figure 3.1).

In both forms of thyroiditis, there is also fibrosis, but this is far more prominent in atrophic thyroiditis, in which the lymphocytic infiltrate may be

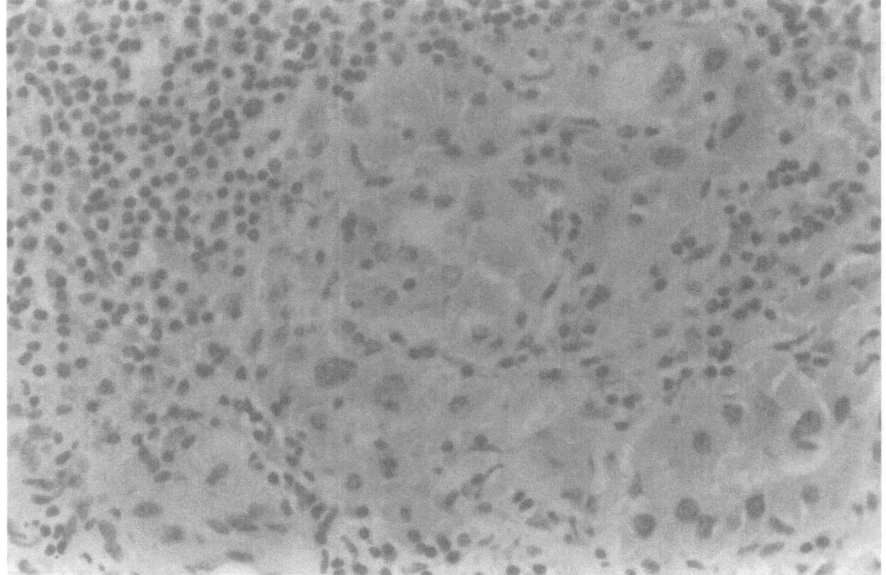

Figure 3.1 Lymphocytic infiltrate and Askenazy cell change in the thyroid follicular cells in Hashimoto's thyroiditis (photo courtesy of Dr. Judith Channer; original magnification ×400)

rather modest (Figure 3.2). There is no good evidence that goitrous thyroiditis precedes the atrophic form. Although goitre usually reduces with T_4 treatment, histological features remain remarkably stable over 20 years [10]. Rarely, histological changes of Graves' disease may also be seen ('hashitoxicosis') and clinically such patients may fluctuate rapidly from thyrotoxicosis to hypothyroidism or vice versa.

PREDISPOSING FACTORS

Immunogenetics

As with autoimmune diseases in general, predisposition to autoimmune hypothyroidism depends on the interplay between genetic, endogenous and environmental factors. The relative contribution of each is not clearly defined and in any case varies between patients. This is most clearly shown in juvenile autoimmune hypothyroidism, in which the strength of the genetic contribution is far more clearly evident than in the commoner adult form of the disease [11]. As the influence of environmental factors clearly depends on an individual's exposure, such factors are more likely to be important in older patients, and perhaps in those with no family history. There have been no properly conducted monozygotic twin surveys in autoimmune thyroiditis, and variable disease penetrance over a long time period poses a particular problem in organizing

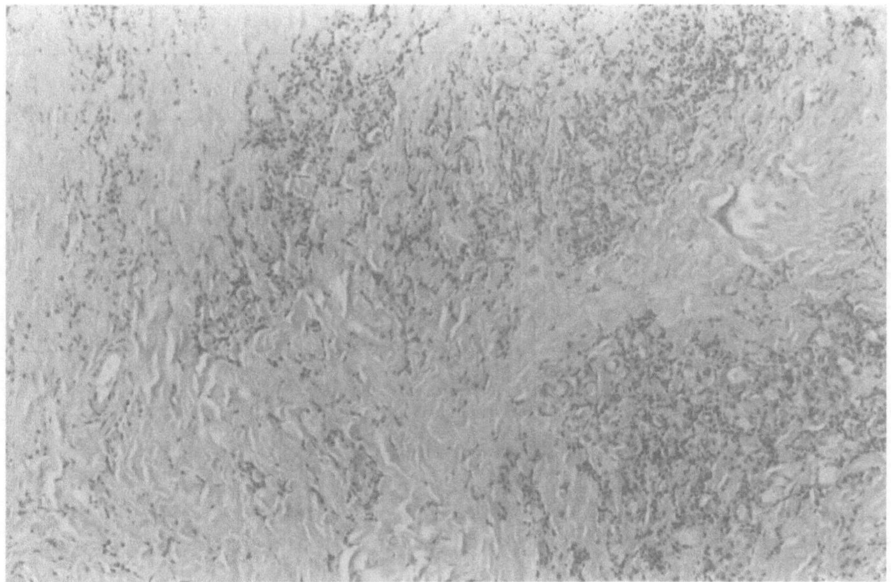

Figure 3.2 Prominent fibrosis and moderate lymphocytic infiltrate in atrophic thyroiditis (photo courtesy of Dr. Judith Channer; original magnification ×100)

such a study. However, by analogy with Graves' disease (Chapter 4), which shares many of the immunological features of autoimmune hypothyroidism, only around 30% of such twins would be expected to be concordant. Siblings of adult patients with Hashimoto's thyroiditis have around a 50% chance of developing thyroid autoantibodies [12]. When examined using modern assays, no clear pattern of inheritance for autoantibody production can be discerned, despite initial suggestions of it being an autosomal dominant trait [13].

HLA genes have received the most attention as potential susceptibility genes, although their influence in autoimmune hypothyroidism seems much less important than other disorders, such as Graves' disease and type 1 diabetes mellitus (Chapters 4 and 8). Initial studies showed no clear HLA associations with autoimmune hypothyroidism overall, but primary myxoedema was found to have an association with HLA-B8 and -DR3, which of course are in linkage disequilibrium [14,15]. Subsequently, Hashimoto's thyroiditis was associated with HLA-DR5 [16] and in both types of disease, the HLA alleles conferred a relative risk of around 3.5. This dichotomy in HLA association provided strong evidence that these two diseases were separate entities, but subsequent studies have failed to confirm the split. A summary of the results in Hashimoto's thyroiditis is provided in Table 3.2. In German patients with primary myxoedema, the clearest association was with HLA-DR5 (relative risk 4.6) and there was no association with HLA-DR3 [25].

Table 3.2 Association of HLA-DR types with Hashimoto's thyroiditis in Caucasians

Reference	*Country*	*Association*	*Relative risk*
17	Denmark	Dw5	2.2
18	Canada	DR4	5.0
19	Hungary	DR3	3.3
20	Canada	DR5	4.2
21	Canada+UK	DR4+DR5	2.9+3.8
22	UK	DR3	2.2
23	USA	None	None
24	UK*	None	None

*A meta analysis included in this paper concluded that the strongest association was with HLA-DR3 (relative risk 2.3) and HLA-DR4 (relative risk 1.6); there was no significant association with HLA-DR5

Part of the reason for these heterogeneous results lies in the quality of serological reagents used for typing in the earlier studies; up to 25% of such types may be incorrect. Modern molecular methods are superior in this regard. It is also likely that even within Caucasian populations there is genetic variation in susceptibility, and of course this may also have altered over time. Certainly, HLA associations with autoimmune hypothyroidism are very different in other races. HLA-Bw46 and -DR9 are associated with Hashimoto's thyroiditis in Chinese patients from Hong Kong [26], whereas in Japanese the strongest association is with HLA-DRw53, and -DR9 to a lesser extent [27]. Another recent Japanese series found an association with HLA-DQw4 [28]. In Korean patients with TSHR blocking antibodies and atrophic thyroiditis there is a significant association with HLA-DR8 and HLA-DQB1*0302 [29].

Clearly, no one HLA specificity confers susceptibility for autoimmune hypothyroidism and it is also obvious that the relative risks involved are small, implicating genetic loci outside of the HLA region. The association of both primary myxoedema and Hashimoto's thyroiditis with HLA-DR3 is similar to the association found with other autoimmune disorders, including endocrinopathies, and may reflect a non-specific enhancing effect that DR3 (or an allele in linkage disequilibrium with it) has on the autoimmune response in general.

The non-HLA genes which contribute to susceptibility are unknown. Several candidates have been proposed, including genes encoding immunoglobulins and T cell receptors (TCR), but these associations have not been substantiated [23]. A high prevalence of autoimmune hypothyroidism has been reported in Down's syndrome and in kindreds with familial Alzheimer's disease, implicating the influence of a gene on chromosome 21 [30]. As with Graves' disease, there is an association between a polymorphism of the CTLA-4 gene on chromosome 2q33 and autoimmune hypothyroidism in English Caucasians [31]; this remains to be confirmed in other groups of patients. Autoimmune thyroiditis is found in 21–88% of patients with Turner's syndrome, with an inconsistent association with the 46 XiXq form [32]. This suggests a role for a gene on the X chromosome but its identity and effect are unknown. The best approach to solving the puzzle of the immunogenetics of autoimmune hypothyroidism will be to perform linkage studies on large numbers of multiply affected families, initially using microsatellite polymorphisms to identify chromosomal regions of potential importance. Automated molecular techniques have greatly facilitated such an approach and several groups are already proceeding with such an analysis.

Non-genetic factors

The female prevalence of autoimmune hypothyroidism seems most likely to be due to the influence of sex hormones, based on the results from studies of their influence on animal models of autoimmune disease [33]. Hormonal changes in pregnancy seem to predispose to a later exacerbation in the severity of autoimmune thyroiditis (Chapter 5). Prolactin, as well as sex hormones, may play a role, as asymptomatic autoimmune thyroiditis is more common in women with hyperprolactinaemia [34]. Another potential endogenous influence is low birthweight, which is associated with an increased prevalence of thyroid autoantibodies in middle age [35]. Hormonal influences again seem likely to account for this effect.

Of the candidate environmental factors, dietary iodide seems the most clearly established, although again the best evidence comes from animals with spontaneous or experimental autoimmune thyroiditis [36]. However, epidemiological surveys do implicate iodide in the human disorder. For instance, the introduction of iodization programmes into iodine-deficient regions is associated with a subsequent increase in the prevalence of thyroid autoantibodies and lymphocytic thyroiditis [37,38]. Iodide is toxic to iodide-deprived thyroid cells, possibly by forming toxic oxidized iodide compounds, although more general immunomodulatory effects are also possible.

There is no clear evidence that infection plays a role in susceptibility, although equally there is nothing definitive to rule this out [39]. However, viral infections of the gland (subacute thyroiditis) are not associated with an increased prevalence of autoimmune thyroiditis. Autoimmune hypothyroidism was more frequent than expected in the survivors of the atomic bomb in Nagasaki, and there is supporting evidence that other types of low dose irradiation may also predispose individuals to the development of thyroid autoimmunity [40]. Exacerbation of pre-existing autoimmune thyroiditis follows the administration of α-interferon (α-IFN) and other cytokines for malignancy or hepatitis [41]. Whilst the doses of cytokines used are massive, it is possible that other events (e.g. stress, infection) could non-specifically perturb cytokine levels and precipitate autoimmune thyroiditis in otherwise predisposed individuals. The only other drug which clearly exacerbates autoimmune thyroiditis is lithium, probably by a direct effect on regulatory T cells [42].

T CELLS

It is clear from animal models of autoimmune thyroiditis that autoreactive T cells play a major role in the immunopathology [43] and there is abundant evidence for a parallel function in chronic thyroiditis. The thyroid itself represents the key site of autoreactivity though autoimmune responses can be detected at other locations including the draining lymph nodes, bone marrow, and the peripheral circulation [44]. The majority of the T cell phenotypic and functional studies described below have been performed on the more readily available peripheral blood population and it remains unclear to what extent these studies reflect the immune processes to be found within the target tissue.

T cell phenotypes

Studies of circulating T cell subsets in Hashimoto's thyroiditis have produced conflicting results, with an increased, decreased, and normal $CD4^+$:$CD8^+$ ratio being reported [45–50]. There is a consensus that activated (HLA-DR^+) T cells are increased in the circulation in autoimmune thyroiditis. Within the thyroid infiltrate, $CD4^+$ cells are in the majority and many of these are DR^+ [51–53]. Most of the intrathyroidal T cells express the αβ T cell antigen receptor (TCR). A minority of T cells expressing the γδ TCR have been detected in thyroid infiltrates in Hashimoto's thyroiditis [54,55], but results have been conflicting [56], and their immunopathological function remains unclear. However, the recent description of a γδ TCR^+ thyroid cell-specific cytotoxic T cell clone derived from the thyroid infiltrating lymphocytes in Graves' disease suggests a role for this class of T cells in autoimmune thyroiditis [56].

Restriction of the TCR repertoire at the site of autoimmune attack would suggest a role for a selected subpopulation of T cells in the disease aetiology and would have important therapeutic implications [57]. The question of T cell restriction in autoimmune thyroid disease remains controversial. In the case of TCR Vβ gene usage there is no apparent restriction of gene usage. However, studies based on Vα gene reverse transcription-polymerase chain reaction (RT-PCR) demonstrated some evidence of restriction (4–5 of 18 Vα families) in intrathyroidal T cells in Graves' disease and Hashimoto's thyroiditis [58,59]. This restriction was still evident, though less marked (12–17 of 18 Vα families), when the same approach was used to analyse TCR gene usage in fine needle aspirates from Hashimoto patients [60]. These results have not been confirmed by others even when the analysis was limited to the activated (IL-2 receptor positive) population [61,62]. While it is reasonable to assume, *a priori*, that early in the autoimmune response there may be a pauciclonal or even monoclonal T cell response, by the time of clinical presentation this process is likely to have diversified by epitope spreading to produce a polyclonal pattern of TCR V gene usage [63]. However, the recent description of restriction in the intrathyroidal $CD8^+$ population in Hashimoto patients [64] suggests that there may be important differences in the selective accumulation of different T cell phenotypes even during the course of a chronic autoimmune process, though the possible immunopathological role of this subpopulation remains to be fully explored.

Functional studies

Thyroid-reactive T cells have been readily detected in the periphery and thyroid infiltrate using assays based on measuring T cell proliferation and the production of a cytokine, migration inhibition factor (MIF). The identification of a defect in thyroid-antigen -specific suppressor T cells was based on the extensive use of the MIF assay [reviewed in Reference 65]. A central piece of evidence for this defect was the inhibition of MIF release from Hashimoto T cells, stimulated by thyroid antigens, when co-cultured with normal T cells, the suggested source of an active suppressor T cell population [66,67]. However the assay has been difficult to reproduce [68], and the use of allogeneic T cells in the co-culturing experiments does not serve to clarify the specificity and mechanism of any suppressive effect. Similar suppressive effect have been described in other cell mixing experiments, using mitogen-driven autoantibody production as an index of stimulation [69,70], though the physiological relevance of these phenomena remains unclear, and the evidence suggests that any defect in suppressor activity appears to be non-specific [71,72]. The suggestion that a specific defect in T cell suppressor activity may contribute to the pathogenesis of autoimmune thyroiditis presents an interesting possibility, but given the dearth of conclusive evidence remains an area of some controversy [73,74].

Relatively weak T cell proliferative responses against TG and TPO can be observed in many patients and these can, generally, be increased by the removal of $CD8^+$ cells from cultures, where they exhibit a non-specific suppressor activity [75,76]. Attempts to identify the key T cell epitopes for TPO have centred around the use of overlapping peptides and recombinant TPO fusion proteins to stimulate circulating T cells from autoimmune thyroiditis patients. A dominant epitope has not been identified and there is considerable heterogeneity in responses both within and between different patients [77–81]. The relevance of these studies to the aetiology of autoimmune thyroid disease remains to be demonstrated, and it is clear that, in the case of TPO, the means by which antigen is supplied, either exogenously or endogenously (by thyroid follicular cells or transfected cell lines), can have profound effects upon the proteolytic processing of antigen and subsequent peptide epitope presentation [82].

A number of studies has demonstrated the production of cytokines by intrathyroidal T cells. *In vitro* cultures of Hashimoto T cells show a high potential for the release of tumour necrosis factor-α (TNF-α) and γ-IFN [83–85]. In addition, T cell clones derived from Hashimoto glands exhibit low levels of IL-4 production, suggesting the predominance of a T_H1 pattern of cytokine expression but others have found no specific pattern of T_H1 or T_H2 cytokine secretion [86]. The subsequent development of the RT-PCR technique enabled the detection of *in vivo* cytokine gene expression with high sensitivity, and has been used to demonstrate a mixed T_H1 and T_H2 cytokine expression profile in Hashimoto tissue [87,88] while another, quantitative study demonstrated a predominately T_H1 cytokine profile [89]. The role of T cells in thyroid injury is discussed below.

B CELLS

The antibody (Ab) response in autoimmune hypothyroidism can readily be divided by the antigens recognized. Most patients have serum Ab to TG and TPO, and more rarely, TSH-R; these antigens are considered in Chapter 2.

Epidemiology and pathology

Anti-TG Ab were the first human autoantibodies to be delineated [90] and for many years, haemagglutination remained the method of choice for their detection. Recently, enzyme-linked immunoassays (ELISA) and sensitive radioimmunoassays have been developed which provide more quantitative data and are more sensitive [91], although these have no major clinical advantage over haemagglutination. The type of assay employed determines the frequency of anti-TG Ab in various study populations: around 5–10% of healthy women are Ab positive by haemagglutination or ELISA, whereas 15–20% are positive by radioimmunoassay; the frequency in men is 10-fold lower [4,91]. In such individuals, there is a close association with focal thyroiditis, and a proportion will progress to overt hypothyroidism over a 20 year period [3,4]. TG Ab are found in the majority of patients with autoimmune hypothyroidism, but almost always in association with TPO Ab; in contrast, TPO Ab may be positive without TG Ab being positive. The pathogenic role of TG Ab remains unclear. They do not fix complement, due to the wide spacing between the major epitopes on TG, which prevents IgG cross-linking. They may play a role in antibody-dependent cell-mediated cytotoxicity, as this can be demonstrated *in vitro* [92]. Some TG Ab also bind to TPO, so-called TGPO Ab [93], and these may reflect a degree of antigenic cross-reactivity which could explain the frequent association between TG and TPO autoreactivity.

Unlike TG Ab, TPO Ab can fix complement and there is abundant complement activation in the thyroids of patients with autoimmune thyroid disease [94], suggesting that this is a major pathogenetic mechanism for thyroid injury. However, the TPO antigen is sequestered, being localized to the follicular luminal border of thyroid cells, and therefore access to TPO by Ab presumably depends on some other type of injury, such as T cell-mediated damage, before TPO Ab can participate in antibody-dependent cell-mediated cytotoxicity [92]. Finally, some TPO Ab can inhibit TPO enzymatic function *in vitro*, which could contribute to hypothyroidism, but the importance of this has been questioned [95].

TSHR Ab are classically associated with Graves' disease, stimulating cyclic AMP accumulation and leading to hyperthyroidism and goitre (Chapter 4).

However, some patients with autoimmune hypothyroidism also display reactivity towards the TSHR, causing inhibition of binding of TSH or inhibition of receptor function [96,97]. TSH-binding inhibiting immunoglobulins (TBII) are detected by a radioligand assay, measuring the inhibition of binding of labelled TSH to the TSHR after binding of patient IgG. Some Ab inhibit TSH activity *in vivo* and *in vitro*; these are termed TSH-stimulating-blocking Ab (TSBAb). Whereas some TSBAb have TBII activity (i.e. act through blocking TSH binding), others do not and appear to block steps subsequent to TSH binding; this latter activity has been partially characterized using rabbit polyclonal sera to TSHR peptides [98], and by other methods (see below). TSBAb may cause or contribute to hypothyroidism [99], and are polyclonal in origin [100].

Molecular analysis

Molecular analysis of the Ab response to TG has been somewhat limited to date because of the lack of a convincing pathological role for these Ab. Historically, the molecular analysis of TG Ab, like that of TPO and TSHR Ab, has followed three phases; analysis of serum TG Ab subclass and light chain restriction, production of TG Ab-secreting B cell hybridomas, and the use of phage display combinatorial libraries. Sequencing analysis of IgG TGAb has been reported from peripheral blood, thyroid tissue and cervical (thyroid draining) lymph node B cells in several patients with Hashimoto's thyroiditis, using both hybridoma and phage display techniques [101–103]. The somewhat limited number of sequences reported to date indicate a moderate degree of restriction, with members of the heavy chain (V_H) 3 and V_H4, kappa chain (V_κ) I and $V_\kappa III$, and lambda chain (V_λ) I forming the majority of sequences. However, these are among the most commonly found families in the normal adult repertoire. There is evidence for somatic hypermutation in many of the TG Ab sequences reported, indicating an antigen-driven immune response. A correlation between the amount of somatic hypermutation and the affinity of TG Ab from the lymph node of a patient with Hashimoto's thyroiditis has been described, emphasizing this point [103].

The molecular nature of the Ab response to TPO is the best characterized among the thyroid autoantigens, with the majority of sequences derived from combinatorial libraries from Graves' patients [reviewed in Reference 104]. However, the similarity of these sequences with those from Hashimoto patient-derived combinatorial libraries ([105] McIntosh *et al.*, submitted), and a single Hashimoto patient-derived monoclonal Ab [106], together with the similarity in behaviour of TPO Ab from various patient groups, suggests that their derivation and activity are comparable. The great majority of sequences reported to date are from IgGκ Ab; a much lower apparent titre of IgGλ than IgGκ TPO Ab appears to be a common pattern in patients with autoimmune thyroid disease [92,104]. TPO Ab are restricted mainly to V_H1, V_H3, $V_\kappa I$ and $V_\kappa III$ family members; as in the TG repertoire, these are among the most common V families. Despite this, certain V regions are 'over-represented' in the repertoire described to date; in particular, V_H1-2, V_H1-3 and $V_\kappa O12$ (from the $V_\kappa I$ family) have been isolated from a number of different patients. Although the $V_\kappa O12$ region is frequently found in the TPO Ab repertoire, and is associated with reactivity to a single epitope on TPO (see below), the frequency of the $V_\kappa O12$ region in unselected phage display libraries indicates only a small fraction of $V_\kappa O12$-containing phage bind TPO. This emphasizes the point that V region analysis alone has not been sufficient to elucidate the features of TPO Ab reactivity.

Analysis of cloned Ab to the TSHR will more readily allows discrimination between the various TSHR Ab activities. Several reports detailing the cloning of human Ab to the TSHR have been published, but sequence data are only provided in two of these reports, both dealing with material from Graves' patients. In two other reports, TSHR Ab from patients with primary myxoedema are described [107,108]. Interestingly, although B cell lines rather than clones formed the bulk of the material in one of these studies, the two lines from a primary myxoedema patient both displayed TSAb activity, whilst many of the lines from the Graves' patients displayed both TSAb and TSBAb activity [108]. Several of the reports detailing the cloning of TSHR Ab from Graves' patients also indicate that activities other than TSAb are present, and conversely, hypothyroid patients often have detectable TSAb activity [109]. It therefore appears likely that the various TSHR Ab types are shared between different patient groups, and that the relative activities of the different TSHR Ab (rather than simply presence or absence) may be responsible for different presenting symptoms. However, several features of the Ab studied to date suggest that they do not adequately represent the biologically active TSHR Ab repertoire. Most importantly, the concentration of Ab required for *in vitro* functional assays has been orders of magnitude above that anticipated [110]; the cloning of TSHR Ab equivalent to those active *in vivo* in both hypothyroid and hyperthyroid patients has therefore still to be achieved.

Antigenic structure

Although the TG Ab response is somewhat heterogeneous, there is apparent restriction of most patient-derived TG Ab to two or three conformational epitopes [102]. Epitope recognition has been determined for only four of the sequenced TG Ab, with two clones each binding to two different epitopes [102]. In contrast to the TPO Ab response, there is no sequence consensus between these clones and the epitope recognized. Analysis of the inhibition of binding of patient sera TG Ab using the mapped Ab indicates a heterogeneous pattern of binding within patients with Hashimoto's thyroiditis, with similar behaviour exhibited by Graves' patient sera [102]. However, too few examples of TG Ab from patients have been mapped to allow detailed analysis of epitope structure.

A great deal more is known concerning the epitopes present on TPO; as stated above, the similarity in sequences and activities of Ab to native (non-denatured) TPO from Graves' and Hashimoto patients is indicative of a similarity in the Ab response. In contrast, some of the TPO Ab to denatured (linear) fragments of TPO, present in a minority of patients, show differences in binding patterns between Graves' and Hashimoto patients [111]. Two complementary systems defining Ab reactivity to native TPO currently have been reported, one based upon murine mAb and the other on Graves' patient combinatorial library-derived FAb fragments [104,112]. Reagents from both are reported to block the binding of the majority of TPO Ab activity in patient sera, although the two have never been adequately compared. The structure of the major immunodominant region is comprised of two neighbouring domains; Ab containing the $V_{\kappa}O12$ light chain bind only one of these domains. However, the location of the immunodominant region on native TPO is still a matter of conjecture [104].

Although unequivocal dissection of the various TSHR Ab activities will result from cloning studies, progress has been made in separating the various activities using mutated forms of the TSHR. Several regions of the large N-terminal extracellular domain of the TSHR have been investigated to determine the binding sites of TSH and TSHR Ab [97]. This work has been carried out using TSHR mutants in which regions or residues have been mutated or replaced with sequence from the homologous luteinizing hormone receptor. A large body of work indicates that TSH binding is affected by mutation of residues at various sites in the first extracellular domain whereas TSAb activity and TSBAb activity appear to act respectively at N-terminal and C-terminal sites within this region [109,113,114].

THYROID FOLLICULAR CELLS (TFC)

Role of HLA class II molecule expression

The discovery that TFC express HLA class II molecules in autoimmune thyroid diseases, but not under normal circumstances, led to the hypothesis that this could initiate or perpetuate the autoimmune response, with the TFC under these circumstances acting as antigen presenting cells [115]. However, γ-IFN is the key regulator of class II expression, and the close correlation between the presence of γ-IFN-containing T cells and class II^+ TFC demonstrates that a lymphocytic thyroiditis is required for class II to be expressed by TFC [116]. Thus, TFC are unlikely to initiate autoimmune hypothyroidism.

A role in disease maintenance has also been questioned [117], as it is now known that certain (particularly naive) $CD4^+$ T cells require a costimulatory or second signal in addition to the recognition of class II molecule plus peptide by the T cell receptor. The best defined costimulatory signals are B7-1 (CD80) and B7-2 (CD86) which signal through CD28 or CTLA-4 molecules on the T cell surface. TFC fail to express either B7 molecule, even after γ-IFN stimulation [118,119].

We have recently re-examined the potential for class II^+ TFC to present antigen, using a model system based on presentation of influenza virus haemagglutinin peptide to T cells by HLA-DR-matched TFC [119]. For clones which were dependent on B7 co-stimulation, class II^+ TFC were unable to act as antigen presenting cells. In contrast, two T cell clones did not require the B7 costimulatory signal and could be stimulated by class II^+ TFC, albeit less well than by conventional antigen presenting cells. Furthermore, co-culture of the B7-dependent T cells overnight with class II^+ TFC plus antigen induced specific anergy. Subsequently, we have shown in alloresponses that such anergy is Fas-dependent for $CD45RA^+$ T cells, but Fas-independent for the $CD45R0^+$ population, in which anergy can instead by reversed by IL-2 (Marelli-Berg *et al.*, submitted).

Thus, the role of class II expression by TFC can be viewed teleologically as a mechanism to induce peripheral tolerance in naive and memory T cells which would otherwise be capable of autoreactivity. For instance, γ-IFN released during an episode of subacute thyroiditis induces class II expression on TFC, which is protective in those individuals who are predisposed to thyroid autoimmunity because they have less rigorously imposed central tolerance (Figure 3.3). However, once thyroid autoimmunity is firmly established, via conventional antigen presenting cells, B7-dependence may not be an issue, in which case class II^+ TFC could present autoantigens and perpetuate the response. In addition, high local concentrations of IL-2 could overcome the TFC-induced anergy in $CD45R0^+$ T cells. In support of this possibility, intrathyroidal T cells appear to be resistant to tolerance induction *in vitro* [120].

Other immunologically relevant molecules

TFC may also interact with the immune system by their expression of a number of other molecules. Under normal conditions, TFC do not express the intercellular adhesion molecule ICAM-1 (CD54), but this can be induced by stimulation with γ-IFN, IL-1 and TNF, and immunohistochemistry reveals striking ICAM-1 expression by the remaining TFC in Hashimoto's thyroiditis [121,122]. Such ICAM-1 expression is associated with an enhanced capacity to bind T cells (via LFA-1) and, as a result, increased susceptibility to T cell-mediated cytotoxicity. TFC do not express ICAM-2 but do express LFA-3 which binds to CD2 on the T cell surface and thus acts as another molecule for T cell adhesion [122,123]. $CD8^+$ T cell clones and lines have been established from patients with Hashimoto's thyroiditis and animals with experimental autoimmune thyroiditis which are capable of killing autologous TFC in an HLA class I-restricted fashion [124,125]. In addition, there are abundant intrathyroidal $CD8^+$ T cells in Hashimoto's thyroiditis containing perforin, which is a marker for functionally activated T cells *in situ* [126]. Minor infiltrating populations of $CD4^+$ and $\alpha\beta^+$ $CD4^-$ $CD8^-$ T cells in Hashimoto's thyroiditis also contain perforin, indicating a diversity of potentially cytotoxic T cells, whose potential for injury will be enhanced by TFC adhesion molecule expression.

Although the infiltrate is the major source of intrathyoidal cytokines, as

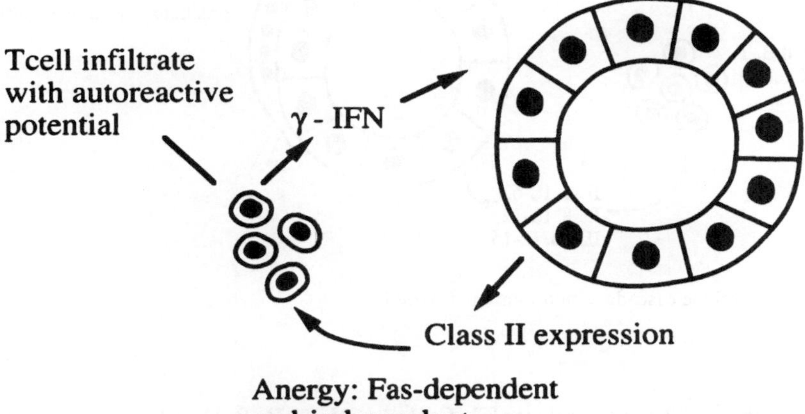

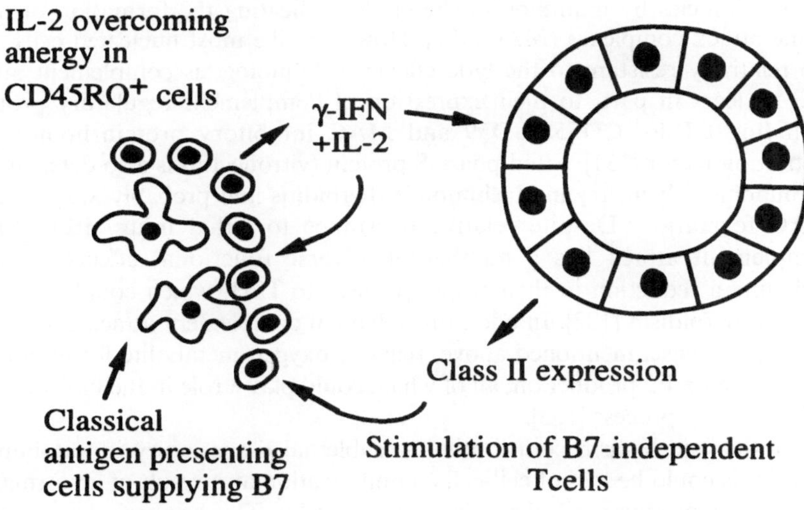

Figure 3.3 Possible outcomes following expression of HLA class II molecules by thyroid follicular cells

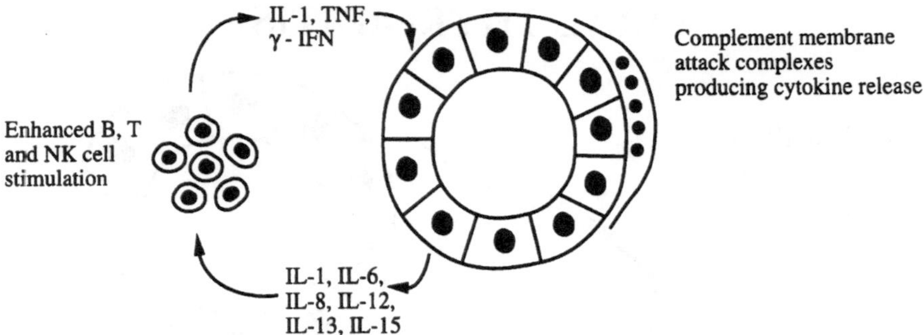

Figure 3.4 Cytokine cascade in autoimmune thyroiditis.

discussed above, TFC also release TNF, IL-1α, IL-6, IL-8, IL-12, IL-13 and IL-15 [127–130]. Production of these cytokines is enhanced by γ-IFN, IL-1 and TNF, so that a cascade may exist whereby a small lymphocytic infiltrate releasing cytokines could stimulate the production of cytokines by TFC, which in turn would increase the size and activity of the infiltrate and so on (Figure 3. 4).

Sublethal complement attack is another stimulator of cytokine production by TFC. Increased circulating levels of terminal complement complexes are found in Hashimoto's thyroiditis, and complexes can also be visualized around the thyroid follicles by immunohistochemistry, indicating the formation of membrane attack complexes (MAC) [94]. However, like most nucleated cells, TFC are relatively resistant to the lytic effects of homologous complement attack, due, at least in part, to their expression of complement regulatory proteins, including CD46, CD55, CD59 and MAC inhibitory protein/homologous restriction factor [131]. Fluid-phase S protein (vitronectin) is also detectable by immunohistochemistry in Hashimoto's thyroiditis and probably also regulates MAC formation. Despite relative resistance to lethal injury from MAC, complement attack has a number of adverse functional effects on TFC, including a reduction in their responsiveness to TSH, which could contribute to hypothyroidism [132]. In addition, sublethal complement attack causes IL-1 and IL-6 release, mentioned above, reactive oxygen metabolite formation and prostaglandin E2 production, all of which could play a role in the intrathyroidal inflammatory process [133].

Another mechanism contributing to sublethal tissue injury in autoimmune thyroiditis could be loss of cell-cell communication as a result of abnormalities in connexin production and gap junction assembly. This has been demonstrated in experimental autoimmune thyroiditis [134], although the events leading up to these connexin abnormalities have not been elucidated: candidates include T cell-derived cytokines, but the abnormalities are maintained on subsequent culture of the isolated TFC, which argues against such a simple explanation. Extension of this work to the human counterpart may provide fresh insights into the pathogenesis of autoimmune hypothyroidism.

SUMMARY

It is now 40 years since the first recognition of autoimmune thyroiditis in its experimentally-induced and spontaneous forms. A vast body of research has been undertaken on this prototypic organ-specific autoimmune disease, which we have summarized in detail elsewhere [135,136]. The application of modern techniques promises at last to unravel the immunogenetics of autoimmune hypothyroidism; it now seems clear that the HLA region plays only a minor role in susceptibility and the new knowledge derived from the planned linkage studies should be important in our understanding of the aetiology of both this disease and the other disorders frequently associated with autoimmune hypothyroidism. It will be more difficult to identify which environmental and endogenous factors are responsible for susceptibility. These will differ between individuals and may well have operated at a distant time.

A spectacular development in the last 10 years has been the molecular definition of the three main thyroid autoantigens, which now permits detailed studies of the T cell and antibody response in autoimmune thyroiditis. Although both T and B cell responses are polyclonal at presentation, it seems intuitive that initially there is an oligoclonal response; identifying this would shed new light on pathogenesis. With regard to effector mechanisms, a plethora have now been identified and it seems likely that the TFC themselves play a role in these intrathyroidal events by expression of HLA, adhesion and complement regulatory molecules and production of cytokines. The relative importance of each of these, especially in relation to the evolution of thyroid dysfunction, remains to be established.

References

1. Williams ED, Doniach I. The post-mortem incidence of focal thyroiditis. J Pathol Bacteriol. 1962;83:255–64.
2. Okayasu I, Hara Y, Nakamura K, Rose NR. Racial and age-related differences in incidence and severity of focal autoimmune thyroiditis. Am J Clin Pathol. 1994;101:698–702.
3. Yoshida H, Amino N, Yagawa K et al. Association of serum antithyroid antibodies with lymphocytic infiltration of the thyroid gland: studies of seventy autopsied cases. J Clin Endocrinol Metab. 1978;46:859–62.
4. Vanderpump MPJ, Tunbridge WMG, French JM et al. The incidence of thyroid disorders in the community: a twenty year follow-up of the Whickham Survey. Clin Endocrinol. 1995;43: 55–68.
5. Mariotti S, Sansoni P, Barbesino G et al. Thyroid and other organ-specific autoantibodies in healthy centenarians. Lancet. 1992;339:1506–8.
6. Matsuzuka F, Miyauchi A, Katayama S et al. Clinical aspects of primary thyroid lymphoma: diagnosis and treatment based on our experience of 119 cases. Thyroid. 1993;3: 93–9.
7. Zimmerman RS, Brennan MD, McConahey WM, Goellner JR, Gharib H. Hashimoto's thyroiditis: an uncommon cause of painful thyroid unresponsive to corticosteroid therapy. Ann Intern Med. 1986;104:355–7.

8. Takasu N, Yamada Y, Takasu M et al. Disappearance of thyrotropin-blocking antibodies and spontaneous recovery from hypothyroidism in autoimmune thyroiditis. New Engl J Med. 1992;326:513–18.
9. Li Volsi VA. Pathology of thyroid disease. In: Falk SA, ed. Thyroid Disease: Endocrinology, Surgery, Nuclear Medicine and Radiotherapy. New York: Raven Press; 1990:127–75.
10. Hayashi Y, Tamai H, Fukata S et al. A long term clinical, immunological, and histological follow-up study of patients with goitrous chronic lymphocytic thyroiditis. J Clin Endocrinol Metab. 1985;61:1172–7.
11. Burek CL, Hoffman WH, Rose NR. The presence of thyroid autoantibodies in children and adolescents with autoimmune thyroid disease and in their siblings and parents. Clin Immunol Immunopathol. 1982;25:395–404.
12. Hall R, Owen SG, Smart GS. Evidence for genetic predisposition to formation of thyroid autoantibodies. Lancet. 1964;ii:187–8.
13. Phillips DIW, Shields DC, Dugoujon JM, Prentice L, McGuffin P, Rees Smith B. Complex segregation analysis of thyroid autoantibodies:are they inherited as an autosomal dominant trait? Hum Hered. 1993;43:141–6.
14. Irvine WJ. The immunology and genetics of autoimmune endocrine disease. In: N.R. Rose, P.E. Bigazzi, N.L. Warner, eds. Genetic Control of Autoimmune Disease. Amsterdam: Elsevier; 1978:77–97.
15. Moens H, Farid NR. Hashimoto's thyroiditis is associated with HLA-DRw3. New Engl J Med. 1978;299:133–4.
16. Weissel M, Hofer R, Zasmeta H, Mayr WR. HLA-DR and Hashimoto's thyroiditis. Tissue Antigens. 1980;16:256–9.
17. Thomsen M, Ryder LP, Bech K et al. HLA-D in Hashimoto's thyroiditis. Tissue Antigens. 1983;21:173–5.
18. Thompson C, Farid NR. Post-partum thyroiditis and goitrous (Hashimoto's) thyroiditis are associated with HLA-DR4. Immunol Lett. 1985;11:301–3.
19. Stenszky V, Balazs C, Kraszits E et al. Association of goitrous autoimmune thyroiditis with HLA-DR3 in eastern Hungary. J Immunogenet. 1987;14:143–8.
20. Vargas MT, Briopnes-Urbina R, Gladman D, Papsin FR, Walfish PG. Antithyroid microsomal autoantibodies and HLA-DR5 are associated with postpartum thyroid dysfunction: evidence supporting an endocrine pathogenesis. J Clin Endocrinol Metab. 1988;67:327–33.
21. Badenhoop K, Schwarz G, Walfish PG et al. Susceptibility to thyroid autoimmune disease:molecular analysis of HLA-D region genes identifies new markers for goitrous Hashimoto's thyroiditis. J Clin Endocrinol Metab. 1990;71:1131–7.
22. Tandon N, Zhang L, Weetman AP. HLA associations with Hashimoto's thyroiditis. Clin Endocrinol. 1991;34:383–6.
23. Mangklabruks A, Cox N, De Groot LJ. Genetic factors in autoimmune thyroid disease analyzed by restriction fragment length polymorphisms of candidate genes. J Clin Endocrinol Metab. 1991;73:236–44.
24. Jenkins D, Penny MA, Fletcher JA et al. MC. HLA class II gene polymorphism contributes little to Hashimoto's thyroiditis. Clin Endocrinol. 1992;37:141–5.
25. Bogner U, Badenhoop K, Peters H et al. HLA-DR/DQ gene variation in nongoitrous autoimmune thyroiditis at the serological and molecular level. Autoimmunity. 1992;14:155–8.
26. Hawkins BR, Lam KSL, Ma JTC, Wang C, Yeung RTT. Strong association between HLA-DRw9 and Hashimoto's thyroiditis in Southern Chinese. Acta Endocrinol. 1987;114:543–6.
27. Honda K, Tamai J, Morita T, Kuma K, Nishimura Y, Sasazuki T. Hashimoto's thyroiditis and HLA in Japanese. J Clin Endocrinol Metab. 1989;69:1268–73.
28. Inoue D, Sato K, Enomoto T et al. Correlation of HLA types and clinical findings in Japanese patients with hyperthyroid Graves' disease: evidence indicating the existence of four subpopulations. Clin Endocrinol. 1992;36:75–82.
29. Cho BY, Chung JH, Shong YK et al. A strong association between thyrotropin receptor-blocking antibody-positive atrophic autoimmune thyroiditis and HLA-DR8 and HLA-DQB1*0302 in Koreans. J Clin Endocrinol Metab. 1993;77:611–15.
30. Ewins DL, Rossor MN, Butler J, Roques PK, Mullan MJ, McGregor AM. Association between autoimmune thyroid disease and familial Alzheimer's disease. Clin Endocrinol. 1991;35:93–6.
31. Kotsa K, Watson PF, Weetman AP. A CLTA-4 gene polymorphism is associated with both Graves' disease and Hashimoto's thyroiditis. Clin Endocrinol. 1997;46:551–4.

32. Hayward PAR, Satsangi J, Jewell DP. Inflammatory bowel disease and the X chromosome. Q J Med. 1996;89:713–18.
33. Olsen NJ, Kovacs WJ. Gonadal steroids and immunity. Endocrine Rev. 1996;17:369–84.
34. Ferrari C, Boghen M, Paracchi A et al. Thyroid autoimmunity in hyperprolactinaemic disorders. Acta Endocrinol. 1983;104:35–41.
35. Phillips DIW, Cooper C, Fall C et al. Fetal growth and autoimmune thyroid disease. Q J Med. 1993;86:247–53.
36. Many M-C, Maniratunga S, Varis J, Dardenne M, Drexhage HA, Denef J-F. Two-step development of Hashimoto-like thyroiditis in genetically autoimmune prone non-obese diabetic mice: effects of iodine-induced cell necrosis. J Endocrinol. 1995;147:311–20.
37. Boukis IA, Koutras DA, Souvantzoglou A, Evangelopolou A, Vrontakis A, Moulopoulos SD. Thyroid hormone and immunological studies in endemic goitre. J Clin Endocrinol Metab. 1983;57:859–62.
38. Harach HR, Escalante DA, Onativia A, Lederer Outes J, Saravia Day E, Williams ED. Thyroid carcinoma and thyroiditis in an endemic goitre region before and after iodine prophylaxis. Acta Endocrinol. 1985;108:55–60.
39. Weetman AP. Infection and endocrine autoimmunity. In: H. Friedman, NR Rose, M Bendinelli, eds. Microorganisms and Autoimmune Disease. Plenum Press: New York; 1996: 257–75.
40. Nagataki S, Shibata Y, Inoue S, Yokoyama N, Izumi M, Shimaoka K. Thyroid diseases amongst atomic bomb survivors in Nagasaki. J Am Med Assoc. 1994;272:364–70.
41. Marazuela M, Garcia-Buey L, Gonzalez-Fernandez B et al. Thyroid autoimmune disorders in patients with chronic hepatitis C before and during interferon-α therapy. Clin Endocrinol. 1996;44:635–42.
42. Lazarus JH, John R, Bennie EH, Chalmers RJ, Crockett G. Lithium therapy and thyroid function:a long-term study. Psychol Med. 1981;11:85–92.
43. Rose NR, Kong YM, Okayasu I, Giraldo AA, Beisel K, Sundick RS. T-cell regulation in autoimmune thyroiditis. Immunol Rev. 1981;55:299–314.
44. Weetman AP, McGregor AM, Wheeler MH, Hall R. Extrathyroidal autoantibody synthesis in Graves' disease. Clin Exp Immunol. 1984;56:330–36.
45. Thielemans C, Vanhaelst L, De Waele M, Jonckheer M, Van Camp B. Autoimmune thyroiditis: a condition related to a decrease in T-suppressor cells. Clin Endocrinol. 1981;15: 259–63.
46. Fournier C, Chen H, Leger A, Charreire J. Immunological studies of autoimmune thyroid disorders: abnormalities in the inducer T cell subset and proliferative responses to autologous and allogeneic stimulation. Clin Exp Immunol. 1983;54:539–46.
47. Chan JYC, Walfish PG. Activated (Ia) T-lymphocytes and their subsets in autoimmune thyroid diseases: analysis by dual laser flow microfluoricytometry. J Clin Endocrinol Metab. 1989;62:403–9.
48. Ohashi H, Okugawa T, Itoh M. Circulating activated T-cell subsets in autoimmune thyroid diseases – differences between untreated and treated patients. Acta Endocrinol. 1991;125:502–9.
49. Gessl A, Wilfing A, Agis H, Steiner G, Czernin S, Boltznitulescu G, Vierhapper H, Waldhausl W. Activated naive $CD4(^{+})$ peripheral-blood T-cells in autoimmune thyroid disease. Thyroid. 1995;5:117–23.
50. Jansson R, Karlsson A, Forsum U. Intrathyroidal HLA-DR expression and T lymphocyte phenotypes in Graves' thyrotoxicosis, Hashimoto's thyroiditis, and nodular colloid goitre. Clin Exp Immunol. 1984;58:264–72.
51. Canonica GW, Caria M, Torre G et al. Autoimmune thyroid disease: purification and phenotypic analysis of intrathyroidal T cells. J Endocrinol Invest. 1984;7:641–5.
52. Aichinger G, Fill H, Wick G. In situ immune complexes, lymphocyte subpopulations and HLA-DR positive epithelial cells in Hashimoto's thyroiditis. Lab Invest. 1985;52:132–40.
53. Teng WP, Cohen SB, Posnett DN, Weetman AP. T cell receptor phenotypes in autoimmune thyroid disease. J Endocrinol Invest. 1990;13:339–42.
54. Iwatani Y, Amino N, Hidaka Y et al. Decreases in αβ T cell receptor negative T cells and $CD8^{+}$ cells, and an increase in $CD4^{+}$ $CD8^{+}$ cells in active Hashimoto's disease and subacute thyroiditis. Clin Exp Immunol. 1992;87:444–9.
55. Paolieri F, Pronzato C, Battifora M, Fiorino N, Canonica GW, Bagnasco M. Infiltrating gamma/delta T-cell receptor-positive lymphocytes in Hashimoto's thyroiditis, Graves' disease, and papillary thyroid cancer. J Endocrinol Invest. 1995;18:295–8.

56. Catalfamo M, Roura Mir C, Sospedra M et al. Self-reactive γδ T lymphocytes in Graves' disease specifically recognise thyroid epithelial cells. J Immunol. 1996;156:804–11.
57. Adorini L, Guery J-C, Rodriguez-Tarduchy G, Trembleau S. Selective immunosuppression. Immunol Today. 1993;14:285–9.
58. Davies TF, Martin A, Concepcion ES, Graves P, Cohen L, Ben Nun A. Evidence for limited variability of antigen receptors on intrathyroidal T cells in autoimmune thyroid disease. New Engl J Med. 1991;325:238–44.
59. Davies TF, Martin A, Concepcion ES et al. Evidence for selective accumulation of intrathyroidal T lymphocytes in human autoimmune thyroid disease based on T cell receptor V gene usage. J Clin Invest. 1992;89:157–62.
60. Davies TF, Concepcion ES, Ben-Nun A, Graves P, Tarjan G. T-cell receptor gene use in autoimmune thyroid disease: direct assessment by thyroid aspiration. J Clin Endocrinol Metab. 1993;76:660–6.
61. McIntosh RS, Tandon N, Pickerill AP, Davies R, Barnett D, Weetman AP. IL-2 receptor-positive intrathyroidal lymphocytes in Graves' disease: analysis of Vα transcript microheterogeneity. J Immunol. 1993;91:3884–93.
62. Caso-Pelaez E, McGregor AM, Banga JP. A polyclonal T cell repertoire of V-α and V-β T cell receptor gene families in intrathyroidal T lymphocytes of Graves' disease patients. Scand J Immunol. 1995;41:141–7.
63. Lehmann PV, Sercarz EE, Forsthuber T, Dayan CM, Gammon G. Determinant spreading and the dynamics of the autoimmune T-cell repertoire. Immunol Today. 1993;14:203–12.
64. McIntosh RS, Watson PF, Weetman AP. Analysis of the T cell receptor Vα repertoire in Hashimoto's thyroiditis: evidence for the restricted accumulation of $CD8^+$ T cells in the absence of $CD4^+$ T cell restriction. J Clin Endocrinol Metab. 1997;82:1140–6.
65. Volpé R. The immunoregulatory disturbance in autoimmune thyroid disease. Autoimmunity. 1988;2:55–72.
66. Okita N, Kidd A, Row VV, Volpé R. Sensitisation of T-lymphocytes in Graves' and Hashimoto's disease. J Clin Endocrinol Metab. 1980;51:316–20.
67. Topliss DJ, Okita N, Lewis M et al . Allosuppressor T lymphocytes abolish migration inhibition factor production in autoimmune thyroid disease. Clin Endocrinol. 1981;15:335–41.
68. Ludgate ME, Ratanachaiyavong S, Weetman AP, Hall R, McGregor AM. Failure to demonstrate cell-mediated immune responses to thyroid antigens in Graves' disease using in vitro assays of lymphokine-mediated migration inhibition. J Clin Endocrinol Metab. 1985; 60:98–102.
69. Tao TW, Gatenby PA, Leu SL, Pham H, Kriss JP. Helper and suppressor activities of lymphocytes on anti-thyroglobulin production in vitro. J Clin Endocrinol Metab. 1985;61: 520–4.
70. Iitaka M, Aguayo JF, Iwatani Y, Row VV, Volpé R. Studies of the effect of suppressor T lymphocytes on the induction of antithyroid microsomal antibody-secreting cells in autoimmune thyroid disease. J Clin Endocrinol Metab. 1988;66:708–14.
71. Mori H, Hamada N, DeGroot LJ. Studies on thyroglobulin-specific suppressor T cell function in autoimmune thyroid disease. J Clin Endocrinol Metab. 1985;61:306–12.
72. Davies TF, Platzer M. The T cell suppressor defect in autoimmune thyroiditis: evidence for a high set 'autoimmunostat'. Clin Exp Immunol. 1985;63:73–9.
73. Volpé R. Immunoregulation in autoimmune thyroid disease. Thyroid. 1994;4:373–7.
74. Martin A, Davies TF. T cells in human autoimmune thyroid disease. Emerging data shows lack of need to invoke suppressor T cell problems. Thyroid. 1992;2:247–61.
75. Aoki N, DeGroot J. Lymphocyte blastogenic response to human thyroglobulin in Graves' disease, Hashimoto's thyroiditis, and matastatic thyroid cancer. Clin Exp Immunol. 1979;38: 523–30.
76. Canonica GW, Cosulich ME, Croci R et al. Thyroglobulin-induced T cell in vitro proliferation in Hashimoto's thyroiditis: identification of the responsive subset and effect of monoclonal antibodies directed to Ia antigens. Clin Immunol Immunopathol. 1984;32:132–41.
77. Fukuma N, McLachlan SM, Rapoport B et al. Thyroid autoantigens and human T cell responses. Clin Exp Immunol. 1990;82:275–83.
78. Tandon N, Freeman M, Weetman AP. T cell responses to synthetic thyroid peroxidase peptides in autoimmune thyroid disease. Clin Exp Immunol. 1991;86:56–60.

79. Dayan CM, Londei M, Corcoran AE et al. Autoantigen recognition by thyroid-infiltrating T cells in Graves' disease. Proc Natl Acad Sci USA. 1991;88:7415–9.
80. Ewins CL, Barnett PS, Ratanchaiyavong S et al. Antigen-specific T cell recognition of affinity-purified and recombinant thyroid peroxidase in autoimmune thyroid disease. Clin Exp Immunol. 1992;90:93–8.
81. Fisfalen ME, Soliman M, Okamoto Y, Soltani K, DeGroot LJ. Proliferative responses of T-cells to thyroid antigens and synthetic thyroid peroxidase peptides in autoimmune thyroid disease. J Clin Endocrinol Metab. 1995;80:1597–604.
82. Quaratino S, Feldmann M, Dayan CM, Acuto O, Londei M. Human self-reactive T cell clones expressing identical T cell receptor beta chains differ in their ability to recognize a cryptic self-epitope. J Exp Med. 1996;183:349–58
83. Del Prete GF, Tiri A, Mariotti S, Pinchera A, Ricci M, Romagnani S. Enhanced production of γ-interferon by thyroid-derived T cell clones from patients with Hashimoto's thyroiditis. Clin Exp Immunol. 1987;69:323–31.
84. Del Prete GF, Tiri A, De Carli M et al. High potential for tumor necrosis factor α (TNF-α) production of thyroid infiltrating T lymphocytes in Hashimoto's thyroiditis: a peculiar feature of destructive thyroid autoimmunity. Autoimmunity. 1989;4:267–76.
85. Mariotti S, Del Prete GF, Chiovato L et al. Cytokines and thyroid autoimmunity. Int J Immunopath Pharmacol. 1992;5:103–13.
86. Grubeck-Loebenstein B, Turner M, Pirich K et al. $CD4^+$ T-cell clones from autoimmune thyroid tissue cannot be classified according to their lymphokine production. Scand J Immunol. 1990;32:433–40.
87. Paschke R, Schuppert F, Taton M, Velu T. Intrathyroidal cytokine gene expression profiles in autoimmune thyroiditis. J Endocrinol. 1994;141:309–15.
88. Ajjan RA, Watson PF, McIntosh RS, Weetman AP. Intrathyroidal cytokine gene expression in Hashimoto's thyroiditis. Clin Exp Immunol. 1996;105:523–8.
89. Hueur M, Aust G, Odehakim S, Scherbaum WA. Different cytokine messenger RNA profiles in Graves' disease, Hashimoto's thyroiditis, and non-autoimmune thyroid disorders determined by quantitative reverse transcriptase polymerase chain reaction (RT-PCR). Thyroid. 1996;6:97–106.
90. Roitt IM, Doniach D, Campbell PN, Vaughan Hudson R. Autoantibodies in Hashimoto's disease (lymphadenoid goitre). Lancet. 1956;ii:820–1.
91. Beever K, Bradbury J, Phillips D et al. Highly sensitive assays of autoantibodies to thyroglobulin and to thyroid peroxidase. Clin Chem. 1989;35:1949–54.
92. Weetman AP, Black CM, Cohen SB, Tomlinson R, Banga JP, Reimer CB. Affinity purification of IgG subclasses and the distribution of thyroid autoantibody reactivity in Hashimoto's thyroiditis. Scand J Immunol. 1989;30:73–82.
93. Weetman AP, Cohen SB, Oleesky DA, Morgan BP. Terminal complement complexes and C1/C1 inhibitor complexes in autoimmune thyroid disease. Clin Exp Immunol. 1989;77:25–30.
94. Ruf J, Feldt-Rasmussen U, Hegedüs L, Ferrand M, Carayon P. Bispecific thyroglobulin and thyroperoxidase autoantibodies in patients with various thyroid and autoimmune diseases. J Clin Endocrinol Metab. 1994;79:1404–9.
95. Saller B, Hörmann R, Mann K. Heterogeneity of autoantibodies against thyroid peroxidase in autoimmune thyroid disease: evidence against antibodies directly inhibiting peroxidase activity as regulatory factors in thyroid hormone metabolism. J Clin Endocrinol Metab. 1991;72:188–95.
96. Rees Smith B, McLachlan SM, Furmaniak J. Autoantibodies to the thyrotropin receptor. Endocr Rev. 1988;9:106–21.
97. Paschke R, van Sande J, Parma J, Vassart G. The TSH receptor and thyroid diseases. Ballière's Clin Endocrinol Metab. 1996;10:9–27.
98. Dallas JS, Cunningham SJ, Patibandla SA et al. Thyrotropin (TSH) receptor antibodies (TSHrAb) can inhibit TSH-mediated cyclic adenosine 3′,5′-monophosphate production in thyroid cells by either blocking TSH binding or affecting a step subsequent to TSH binding. Endocrinology. 1996;137:3329–39.
99. Drexhage HA. Autoimmunity and thyroid growth. Where do we stand? Eur J Endocrinol. 1996;135:39–45.
100. Kraiem Z, Cho BY, Sadeh O, Shong MH, Pickerill P, Weetman AP. The IgG subclass distribution of TSH receptor blocking antibodies in primary hypothyroidism. Clin Endocrinol. 1992;37:135–40.

101. Hexham JM, Furmaniak J, Pegg C, Burton DR, Rees Smith B. Cloning of a human autoimmune response: preparation and sequencing of a human anti-thyroglobulin autoantibody using a combinatorial approach. Autoimmunity. 1992;12:135–41.
102. Prentice L, Kiso Y, Fukuma N et al. Monoclonal thyroglobulin autoantibodies: variable region analysis and epitope recognition. J Clin Endocrinol Metab. 1995;80:977–86.
103. McIntosh RS, Asghar MS, Watson PF, Kemp EH, Weetman AP. Cloning and analysis of IgGκ and IgGλ anti-thyroglobulin autoantibodies from a patient with Hashimoto's thyroiditis: evidence for in vivo antigen-driven repertoire selection. J Immunol. 1996;157:927–35.
104. McLachlan SM, Rapoport B. Genetic and epitopic analysis of thyroid peroxidase (TPO) autoantibodies: markers of the human thyroid autoimmune response. Clin Exp Immunol. 1995;101:200–6.
105. Hexham JM, Partridge LJ, Furmaniak J et al. Cloning and characterisation of TPO autoantibodies using combinatorial phage display libraries. Autoimmunity. 1994;17:167–79.
106. Hexham JM, Pegg CAS, Burton DR et al. Variable region sequence of a human monoclonal thyroid peroxidase autoantibody. Autoimmunity. 1992;14:169–72.
107. Okuda J, Akamizu T, Sugawa H, Matsuda F, Hua L, Mori T. Preparation and characterization of monoclonal antithyrotropin receptor antibodies obtained from peripheral lymphocytes of hypothyroid patients with primary myxedema. J Clin Endocrinol Metab. 1994;79: 1600–4.
108. Morgenthaler NG, Kim MR, Tremble J et al. Human-immunoglobulin G autoantibodies to the thyrotropin receptor from Epstein Barr virus-transformed B lymphocytes: characterization by immunoprecipitation with recombinant antigen and biological activity. J Clin Endocrinol Metab. 1996;81:3155–61.
109. Kosugi S, Ban T, Akamizu T, Valente W, Kohn LD. Use of thyrotropin receptor (TSHR) mutants to detect stimulating TSHR antibodies in hypothyroid patients with idiopathic myxedema, who have blocking TSHR antibodies. J Clin Endocrinol Metab. 1993;77:19–24.
110. McLachlan SM, Rapoport B. Monoclonal, human autoantibodies to the TSH receptor: the holy grail and why are we looking for it? J Clin Endocrinol Metab. 1996;81:3152–4.
111. Arscott PL, Koenig RJ, Kaplan MM, Glick GD, Baker JR Jr. Unique autoantibody epitopes in an immunodominant region of thyroid peroxidase. J Biol Chem. 1996;271:4966–73.
112. Ruf J, Toubert M-E, Czarnocka B, Durand-Gorde J-M, Ferrand M, Carayon P. Relationship between immunological structure and biochemical properties of human thyroid peroxidase. Endocrinology. 1989;125:1211–18.
113. Kosugi S, Ban T, Akamizu T, Kohn LD. Site-directed mutagenesis of a portion of the extracellular domain of the rat thyrotropin receptor important in autoimmune thyroid disease and nonhomologous with gonadotropin receptors. Relationship of functional and immunogenic domains. J Biol Chem. 1991;266:19413–8.
114. Kosugi S, Ban T, Akamizu T, Kohn LD. Identification of separate determinants on the thyrotropin receptor reactive with Graves' thyroid-stimulating antibodies and with thyroid-stimulating blocking antibodies in idiopathic myxedema: these determinants have no homologous sequence on gonadotropin receptors. Mol Endocrinol. 1992;6:168-80.
115. Bottazzo GF, Pujol-Borrell R, Hanafusa T, Feldmann M. Role of aberrant HLA-DR expression and antigen presentation in induction of endocrine autoimmunity. Lancet. 1983; ii:1115–9.
116. Hamilton F, Black M, Farquharson MA, Stewart C, Foulis AK. Spatial correlation between thyroid epithelial cells expressing class II MHC molecules and interferon-gamma-containing lymphocytes in human thyroid autoimmune disease. Clin Exp Immunol. 1991;83:64–8.
117. Weetman AP. Antigen presentation in the pathogenesis of autoimmune endocrine disease. J Autoimmunity. 1995;8:305–12.
118. Tandon N, Metcalfe R, Barnet D, Weetman AP. Expression of the costimulatory molecule B7/BB1 in autoimmune thyroid disease. Q J Med. 1994;87:231–6.
119. Lombardi G, Arnold K, Uren J et al. Antigen presentation by IFN-γ-treated thyroid follicular cells inhibits IL-2 and supports IL-4 production by B7-dependent human T cells. Eur J Immunol. 1997;27:62–71.
120. Dayan CM, Chu NR, Londei M, Rapoport B, Feldmann M. T cells involved in human autoimmune disease are resistant to tolerance induction. J Immunol. 1993;151:1606–13.
121. Weetman AP, Freeman MA, Borysiewicz LK, Makgoba MW. Functional analysis of intercellular adhesion molecule-1 expressing human thyroid cells. Eur J Immunol. 1990;20: 271–5.

122. Zheng RQH, Abney ER, Grubeck-Loebenstein B, Dayan C, Maini RN, Feldmann M. Expression of intercellular adhesion molecule-1 and lymphocyte function-associated antigen-3 on human thyroid epithelial cells in Graves' and Hashimoto's diseases. J Autoimmunity. 1990;3:727–6.
123. Tandon N, Makgoba MW, Gahmberg CG, Weetman AP. The expression and role in T cell adhesion of LFA-3 and ICAM-2 on human thyroid cells. Clin Immunol Immunopathol. 1992;64:30–5.
124. MacKenzie WA, Schwartz AE, Friedman EW, Davies TF. Intrathyroidal T cell clones from patients with autoimmune thyroid disease. J Clin Endocrinol Metab. 1987;64:818–23.
125. Sugihara S, Fujiwara H, Niimi H, Shearer GM. Self-thyroid epithelial cell (TEC)-reactive $CD8^+$ T cell lines/clones derived from autoimmune thyroiditis lesions. J Immunol. 1995;155: 1619–28.
126. Wu Z, Podack ER, McKenzie JM, Olsen KJ, Zakarija M. Perforin expression by thyroid-infiltrating T cells in autoimmune thyroid disease. Clin Exp Immunol. 1994;98:470–7.
127. Zheng RQH, Abney E, Chu CG et al. Detection of interleukin-6 and interleukin-1 production in human thyroid epithelial cells by non-radioactive in situ hybridization and immunohistochemical methods. Clin Exp Immunol. 1991;83:314–19.
128. Zheng RQH, Abney ER, Chu CQ et al. Detection of in vitro production of tumour necrosis factor-alpha by human thyroid epithelial cells. Immunology. 1992;75:456–62.
129. Weetman AP, Bennett GL, Wong WLT. Thyroid follicular cells produce interleukin-8. J Clin Endocrinol Metab. 1992;75:328–30.
130. Ajjan R, Watson PF, Weetman AP. Detection of IL-12, IL-13 and IL-15 mRNA in the thyroid of patients with autoimmune thyroid disease. J Clin Endocrinol Metab. 1997;82:666–9.
131. Tandon N, Yan SL, Morgan BP, Weetman AP. Expression and function of multiple regulators of complement activation in autoimmune thyroid disease. Immunology. 1994;81:643–7.
132. Tandon N, Morgan BP, Weetman AP. Expression and function of membrane attack complex inhibitory proteins on thyroid follicular cells. Immunology. 1992;75:372.
133. Weetman AP, Tandon N, Morgan BP. Antithyroid drugs and release of inflammatory mediators by complement-attacked thyroid cells. Lancet. 1992;340:633–6.
134. Green LM, La Bue M, Lazarus JP, Jennings JC. Reduced cell-cell communication in experimentally induced autoimmune thyroid disease. Endocrinology. 1996;137:2823–32.
135. Weetman AP, McGregor AM. Autoimmune thyroid disease: developments in our understanding. Endocrine Rev. 1984;5:309–55.
136. Weetman AP, McGregor AM. Autoimmune thyroid disease: further developments in our understanding. Endocrine Rev. 1994;15:788–830.

4
Graves' disease: progress to date and future prospects

A. M. McGREGOR and J.-P. BANGA

The history of Graves' disease can be characterized by four distinct eras: the first, beginning in the 1820s led to the clinical description of the disease by Parry (1825), Graves (1835) and von Basedow (1848). The second era, beginning in the 1940s, saw the introduction of therapeutic strategies using antithyroid drugs [1] and radioactive iodine [2] which were directed specifically at the thyroid and could both modify and cure the disease. The third era began in 1956 with the classic description by Adams and Purves [3] of a factor in the serum of patients with hyperthyroid Graves' disease which stimulated thyroid function; the so called long acting thyroid stimulator (LATS). The fourth and final era, which brings us to the present time began with the cloning of the thyrotropin (TSH) receptor by Vassart and his colleagues in 1989 [4; Chapter 2]. As a result of these crucial observations and the intervening contributions of many other clinicians and scientists we understand far better the clinical disease and its pathogenesis [5,6].

Graves' disease is an organ-specific autoimmune disease which is almost unique in being due to autoantibodies which stimulate thyroid function. These antibodies function by binding to the cell surface membrane of thyroid follicular cells and specifically to the TSH receptors expressed on these cell membranes. The TSH receptor is a member of the 7-transmembrane spanning domain G binding protein coupled receptor family and through its activation by TSH receptor antibodies, stimulation of adenylate cyclase leads to the increase in synthesis of thyroid hormones and the subsequent clinical syndrome of hyperthyroid Graves' disease [7–9]. While there has been considerable progress in our understanding of the disease there is still much to learn. Despite a clear

A.P. Weetman (ed.), Endocrine Autoimmunity and Associated Conditions. 63–81.

understanding of the pathogenetic mechanisms involved in the induction of hyperthyroidism it is disappointing that this knowledge has had absolutely no impact on our management of the disease. Similarly, while we recognize aetiologically that the disease is multifactorial in its origin with major contributions from genetic, constitutional and environmental factors, defining precisely what these factors are and their specific contributions has proved difficult. Finally despite the cloning of the TSH receptor in 1989, we continue to be frustrated in our efforts to express the whole mature TSH receptor and to define the interactions at the molecular level, between determinants of the immune system and the receptor, which are central both to the induction and the maintenance of the disease. Until these issues are resolved and a credible animal model of hyperthyroid Graves' disease is available, prospects for disease prevention or even modification of the disease by treatment directed at the aberrant autoimmune response rather than at the thyroid cell itself look unlikely. This chapter seeks to highlight where the field has reached but also where the gaps remain.

HYPERTHYROID GRAVES' DISEASE

Patients presenting with hyperthyroid Graves' disease exhibit the classical symptoms and signs of hyperthyroidism. The cause of their hyperthyroidism is likely to be Graves' disease when clinical assessment demonstrates diffuse rather than nodular enlargement of the thyroid gland associated with symptoms and signs suggestive of thyroid-associated ophthalmopathy (Chapter 6). Laboratory investigations which demonstrate diffuse uptake of radioisotope on a thyroid isotope scan, coupled with the presence of circulating autoantibodies, particularly to the TSH receptor or to thyroid peroxidase, confirm the diagnosis. A number of other characteristics further define the disease and emphasise its autoimmune nature [5,6].

As an organ-specific autoimmune disease (Table 4.1) it runs in families and may be associated both in the index patient and in his or her family with other organ-specific autoimmune diseases. The disease occurs 7–10 times more frequently in women than in men though when it does occur in men it tends to be both more severe and to be associated with a higher relapse rate following antithyroid drug medication. Occuring in women, it is of interest that the disease tends to remit during pregnancy often with a post-partum exacerbation.

The peak age of occurrence of the disease is during the third and fourth decades of life. It has been reported in all racial groups. Studies in the north-east of England suggest an incidence of hyperthyroidism of 1–2 cases/1000 population/year [10]. In areas of the world were iodine intake is adequate Graves' disease is the most common cause of hyperthyroidism and accounts for about 75% of all patients presenting with hyperthyroidism to an endocrine service. Prior to the introduction of specific treatments for modifying the disease, the natural history of hyperthyroid Graves' disease was one of relapses and remissions, though at least 10% of this untreated population died from the disease.

Table 4.1 Characteristics of Graves' disease

Organ-specific autoimmune disease
Runs in families
HLA associations
Female predominance
Target-organ lymphocytic infiltration
Immune system activation with circulating:
Activated (HLA-DR$^+$) T cells
Thyroid-specific autoantibodies
Autoantibodies transmit disease
No animal model?

AETIOLOGY

As an organ-specific autoimmune disease, the evidence from studies in patients with other diseases in this group such as insulin-dependent diabetes mellitus (IDDM) suggest that Graves' disease is likely to be a member of the group of polygenic multifactorial diseases. Aetiological factors of multifactorial diseases which are likely to require consideration when considering the development of Graves' disease are defined in Table 4.2.

Table 4.2 Elements of multifactorial diseases which need to be considered as contributors towards the development of Graves' disease

Genetic	*Constitutional*	*Environmental*
Genes	Age	Time
Number	Sex	Geography
Specific	Developmental stage	Climate/seasonal changes
Predisposing	Birth weight	Infectious agents
Dose	Homeostatic mechanisms	Socioeconomic status
MHC	Biochemical	Occupation
Non-MHC	Physiological	Education
Twins share	Immunological	Diet (iodine intake)
Genes	Maternal factors	Stressful stimuli
Uterine environment	Ethnic group	Medication
	Temperament	Toxins
	Pregnancy	

Genetic factors

Association studies using polymorphic markers of potential candidate genes and appropriate control populations have had an important role in defining linkage between genetic markers of determinants within the immune system and Graves' disease [5,6,11]. Due to the crucial role of the major histocompatibility complex (MHC) genes and their products in determining the immune response and particularly antigen presentation, much effort has focused on the association between Graves' disease and the genes that encode the HLA antigens in the MHC region on the short arm of chromosome 6. Associations have been sought with genes in the class I, class II and class III regions [12]. The highly polymorphic class II region genes have been defined by direct sequencing and the polymorphisms determined by PCR amplified DNA products using allele-specific oligonucleotide probes. Conventional serological typing has repeatedly defined associations in Caucasians with Graves' disease and the class II HLA-DR3 molecule [5,6]. The relative risk of this association however, has always been disappointingly small and never greater than 4.

Many other HLA associations reported have tended to be weaker and have usually been attributed to linkage disequilibrium. More recently claims for a stronger association with an HLA DQA1*0501 phenotype have been made by some authors [13,14], particularly when studying male patients with Graves' disease [15] but these observations have not been confirmed by others [16]. Of interest, however, in non-Caucasian populations has been the ability to define particular HLA haplotype associations with the presence or absence of antibody activity to the TSH receptor [17,18] and also resistance to autoimmune thyroid disease on the basis of HLA-DQ genetic analysis [19]. All the evidence available to date, however, points to HLA genes playing only a minor role in susceptibility to Graves' disease. Recent studies in families with multiple affected members which have sought evidence of linkage of MHC genes and Graves' disease have either failed to find evidence of linkage [20] or only been able to show linkage with the presence of thyroid autoantibodies rather than with Graves' disease itself [21].

A search for non-MHC genes which might contribute to the development of autoimmune thyroid disease has provided little evidence to support the view that genes for immunoglobulins or the T cell receptor have a major role to play in the development of Graves' disease [6]. Graves' disease has been associated with a polymorphism for an antagonist of the interleukin-1 receptor [22]. Of particular interest have been recent reports of an association with CTLA-4. Like CD28, CTLA-4 binds the B7 molecule on antigen presenting cells and thus is likely to have a crucial role in the co-stimulatory signal transduced by the B7 molecule necessary for regulation of T cell activation. While an initial American study suggested an association between a polymorphism of the CTLA-4 gene and Graves' disease [23] it seems much more likely that this association will be with organ-specific autoimmune diseases in general rather than with Graves' disease in particular [24].

Not surprisingly in the search for genetic linkage, the target autoantigen, the TSH receptor itself, has also attracted attention. Initial claims that a polymorphism in the extracellular coding region of the human TSH receptor gene might be associated with Graves' disease have not been confirmed [25]. In more recent studies using a series of microsatellite markers within the TSH receptor introns, studies with large multiple affected families with Graves' disease failed to show any significant role of the TSH receptor gene locus in the genetics of Graves' disease [26]. Increasingly, workers in the field have begun to recognize that, with the large number of genes likely to be relevant and the disappointing results obtained to date using the candidate gene approach, alternative strategies are necessary. Efforts are increasingly directed towards genome-wide searches that will allow definition of the spectrum of genes that contribute to the development of Graves' disease. With the development of large numbers of highly polymorphic marker loci such as microsatellites, automated genome searching and access to sufficient numbers of sib-pairs from affected families with Graves' disease by multicentre collaboration, prospects for finally defining the genes which contribute to the development of Graves' disease seem more hopeful. How significant the genetic contribution is remains uncertain.

Constitutional factors

The marked prevalence of hyperthyroid Graves' disease in women over men and the difference in disease severity between the two sexes imply that oestrogens and androgens influence disease development and maintenance. Studies in animal models of autoimmune disease show beyond doubt the importance of these sex hormones in modifying autoimmune disease [27]. The role of glucocorticoids is less clear but autoimmune thyroid disease developing after treatment of hypercortisolism is well described [28].

Aberrations in the immune system itself have had a considerable role as potential initiators of the autoimmune response [5,6]. In this context, indirect evidence based on peripheral blood T cell subset numbers and functional assays of so called suppressor T cell function using peripheral blood lymphocytes and crude thyroid antigen preparations have suggested that a suppressor T cell lymphocyte defect underlies the development of Graves' disease. These observations remain controversial and replicating them has proved difficult [5,6]. A further area of intense interest in considering aberration in the immune system as the initial insult in the development of Graves' disease has been the demonstration of the expression of MHC class II antigens on thyroid cells from patients with Graves' disease but not thyroid cells from normal controls [29]. The assumption was that this process would permit the thyroid cell to take on the role of an antigen-presenting cell and, therefore, induce a T cell response. Considerable evidence has accumulated, however, which demonstrates beyond doubt that the expression of MHC class II is a secondary event which relies on the secretion of γ-interferon by T lymphocytes within the thyroid [30,31]. There is evidence to suggest that viral infection of the thyroid may be capable of inducing MHC class II expression on thyroid cells. Whether this would be sufficient to induce autoimmunity is uncertain particularly as we now know that in order for activation to occur, naive T cells not only require the initial signal of MHC class II molecule with an antigenic peptide in its groove presented to the T cell receptor, but in addition need a second co-stimulatory signal via the B7 molecules which bind to the CD28 or CTLA-4 receptor on the T cell. If this second signal is not provided, T cell anergy rather than stimulation (peripheral tolerance) results.

Environmental factors

In animal models of autoimmune thyroid disease where thyroglobulin is the key autoantigen, dietary iodine depletion which results in the production of poorly iodinated thyroglobulin prevents the development of thyroiditis [32; Chapter 1]. In situations of iodine deficiency, humans who have their iodine stores replenished show increased evidence of thyroiditis and the development of thyroid autoantibodies. The mechanisms remains uncertain, although an influence on MHC antigen expression has been suggested [33] and the relevance for the development of Graves' disease is likewise uncertain [5,6]. What is not in doubt, however, is that in studies of the frequency with which Graves' disease is the presenting cause of hyperthyroidism across Europe, hyperthyroid Graves' disease is a more common cause of hyperthyroidism in areas which are iodine replete rather than iodine deficient. Similarly it is of interest that in the UK, where the major source of iodine is from cow's milk, there is considerable variation in the annual human intake of iodine, with the highest levels being achieved during the winter, and the major peak of onset of hyperthyroid Graves' disease seems to follow this peak of iodine intake. Whether this association is coincidence or causal is again uncertain.

A considerable literature has accumulated on the contribution which stressful life events may make to the development of hyperthyroid Graves' disease [34]. In a number of different settings studies of patients with Graves' disease continue to identify stressful precipitating events which were not present in control populations [35]. Trying to prove this association beyond doubt and understanding the mechanism has proved difficult. The well recognized impact of stress on the hypothalamic-pituitary axis and the known interactions between this axis and immune function suggest that relief of acute stress-induced immune suppression may be followed by a rebound of immune hyperactivity which, in those who are predisposed, might result in development of Graves' disease.

The other major environmental factor which has been implicated in the development of autoimmune diseases in general is that of infectious agents [36]. Whilst a considerable literature has accrued there is little firm evidence to support what seems a very likely aetiological agent. Studies are clearly complicated by the fact that an initial insult is likely to pre-date by many months the development of frank clinical hyperthyroidism: at this stage, evidence of infection is unlikely to be obtained either in the peripheral blood or the thyroid which is, in any case, not always accessible for study. Of interest, however, is the fact that attacks of allergic rhinitis, presumably through the production of cytokines, may result in the recurrence of hyperthyroid Graves' disease [37]. Further evidence that cytokines may have the ability to induce autoimmune thyroid disease come from studies in which cytokines have been used in the treatment of malignancies or hepatitis and been shown to induce or exacerbate pre-existing autoimmune thyroiditis [38–40].

THE ROLE OF T LYMPHOCYTES

T lymphocytes have a central role in the normal immune response and their phenotypic subdivision into $CD4^+$ and $CD8^+$ lymphocytes defines functional characteristics, the $CD4^+$ cells being predominantly helper cells and the $CD8^+$ being predominantly cyotoxic. The organ-specific autoimmune diseases are characterized by lymphocytic infiltration of the target organ and the infiltrate is predominantly of T cells. In Graves' disease studies have sought to define phenotypically the T cell distribution both in the peripheral blood and in the thyroid gland [5,6]. Studies initially examining non-specific functional characteristics of these T cells have evolved to examine T cell responsiveness towards putative autoantigens. Phenotypically, within the peripheral blood in patients with untreated hyperthyroid Graves' disease, $CD8^+$ T cell numbers are reduced and levels of HLA-DR^+ (and $CD25^+$, activated) T cells are increased. Interpretation of the phenotype of intrathyroidal T cells is made difficult by the impact of antithyroid medication on the T cell infiltrate. Against this background, the dominant T cell phenotype is $CD4^+$. Functional studies with T cells obtained from the peripheral blood or thyroid glands of patients with Graves' disease have failed to show any single dominant epitope within the TSH receptor against which these T cells might be directed [41–43]. More recently however it has been suggested that recognition of residues 158–176 of the TSH receptor may be a relevant early event in onset of disease [44]. 'Epitope spreading' almost certainly accounts for the fact that, at the stage of the disease at which the T cells are studied, a multitude of epitopes is recognized and these will differ from patient to patient and almost certainly from those relevant at the time of disease induction [45].

In animal models of autoimmune disease, marked restriction of the T cell receptor variable gene repertoire by T cells recognizing relevant autoantigens suggested that these diseases might have an oligoclonal or even a monoclonal basis to their pathogenesis. Considerable effort has therefore been invested by a number of groups in examining the T cell antigen receptor variable region genes of the two non-covalently linked α and β chains of the human T cell receptor. Despite early claims of restricted $V\alpha$ gene usage by intrathyroidal T cells from patients with Graves' disease [46,47], the results have not been confirmed by several other groups [48,49]. This seems hardly surprising: patients with Graves' disease present late, long after the initial insult, and it is to be expected that, through epitope spreading, T cells will have been exposed over time to a number of epitopes from a variety of target autoantigens. Wide usage of T cell receptor genes, with a resulting polyclonal T cell response is, therefore, a much more likely situation. Surprisingly, however, reports of oligoclonal expansion of T cells continue to appear [50].

While T cells are likely to have a direct pathogenetic role in destructive thyroiditis, acting via direct cytotoxic mechanisms [51], through cytokine production [52,53] or even through the induction of apoptosis of thyroid cells by interleukin-1-induced Fas expression on these cells [54], their role in Graves' disease, following antigen recognition, is primarily in helping B cells in autoantibody production. The mechanisms leading to the selection of these relevant intrathyroidal $CD4^+$ T cell populations in Graves' disease are a continuing focus of research [55].

PATHOGENESIS

Following the initial description of the presence in sera of patients with hyperthyroid Graves' disease of LATS [3], a vast literature has accumulated on the characterization and measurement of this activity. The major milestones (Table 4.3) in this process have demonstrated that: (i) the activity is due to an immunoglobulin; (ii) these immunoglobulins stimulate thyroid function in Graves' disease and (iii) this bioactivity is mediated by the binding of these immunoglobulins to the thyroid follicular cell basement membrane TSH receptor. The successful cloning of the TSH receptor, its successful expression in CHO cell lines and the use of assay systems based on these lines has proved beyond doubt that these antibodies stimulate cell function through their interaction with the TSH receptor [75]. The disease is, therefore, due to thyroid-stimulating antibodies (TSAb). The lymphoid cells in the thyroid are only one of a number of sites in which these antibodies are synthesized [77].

Prior to the cloning of the TSH receptor a major limitation in our attempts to understand the pathogenesis of Graves' disease was the lack of sensitivity and specificity of assay systems used to measure the antibody activity. The development of robust and yet sensitive and specific radioreceptor type assays, in which TSAb are assayed by their ability to inhibit the binding of radiolabelled TSH to thyroid membrane preparations, has allowed the development of commercial assay systems [63]. The development of bioassay systems using both human primary thyroid cell culture systems [68] and the rat FRTL5 thyroid cell line [65], and the increased sensitivity achieved with these assay systems with the use of hypotonic medium [70], has clarified the existence of a spectrum of TSH receptor antibody activities which range from antibodies which bind to the TSH receptor and stimulate thyroid function (TSAb) on the one hand, so leading to hyperthyroid Graves' disease, to antibodies which bind to the TSH receptor but fail to stimulate thyroid function and may be associated, by blocking the receptor (TSH receptor-blocking antibodies; TBAb), with the subsequent development of hypothyroidism [71,78,79].

Table 4. 3 Pathogenesis of thyroid stimulation in Graves' disease

1956	Adams DD and Purves HD [3] Long-acting thyroid stimulator (LATS)
1958	McKenzie JM [56,57] Mouse bioassay
1964	Kriss JP *et al.* [58] LATS is an immunoglobulin
1964	McKenzie JM [59] LATS crosses placenta – neonatal hyperthyroidism
1967	Adams DD and Kennedy TH [60] LATS-protector (LATS-P) – human thyroid stimulator
1973	Mehdi SQ and Nussey SS [61] Graves' immunoglobulins inhibit binding of ^{125}I labelled TSH
1974	Smith BR and Hall R [62,63] Radioreceptor assay - thyrotropin binding inhibiting immunoglobulins (TBII)
1974	Adams DD *et al.* [64] LATS-P stimulates human thyroid *in vivo*
1980	Ambesi-Impiombato *et al.* [65,66] FRTL5 rat thyroid cell line
1980	Matsuura N *et al.* [67] Transplacental TBII – neonatal hypothyroidism
1981	Rapoport B *et al.* [68,69] Human thyroid cell bioassay
1982	Kasagi K *et al.* [70] Increased bioassay sensitivity – hypotonic medium
1983	Konishi J *et al.* [71] Blocking antibodies to TSH receptor in primary myxoedema
1983	Zakarija MJ [72,73] TSH receptor antibodies – restricted heterogeneity
1989	Vassart G *et al.* [4,8,74–76] Cloning of TSH receptor

The original self-infusion of sera from patients with hyperthyroid Graves' disease, which induced thyroid stimulation in the recipient [64], and the clear evidence of the induction of transient neonatal hyperthyroidism in the offspring of mothers with hyperthyroid Graves' disease whose TSAb activity was present at sufficient levels to induce transient hyperthyroidism in the offspring due to passage of the antibody across the placenta [59], provide overwhelming evidence of the pathogenetic role of TSAb. With modern assay techniques almost all patients with untreated hyperthyroid Graves' disease have TSAb detectable in their serum. These antibodies are only detectable in patients with autoimmune thyroid disease and are therefore disease specific. They demonstrate immunoglobulin light chain restriction [72] and tend mainly to be of the IgG_1 subclass [73], suggesting that they are oligoclonal. Like TSH itself, these antibodies in patients with Graves' disease cause cyclic AMP-mediated release of thyroid hormone and thyroglobulin, and stimulate iodine uptake, protein synthesis and thyroid growth. In patients treated with antithyroid drugs TSAb activity falls in response to treatment, tends to rise again or fail to respond to treatment in patients who relapse and finally disappears when the disease is cured, usually in response to treatment with radioactive iodine or surgical subtotal thyroidectomy [5,6].

Characterization of the TSH receptor at the molecular level and its successful expression have led to a number of strategies, based on the establishment of mutations and chimeras of the receptor, which seek to examine the structure/function relationships between TSH and receptor antibodies with the TSH receptor [80–86]. These studies, which are discussed in detail in Chapter 2, will in the longer term presumably lead not only to a clear understanding of the interaction of TSH and TSH receptor antibodies with the receptor but also allow discrimination between the sites of interaction of TSAb and TBAb with the extracellular domain of the TSH receptor. Crucial to our understanding of all of these interactions is the need to recognize that the normal functioning TSH receptor is a three-dimensional structure on the cell membrane and that the B cell (antibody) epitopes on this autoantigen which are recognized by TSH receptor antibodies are almost certainly conformational in nature and depend on the three-dimensional structure of the mature whole receptor [87–89]. In this context, any studies seeking to interpret interactions of TSH or these antibodies with the receptor are only of relevance when the correct maturation (e.g. appropriately glycosylated) and conformational nature of the receptor can be assured.

Repeated claims have been made that modification of the TSH receptor as a self-antigen provides a target organ explanation for the development of hyperthyroid Graves' disease. Whilst a number of variants of the TSH receptor have been described, with more careful study most have been shown to be germline and to correspond to polymorphisms which are also present in normal controls [90]. From all of the data accumulated to date it seems much more likely that the primary structure of the TSH receptor expressed on the surface of the Graves' follicular cell is no different from that on the normal follicular cell.

TREATMENT

Treatment of Graves' disease relies on the thionamide group of antithyroid drugs, radioactive iodine or surgical subtotal thyroidectomy [91]. There remains considerable variation amongst thyroidologists across the world as to which modalities of treatment are used and the order in which they are used [92]. Likewise a significant literature has accumulated on the impact which these various modes of therapy may have on the natural history of Graves' disease itself, particularly as assessed by changes in TSH receptor antibody activity in response to treatment [5,6]. These studies have been extended by observations which provide evidence that antithyroid drugs may contribute to the induction of remission in patients with hyperthyroid Graves' disease by acting directly on the immune system [93,94]. The area remains controversial.

Considerable controversy has also surrounded the issue of 'resting the thyroid' as proposed in 1991 by Hashizume and colleagues [95]. They provided evidence to support the view that combining antithyroid drugs with thyroxine initially, and then maintaining thyroxine after stopping the antithyroid drugs, was associated with a continuing reduction of TSH receptor antibody levels and a reduction in the recurrence of hyperthyroidism. Subsequent studies have failed to replicate these results [96–98]. Despite the best efforts to devise appropriate protocols for the use of antithyroid drugs for the management of Graves' disease [99], variables such as dietary iodine intake [100], genetic background, the sex of the patient, the severity of the disease at the time of presentation, and the size of goitre make standard regimens more difficult to define. Evidence continues to accumulate, however, which suggests that the response to treatment of the disease is greatest with higher dosages of antithyroid drugs and that these regimens are associated with higher rates of disease remission [101,102]. The doses recommended would certainly achieve levels of antithyroid drug in the thyroid which would be likely to modify the autoimmune response there. With the cloning of the TSH receptor, evidence has been generated using human TSH receptor transfected CHO cells that the response to antithyroid drug medication may be determined by the epitopes on the receptor which particular patients' TSH receptor antibodies recognize [103]. These preliminary studies on small numbers of patients need both to be extended by the authors themselves and replicated by independent laboratories.

THE FUTURE

As suggested initially we now understand well both the clinical syndrome of hyperthyroid Graves' disease and the TSH receptor antibodies which are responsible for inducing the disease. A number of key issues are being or still need to be addressed (Table 4.4). The critical actions of TSH receptor antibodies, which in binding either block or stimulate the TSH receptor, are the subject of intense current investigation. Whether all of the reagents and assay systems are yet in place to draw definitive conclusions is open to speculation. Understanding of the aetiology of the disease remains disappointing. In the next few years genome-wide screens may well begin to identify those individuals who are at risk. It remains disappointing too that for all the progress in our understanding of this disease, treatment is still largely directed at inhibiting thyroid hormone synthesis or destroying the thyroid. The controversy that surrounds the immunological mechanisms which lead to the development of hyperthyroid Graves' disease and the search for potential aetiological agents such as infectious organisms will continue so long as we fail to recognize the clinical setting of 'pre-Graves' disease'. Definition of those at risk may well help to define this group of individuals who need to be followed clinically, biochemically, immunologically and microbiologically in the period before overt disease develops.

It seems unlikely that characterization of the interactions between T cells and B cells with the TSH receptor,in order to define the T and B cell epitopes on the

Table 4.4 Graves' disease – future directions

Aetiology	
	Who is at risk?
	Genome-wide screen in multiplex families
Pre-Graves' disease	
	Characterize
TSH receptor antibodies	
	Produce human monoclonal antibodies
	Improve assay systems
	Characterise structure/function interactions with TSH receptor
TSH receptor	
	Purify in bulk whole native receptor
	High level expression whole mature receptor
	Obtain crystals (three-dimensional structure)
	Characterize T and B cell epitopes
Animal models	
	Establish truly representative models
	Test beds of therapy
Treatment	
	Prevent onset/treat disease
	Aim to direct it at aberrant autoimmune response

receptor against which the autoimmune response is directed, will be successfully achieved without establishment of the three-dimensional structure of the TSH receptor. Success in achieving the latter goal will require the purification of very large amounts of the native human TSH receptor or success in achieving high level expression of the whole mature solubilized receptor. Attempts to achieve this have to date been disappointing. In this context our own efforts have been directed towards the use of the baculovirus insect expression system [104]. This system is recognized as being ideal for the expression of membrane proteins, achieves high levels of expression, is relatively easy to use and ensures appropriate post-translational processing of the nascent protein so that a mature three-dimensional structure is expressed. While the system has worked well we have only had success in expressing the extracellular domain of the human TSH receptor using the baculovirus system and this has been the experience of others.

With the low level of expression of TSH receptors on the thyroid follicular cell membrane, access to sufficient material for receptor characterization, assay systems, and the bulking up of receptors for structural studies has proved difficult. Attempts to try and address this problem have sought to develop specific monoclonal antibodies directed against the receptor. Although there has been considerable success in establishing mouse monoclonal antibodies directed against the receptor [105], concerns have continued to exist about the relevance of non-species-specific antibodies and on these grounds considerable effort has been expanded on trying to establish human monoclonal antibodies to the TSH receptor. Using the immunoglobulin gene combinatorial library approach, organ-specific, high affinity IgG class autoantibodies directed against a variety of target autoantigens have been successfully cloned [106]. The antibodies which result resemble patient serum autoantibodies in terms of their affinity, specificity and epitope recognition, and the ability to generate such antibodies against the TSH receptor will provide exceedingly important reagents not only for defining the pathogenetically relevant autoantigenic eptiopes but also for defining the structure/function relationships between these antibodies and the TSH receptor. An alternative approach to establish human monoclonal antibodies to the TSH receptor, which has been adopted with some success in our laboratory, has made use of Epstein-Barr virus-transformed B lymphocytes from patients with hyperthyroid Graves' disease [107]. These immortalized peripheral blood B cell lines produce TSH receptor antibodies of the IgG class. This methodology and the products generated offer the potential of crucial reagents for characterization of the antibody-antigen interaction in Graves' disease.

With the cloning of the TSH receptor, further developments in methodology for the detection of TSH receptor antibodies have, not surprisingly, resulted; in addition, the availability of CHO cells expressing either wild type or chimeric human TSH receptors is allowing clearer definition of the spectrum of anti-TSH receptor antibody activities detected in the serum of patients with autoimmune thyroid disease [108]. A sensitive method of *in vitro* transcription and translation which generates nascent TSH receptor polypeptides, with assessment by immunoprecipitation of the binding of TSH receptor autoantibodies, offers a further strategy for detecting these antibodies without the need for bioassay systems [109]. Studies using flow cytometry with CHO cells expressing high numbers of TSH receptors on their surface make clear the very low level of TSH receptor autoantibody activity present in the sera of patients with Graves' disease [110] and, therefore, continues to highlight the need for increasing sensitivity in the assay systems for the detection of this antibody activity.

As is clear from most of the work that has been discussed in this chapter, a major impediment to developments in our understanding of hyperthyroid Graves' disease has been the lack of an appropriate animal model. A great deal of effort has been invested, both historically and since the cloning of the TSH receptor, in this area of research but to date with very little success. Without the establishment of a robust and representative animal model attempts to begin to focus therapeutic strategies on the aberrant immune response rather than on the thyroid gland itself will be hindered. The report recently by Kohn and his colleagues [111] of the induction of a Graves'-like disease in mice immunized with fibroblasts transfected with the TSH receptor and an MHC class II molecule looks as though finally this goal may be achievable, although thyroid lymphocyte infiltration was not detected. On the other hand we have recently established an antibody-mediated model of hypothyroidism using large fragments of the extracellular domain of the TSH receptor. Small variations in the size and subregions of this domain results in the presence or absence of thyroid lymphocytic infiltration. It therefore appears that using animal models it is possible to dissect out distinct events in autoimmune thyroid disease including not only altered thyroid gland function but also whether or not infiltration develops.

In the context of treatment, and ideally prevention of the development of Graves' disease, research strategies will need to focus on early identification of individuals at risk of the development of the disease and of therapies which might then modify or abrogate directly the potential or early autoimmune response. Considerable publicity has been associated, at least in animal models of autoimmune disease, with therapeutic interventions which rely on the concept that prior administration of oral antigen reduces the subsequent response when the animal is re-exposed to the antigen. The induction of 'oral tolerance' [112] in this way may be due to clonal anergy, apoptosis of affected T cells or the induction of inhibitory cytokines. Of great potential interest is the relevance of this form of immune modulation for human autoimmune thyroid disease, in the light of recent animal data on thyroglobulin-induced thyroiditis [113,114].

Despite the relatively benign nature of hyperthyroid Graves' disease, characterization both of the target autoantigen and of the pathogenetic autoantibodies suggests that we are in an excellent position to capitalize on this information over the next few years in furthering our understanding, particularly of the aetiology of the disease, the interaction of TSH receptor antibodies with their target autoantigen and the potential for modifying the disease by directing therapies towards the immune process itself.

References

1. Astwood EB. Treatment of hyperthyroidism with thiourea and thiouracil. J Am Med Assoc. 1943;122:78–89.
2. Chapman EM. History of the discovery and early use of radioactive iodine. J Am Med Assoc. 1983;250:2042–51.
3. Adams DD, Purves HD. Abnormal responses in the assay of thyrotropin. Proceedings of the University of Otago Medical School. 1956;34:11–12.
4. Parmentier M, Libert F, Maenhaut C et al. Molecular cloning of the thyrotropin receptor. Science. 1989;246:1620–2.
5. Weetman AP, McGregor AM. Autoimmune thyroid disease: developments in our understanding. Endocr Rev. 1984;5:309–55.
6. Weetman AP, McGregor AM. Autoimmune thyroid disease: further developments in our understanding. Endocr Rev. 1994;15:788–830.
7. Rees Smith B, McLachlan S M, Furmaniak J. Autoantibodies to the thyrotropin receptor. Endocr Rev. 1988;9:106–21.
8. Nagayama Y, Kaufman KD, Seto P, Rapoport B. Molecular cloning, sequence and functional expression of the cDNA for the human thyrotropin receptor. Biochem Biophys Res Commun. 1989;165:1184–90.

9. McGregor AM. Graves' disease and the thyrotropin (TSH) receptor. In: Edwards CRW, Lincoln DW, eds. Recent Advances in Endocrinology and Metabolism. Churchill Livingstone 1992;4:51–65.
10. Vanderpump MPJ, Tunbridge WM. The epidemiology of thyroid diseases. In: Braverman LE, Utiger RD, eds. Werner and Ingbars The Thyroid. Lippincott-Raven: Philadelphia; 1996:474–82.
11. Mangklabruks A, Cox N, De Groot LJ. Genetic factors in autoimmune thyroid disease analysed by restriction fragment length polymorphisms of candidate genes. J Clin Endocrinol Metab. 1991;73:236–44.
12. Abraham LJ, French MAH, Dawkins RL. Polymorphic MHC ancestral haplotypes affect the activity of tumour necrosis factor-alpha. Clin Exp Immunol. 1993;92:14–18.
13. Yanagawa T, Mangklabruks A, Chang Y-B et al. Human histocompatibility leucocyte antigen-DQA1*0501 allele associated with genetic susceptibility to Graves' disease in a Caucasian population. J Clin Endocrinol Metab. 1993;76:1569–74.
14. Chuang L-M, Wu HP, Chang CC et al. HAL DRB1/DQA1/DQB1 haplotype determines thyroid autoimmunity in patients with insulin dependent diabetes mellitus. Clin Endocrinol. 1996;45:631–6.
15. Yanagawa T, Mangklabruks A, De Groot LJ. Strong association between HLA-DQA1*0501 and Graves' disease in a male Caucasian population. J Clin Endocrinol Metab. 1994;79:227–9.
16. Cuddihy RM, Bahn RS. Lack of an independent association between the human leukocyte antigen allele DQA1*0501 and Graves' disease. J Clin Endocrinol Metab. 1996;81:847–9.
17. Inoue D, Sato K, Sugawa H et al. Apparent genetic difference between hypothyroid patients with blocking-type thyrotropin receptor antibody and those without, as shown by restriction fragment length polymorphism analyses of HLA-D loci. J Clin Endocrinol Metab. 1993;77:606–10.
18. Cho BY, Chung JH, Shong YK et al. A strong association between thyrotropin receptor-blocking antibody – positive atrophic autoimmune thyroiditis and HLA-B8 and HLA-DQB1*0302 in Koreans. J Clin Endocrinol Metab. 1993;77:611–5.
19. Tamai H, Kimura A, Dong R-P et al. Resistance to autoimmune thyroid disease is associated with HLA-DQ. J Clin Endocrinol Metab. 1994;78:94–7.
20. Roman SH, Greenberg D, Rubinstein P, Wallenstein S, Davies TF. Genetics of autoimmune thyroid disease: lack of evidence for linkage to HLA within families. J Clin Endocrinol Metab. 1992;74:496–503.
21. Shields DC, Ratanachaiyavong S, McGregor AM, Collins A, Morton NE. Combined segregation and linkage analysis of Graves' disease with a thyroid autoantibody diathesis. Am J Hum Genet. 1994;55:540–54.
22. Blakemore AIF, Watson PF, Weetman AP et al. Association of Graves' disease with an allele of the Interleukin-1 receptor antagonist gene. J Clin Endocrinol Metab. 1995;80:111–15.
23. Yanagawa T, Hidaka Y, Guimaraes V, Soliman M, De Groot LJ. CTLA-4 gene polymorphism associated with Graves' disease in a Caucasian population. J Clin Endocrinol Metab. 1995;80:41–5.
24. Donner H, Rau H, Walfish PG et al. CTLA4 alanine-17 confers genetic susceptibility to Graves' disease and to type I diabetes mellitus. J Clin Endocrinol Metab. 1997;82:143–6.
25. Kotsa KD, Watson PF, Weetman AP. No association between a thyrotropin receptor gene polymorphism and Graves' disease in the female population. Thyroid. 1997;7:31–3.
26. De Roux N, Shields DC, Misrahi M, Ratanachaiyavong S, McGregor AM, Milgrom E. Analysis of the thyrotropin receptor as a candidate gene in familial Graves' disease. J Clin Endocrinol Metab. 1996;81:3483–6.
27. Ahmed AS, Young PR, Penhale WJ. The effects of female sex hormones on the development of autoimmune thyroiditis in thymectomised and irradiated rats. Clin Exp Immunol. 1983;4:351–8.
28. Takasu N. Komiya I, Nagasawa Y, Aaswa T, Yamada T. Exacerbation of autoimmune thyroid dysfunction after unilateral adrenalectomy in patients with Cushing's syndrome due to an adrenocortical adenoma. N Engl J Med. 1990;322:1708–12.
29. Bottazzo GF, Pujol-Borrell R, Hanafusa T, Feldmann M. Role of aberrant HLA-DR expression and antigen presentation in induction of endocrine autoimmunity. Lancet. 1983;2:1115–9.
30. Hassman R, Solic N, Jasani B, Hall R, McGregor AM. Immunological events leading to destructive thyroiditis in the AUG rat. Clin Exp Immunol. 1988;73:410–16.

31. Hamilton F, Black M, Farquharson MA, Stewart C, Foulis AK. Spatial correlation between thyroid epithelial cells expressing class II MHC molecules and interferon-gamma-containing lymphocytes in human autoimmune thyroid disease. Clin Exp Immunol. 1991;83:64–8.
32. Brown TR, Sundick RS, Dhar A, Sheth D, Bagchi N. Uptake and metabolism of iodine is crucial for the development of thyroiditis in obese strain chickens. J Clin Invest. 1991;88:106–11.
33. Schuppert F, Taniguchi S-I, Schroder S, Dralle H, von Zur Muhlen A, Kohn LD. *In vivo* and *in vitro* evidence for iodide regulation of MHC class I and class II expression in Graves' disease. J Clin Endocrinol Metab. 1996;81:3622–8.
34. Gorman CA. A critical review of the role of stress in hyperthyroidism. In: Drexhage HA, de Vijlder JJM and Wiersinga WM, eds. The Thyroid Gland Environment and Autoimmunity. Amsterdam: Elsevier Science Publishers; 1990:191–200.
35. Winsa B, Adami H, Bergstrom R et al. Stressful life events and Graves' disease. Lancet. 1991; 338:1475–9.
36. Tomer Y, Davies TF. Infection, thyroid disease, and autoimmunity. Endocr Rev. 1993;14: 107–15.
37. Hidaka Y, Amino N, Iwatani Y, Itoh E, Matsunaga M, Tamaki H. Recurrence of thyrotoxicosis after attack of allergic rhinitis in patients with Graves' disease. J Clin Endocrinol Metab. 1993;77:1667–0.
38. Ronnblom LE, Alm GV, Oberg KE. Autoimmunity after alpha-interferon therapy for malignant carcinoid tumours. Ann Intern Med. 1991;115:178–83.
39. Van Liessum PA, De Mulder PHM, Mattijssen EJM, Corstens FHM, Wagener DJT. Hypothyroidism and goitre during interleukin-2 therapy without LAK cells. Lancet. 1989;1: 224.
40. Hoekman K, von Blomberg-Van Der Flier BME, Wagstaff J, Drexhage HA, Pinedo HM. Reverible thyroid dysfunction during treatment with GM-CSF. Lancet. 1991;338:541–2.
41. Tandon N, Freeman MA, Weetman AP. T cell responses to synthetic TSH receptor peptides in Graves' disease. Clin Exp Immunol. 1992;89:468–73.
42. Soliman M, Kaplan E, Yanagawa T, Hidaka Y, Fisfalen M, De Groot LJ. T cells recognise multiple epitopes in the human thyrotropin receptor extracellular domain. J Clin Endocrinol Metab. 1995;80:905–14.
43. Dayan CM, Londei M, Corcoran AE et al. Autoantigen recognition by thyroid-infiltrating T cells in Graves' disease. Proc Natl Acad Sci USA. 1991;88:7415–19.
44. Soliman M, Kaplan E, Guimaraes V, Yanagawa T, de Groot LJ. T cell recognition of residue 158-176 in TSH receptor confers risk for development of thyroid autoimmunity in siblings in a familty with Graves' disease. Thyroid. 1996;6:545–61.
45. Sercarz EE, Lehmann PV, Ametani A et al. Dominance and crypticity of T cell antigenic determinants. Ann Rev Immunol. 1993;11:729–66.
46. Davies TF, Martin A, Concepcion ES, Graves P, Cohen I, Ben-Nun A. Evidence of limited variability of antigen receptors on intrathyroidal T cells in autoimmune thyroid disease. N Engl J Med. 1991;325:238–44.
47. Davies TF, Martin A, Concepcion ES et al. Evidence for selective accumulation of intrathyroidal T lymphocytes in human autoimmune thyroid disease based on T cell receptor V gene usage. J Clin Invest. 1992;89:157–62.
48. McIntosh RS, Tandon N, Pickerill AP, Davies R, Barnett D, Weetman AP. IL-2 receptor-positive intrathyroidal lymphocytes in Graves' disease: analysis of Va transcript microheterogeneity. J Immunol. 1993;91:3884–93.
49. Caso-Pelaez E, McGregor AM, Banga JP. A polyclonal T cell repertoire of V-alpha and V-beta T cell receptor gene families in intrathyroidal T lymphocytes of Graves' disease patients. Scand J Immunol. 1995;41:141–7.
50. Heufelder AE, Wenzel BE, Scriba PC. Antigen receptor variable region repertoires expressed by T cells infiltrating thyroid retroorbital and pretibial tissue in Graves' disease. J Clin Endocrinol Metab. 1996;81:3733–9.
51. Sugihara S, Fujiwara H, Niimi H, Shearer GM. Self-thyroid epithelial cell (TEC)-reactive $CD8^+$ T cell lines/clones derived from autoimmune thyroiditis lesions. J Immunol. 1995;155: 1619–28.
52. Watson PF, Pickerill P, Davies R, Weetman AP. Analysis of cytokine gene expression in Graves' disease and multinodular goitre. J Clin Endocrinol Metab. 1994;79:355–60.
53. Nishikawa T, Yamashita S, Namba H et al. Interferon-gamma inhibition of human thyrotropin receptor gene expression. J Clin Endocrinol Metab. 1993;77:1084–9.

54. Giordano C, Stassi G, de Maria R et al. Potential involvement of Fas and its ligand in the pathogenesis of Hashimoto's thyroiditis. Science. 1997;275:960–3.
55. Nakashima M, Martin A, Davies TF. Intrathyroidal T cell accumulation in Graves' disease:delineation of mechanisms based on in situ T cell receptor analysis. J Clin Endocrinol Metab. 1996;81:3346–51.
56. McKenzie JM. The bioassay of thyrotropin in serum. Endocrinology. 1958;63:372–82.
57. McKenzie JM. Delayed thyroid response to serum from thyrotoxic patients. Endocrinology. 1958;63:865–8.
58. Kriss JP, Pleshakov V, Chien JR. Isolation and identification of the long-acting thyroid stimulator and its relation to hyperthyroidism and circumscribed pretibial myxoedema. J Clin Endocrinol Metab. 1964;24:1005–28.
59. McKenzie JM. Neonatal Graves' disease. J Clin Endocrinol Metab. 1964;24:660–8.
60. Adams DD, Kennedy TH. Occurrence in thyrotoxicosis of a gamma globulin which protects LATS from neutralisation by an extract of thyroid gland. J Clin Endocrinol Metab. 1967;27: 173–7.
61. Mehdi SQ, Nussey SS. A radio-ligand receptor assay for the long-acting thyroid stimulator. Biochem J. 1975;145:105–11.
62. Smith BR, Hall R. Thyroid-stimulating immunoglobulins in Graves' disease. Lancet. 1974;2: 427–30.
63. Southgate K, Creagh FM, Teece M, Kingswood C, Rees Smith B. A receptor assay for the measurement of TSH receptor antibodies in unextracted serum. Clin Endocrinol. 1984;20: 539–48.
64. Adams DD, Fastier FN, Howie JB, Kennedy TH, Kilpatrick JA, Stewart RDH. Stimulation of the human thyroid by infusions of plasma containing LATS protector. J Clin Endocrinol Metab. 1974;39:826.
65. Ambesi-Impiombato FS, Parks LAM, Coon HG. Culture of hormone-dependent epithelial cells from rat thyroids. Proc Natl Acad Sci USA. 1980;77:3455–9.
66. Vitti P, Rotella CM, Valente WA et al. Characterisation of the optimal stimulatory effects of Graves' monoclonal and serum immunoglobulin G on adenosine 3′5′-monophosphate production in FRTL5 thyroid cells. A potential clinical assay. J Clin Endocrinol Metab. 1983;57:782–91.
67. Matsuura N, Yamada Y, Nohara Y et al. Familial neonatal transient hypothyroidism due to maternal TSH-binding inhibitor immunoglobulins. N Eng J Med. 1980;303:738–41.
68. Hinds WE, Takai N, Rapoport B, Filetti S, Clark OH. Thyroid-stimulating immunoglobulin bioassay using cultured human thyroid cells. J Clin Endocrinol Metab. 1981;52:1204–10.
69. Rapoport B, Greenspan FS, Filetti S, Pepitone M. Clinical experience with a human thyroid cell bioassay for thyroid stimulating immunoglobulin. J Clin Endocrinol Metab. 1984;58: 332–8.
70. Kasagi K, Konishi J, Iida Y et al. A new in vitro assay for human thyroid stimulator using cultured thyroid cells: effect of sodium chloride on adenosine 3′5′-monophosphate increase. J Clin Endocrinol Metab. 1982;54:108–14.
71. Konishi J, Iida Y, Endo K et al. Inhibition of thyrotropin-induced adenosine 3′5′-monophosphate increase by immunoglobulins from patients with primary myxoedema. J Clin Endocrinol Metab. 1983;57:544-9.
72. Zakarija MJ. Immunochemical characterisation of the thyroid-stimulating antibody (TSAb) of Graves' disease: evidence for restricted heterogeneity. J Clin Lab Immunol. 1983;10:77.
73. Weetman AP, Yateman ME, Ealey PA et al. Thyroid-stimulating antibody activity between different immunoglobulin G subclasses. J Clin Invest. 1990;86:723.
74. Libert F, Lefort A, Gerard C et al. Cloning, sequencing and expression of the human thyrotropin (TSH) receptor: evidence for binding of autoantibodies. Biochem Biophys Res Commun. 1989;165:1250–5.
75. Nagayama Y, Rapoport B. The thyrotropin receptor 25 years after its discovery: new insights after its molecular cloning. Mol Endocrinol. 1992;6:145–56.
76. Perret J, Ludgate M, Libert F et al. Stable expression of the human TSH receptor in CHO cells and characterisation of differentially expressing clones. Biochem Biophys Res Commun. 1990;171:1044–50.
77. Weetman AP, McGregor AM, Wheeler MH, Hall R. Extrathyroidal sites of autoantibody synthesis in Graves' disease. Clin Exp Immunol. 1984;56:330–6.

78. Cho BY, Shong YK, Lee HK, Koh C-S, Min HK. Graves' hyperthyroidism following primary hypothyroidism: sequential changes in various activities of thyrotropin receptor antibodies. Acta Endocrinol (Copenh.) 1989;120:447–50.
79. Chiovato L, Vitti P, Santini F et al. Incidence of antibodies blocking thyrotropin effect in vitro in patients with euthyroid or hypothyroid autoimmune thyroiditis. J Clin Endocrinol Metab. 1990;71:40–5.
80. Chazenbalk GD, Nagayama Y, Russo D, Wadsworth HL, Rapoport B. Functional analysis of the cytoplasmic domains of the human thyrotropin receptor by site-directed mutagenesis. J Biol Chem. 1990;265:20970–5.
81. Russo D, Chazenbalk GD, Nagayama Y, Wadsworth HL, Rapoport B. Site-directed mutagenesis of the human thyrotropin receptor: Role of asparagine-linked oligosaccharides in the expression of a functional receptor. Mol Endocrinol. 1991;5:29–33.
82. Nagayama Y, Wadsworth HL, Chazenbalk GD, Russo D, Seto P, Rapoport B. Thyrotropin-luteinizing hormone/chorionic gonadotropin receptor extracellular domain chimeras as probes for thyrotropin receptor function. Proc Natl Acad Sci USA. 1991:88:902–5.
83. Wadsworth HL, Russo D, Nagayama Y, Chazenbalk GD, Rapoport B. Studies on the role of amino acids 38-45 in the expression of a functional thyrotropin receptor. Mol Endocrinol. 1992;6:394–8.
84. Nagayama Y, Rapoport B. Thyroid stimulatory autoantibodies in different patients with autoimmune thyroid disease do not all recognise the same components of the human thyrotropin receptor: Selective role of receptor amino acids Ser 25-Glu 30. J Clin Endocrinol Metab. 1992;75:1425–30.
85. Costagliola S, Swillens S, Niccoli P, Dumont JE, Vassart G, Ludgate M. Binding assay for thyrotropin receptor autoantibodies using the recombinant receptor protein. J Clin Endocrinol Metab. 1992;75:1540–4.
86. Kosugi S, Ban T, Akamizu T, Valente W, Kohn LD. Use of thyrotropin receptor (TSHR) mutants to detect stimulating TSHR antibodies in hypothyroid patients with idiopathic myxoedema, who have blocking TSHR antibodies. J Clin Endocrinol Metab. 1993;77:19–24.
87. Graves PN, Vlase H, Davies TF. Folding of the recombinant human TSH receptor extracellular domain: identification of folded monomeric and tetrameric complexes that bind TSH receptor autoantibodies. Endocrinology. 1995;136:521–7.
88. Rapoport B, McLachlan SM, Kakinuma A, Chazenbalk GD. Critical relationship between autoantibody recognition and TSH receptor maturation as reflected in the acquisition of complex carbohyrdrate. J Clin Endocrinol Metab. 1996;81:2525–33.
89. Park JY, Kim IJ, Lee MH et al. Identification of the peptides that inhibit the stimulation of TSH receptor by Graves' immunoglobulin G from peptide libraries. Endocrinology. 1997; 138:617–26.
90. Tonacchera M, Van Sande J, Parma J, Duprez L. TSH receptor and disease. Clin Endocrinol. 1996;44:621–33.
91. Vanderpump MPJ, Ahlquist JAO, Franklyn JA, Clayton RN. Consensus statement for good practice and audit measures in the management of hypothyroidism and hyperthyroidism. Br Med J. 1996;313:539–44.
92. Wartofsky L, Glinoer D, Solomon B et al. Differences and similarities in the diagnosis and treatment of Graves' disease in Europe, Japan and the United States. Thyroid. 1991;1:129–35.
93. McGregor AM, Petersen MM, McLachlan SM, Rooke P, Rees Smith B, Hall R. Carbimazole and the autoimmune response in Graves' disease. N Engl J Med. 1980;303;302–7.
94. Ratanachaiyavong S, McGregor AM. Immunosuppressive effects of antithyroid drugs. Clin Endocrinol Metab. 1985;14:449–66.
95. Hashizume K, Ichikawa K, Sakurai A et al. Administration of thyroxine in treated Graves' disease: effects on the level of antibodies to thyroid-stimulating hormone receptors and on the risk of recurrence of hyperthyroidism. N Engl J Med. 1991;324:947–53.
96. Tamai H, Hayaki I, Kawai K et al. Lack of effect of thyroxine administration on elevated thyroid stimulating hormone receptor antibody levels in treated Graves' disease patients. J Clin Endocrinol Metab. 1995;80:1481–4.
97. McIver B, Rae P, Beckett G, Wilkinson E, Gold A, Toft A. Lack of effect of thyroxine in patients with Graves' hyperthyroidism who are treated with an antithyroid drug. N Engl J Med. 1996;334:220–4.
98. Rittmaster RS, Zwicker H, Abbott EC et al. Effect of methimazole with or without exogenous L-thyroxine on serum concentrations of TSH receptor antibodies in patients with Graves' disease. J Clin Endocrinol Metab. 1996;81:3283–8.

99. Benker G, Vitti P, Kahaly G, Raue F, Tegler F, Hirche H, Reinwein D and European Mutlicenter Study Group. Response to methimazole in Graves' disease. Clin Endocrinol. 1995;43:257–63.
100. Solomon B, Evaul JE, Burman KD, Wartofsky L. Remission rates with antithyroid drug therapy: continuing influence of iodine intake? Ann Int Med. 1987;107:510–12.
101. Weetman AP, Pickerill AP, Watson P, Chatterjee VK, Edwards OM. Treatment of Graves' disease with the block-replace regimen of antithyroid drugs: the effect of treatment duration and immunogenetic susceptibility on relapse. Q J Med. 1994;87:337–41.
102. Wilson R, Buchanan L, Fraser WD, McKillop JH, Thomson JA. Do higher doses of carbimazole improve remission in Graves' disease? Q J Med. 1996;89:381–5.
103. Kim WB, Cho BY, Park HY et al. Epitopes for thyroid-stimulating antibodies in Graves' sera: A possible link of heterogeneity to differences in response to antithyroid drug treatment. J Clin Endocrinol Metab. 1996;81:1758–67.
104. Huang GC, Page MJ, Nicholson LB, Collison KS, McGregor AM, Banga JP. The thyrotropin hormone receptor of Graves' disease:overexpression of the extracellular domain in insect cells using recombinant baculovirus, immunoaffinity purification and analysis of autoantibody binding. J Mol Endocrinol. 1993;10:127–42.
105. Nicholson LB, Vlase H, Graves P et al. Monoclonal antibodies to the human TSH receptor:epitope mapping and binding to the native receptor on the basolateral plasma membrane of thyroid follicular cells. J Mol Endocrinol. 1996;16:159–70.
106. Rapoport B, Portolano S, McLachlan SM. Combinatorial libraries:new insights into human organ-specific autoantibodies. Immunol Today. 1995;16:43–9.
107. Morgenthaler NG, Kim MR, Tremble J et al. Human immunoglobulin G autoantibodies from EB virus-transformed B lymphocytes: characterisation by immune precipitation with recombinant antigen and biological activity. J Clin Endocrinol Metab. 1996;81:3155–61.
108. Watanabe Y, Tahara K, Hirai A, Tada H, Kohn LD, Amino N. Subtypes of anti-TSH receptor antibodies classified by various assays using CHO cells expressing wild type or chimeric human TSH receptor. Thyroid. 1997;7:13–9.
109. Morgenthaler NG, Tremble J, Huang GC, Scherbaum WA, McGregor AM, Banga JP. Binding of antithyrotropin receptor autoantibodies in Graves' disease serum to nascent, in vitro translated TSH receptor: ability to map epitopes recognised by antibodies. J Clin Endocrinol Metab. 1996;81:700–6.
110. Jaume JC, Kakinuma A, Chazenbalk GD, Rapoport B, McLachlan SM. Thyrotropin receptor autoantibodies in serum are present at much lower levels than thyroid peroxidase autoantibodies: analysis by flow cytometry. J Clin Endocrinol Metab. 1997;82:500–7.
111. Shimojo N, Kohno Y, Yamaguchi K-I et al. Induction of Graves'-like disease in mice by immunisation with fibroblasts transfected with the TSH receptor and a class II molecule. Proc Natl Acad Sci USA. 1996;93:11074–9.
112. Weiner HL. Oral tolerance for the treatment of autoimmune disease. Ann Rev Med. 1997;48: 341–51.
113. Guimaraes VC, Quintans J, Fisfalen M et al. Suppression of development of experimental autoimmune thyroiditis by oral administration of thyroglobulin. Endocrinology. 1995;136: 3353–9.
114. Guimaraes VC, Quintans J, Fisfalen M-E et al. Immunosuppression of thyroiditis. Endocrinology. 1996;137:2199–207.

5
Postpartum thyroiditis

J. H. LAZARUS, L. D. K. E. PREMAWARDHANA and A. B. PARKES

In 1948 H.E.W. Roberton, a general practitioner in New Zealand, described the occurrence of lassitude and other symptoms of hypothyroidism relating to the postpartum period [1]. These complaints were treated successfully with thyroid extract. The syndrome remained generally unrecognized until the 1970s, when reports from Japan [2] and Canada [3] rediscovered the existence of postpartum thyroid disease (PPTD) and recognized the immune nature of the condition. A number of reviews of the condition are available [4–7].

CLINICAL FEATURES

Postpartum thyroiditis is characterized by the development of transient thyrotoxicosis and/or hypothyroidism during the first 6 months of the postpartum period. Hypothyroidism is permanent in up to 25–30% of women.

Prevalence

A variable prevalence (from 3 to 17%) has been reported worldwide because of wide variations in the number of women studied, the frequency of thyroid assessment postpartum, diagnostic criteria employed and differences in hormone assay methodology [8–13]. However, there is a general consensus that the disease occurs in 5–9% of unselected postpartum women [6,14]. Recent studies have emphasized that women with type I diabetes have a three-fold incidence of PPT over non-diabetics [15]. In these cases there is a strong association with thyroid antibodies. PPT is also more likely to occur in a woman who has had a previous episode, as discussed below.

A.P. Weetman (ed.), Endocrine Autoimmunity and Associated Conditions. 83–97.

Clinical spectrum

Transient thyrotoxicosis presents at about 14 weeks postpartum followed by transient hypothyroidism at a median of 19 weeks. Very occasionally the hypothyroid state is seen before the thyrotoxicosis. PPT is usually associated with the presence of thyroid antibodies. In one series from Wales [16], the condition was not seen in thyroid antibody-negative women. Thyroid peroxidase (TPO) antibodies are normally found, occasionally accompanied by thyroglobulin (TG) antibodies. In less than 5%, TG antibodies are the only marker. PPT occurred in 50% of 152 TPO Ab women (as ascertained at 16 weeks gestation), compared with 239 control women and studied monthly for 12 months postpartum. Of the antibody-positive patients, 19% were thyrotoxic alone, 49% hypothyroid alone and the remaining 32% had thyrotoxicosis followed by hypothyroidism (Figure 5.1). Although the clinical manifestations of the thyrotoxic state are not usually severe in PPT, lack of energy and irritability are particularly prominent even in antibody-positive women who do not develop thyroid dysfunction. In contrast, the symptomatology of the hypothyroid phase may be profound. Many classic hypothyroid symptoms occur before the onset of thyroid hormone reduction and persist following

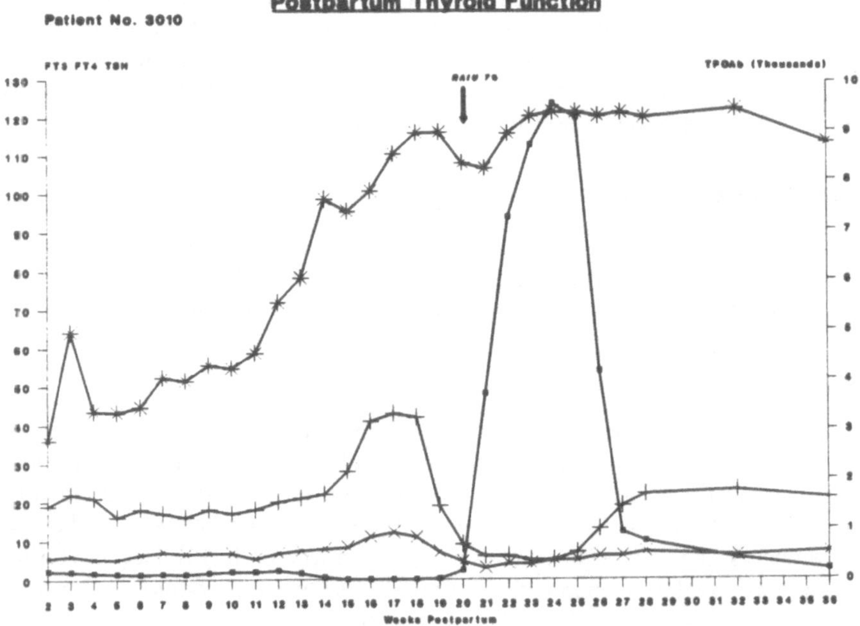

Figure 5.1 Postpartum thyroid dysfunction showing modest transient thyrotoxicosis followed by severe transient hypothyroidism. Blood samples were obtained weekly. Note significant postpartum rise in TPO antibody. RAIU, radioiodine uptake. +, FT4 pmol/L; -×-, FT3 pmol/L; -■-, TSH mU/L; *, TPOAb U/ml

recovery of hormone levels. Early accounts of PPT noted an anecdotal association of depression with thyroid dysfunction in the postpartum period. More recently, depressive symptomatology has been quantitated by Harris *et al.* [17] in a large number of postpartum, TPO antibody-positive women and compared with an age-matched control group of TPO antibody-negative postpartum women. The data clearly show an increase of mild to moderate depression in the antibody-positive women irrespective of thyroid status. Some indication of the excess of depressive symptomatology was seen as early as 6 weeks postpartum. There is no clear explanation for these findings but it is possible that antibodies modulate neurotransmitter function, and it is known that there are cytokine receptors in the brain [18]. The possibility that thyroid antibodies are a marker for a specific genotype related to depression also requires investigation. A large double-blind randomized placebo controlled trial of thyroxine (T_4) 100 μg per day, administered from 6 weeks to 24 weeks in TPO antibody-positive women (as ascertained at 16 weeks gestation), failed to show any significant effect of T_4 on the frequency and severity of depressive symptomatology [19].

Diagnosis

Many changes can occur in thyroid function after pregnancy. In women with a previous history of thyroid dysfunction, such as Graves' disease or Hashimoto's disease, an exacerbation of these conditions may be seen. Postpartum thyroiditis is associated with an immune rebound in women with pre-existing thyroid antibodies. The reason for the dramatic increase in antibody titres is not clear but is presumably related to removal of the so-called immunosuppression observed during normal pregnancy. Thyrotoxicosis in the postpartum period may be due to a recurrence or the development of new Graves' disease or to the thyrotoxic phase of postpartum thyroiditis. Symptoms of thyrotoxicosis are much more evident in Graves' disease. As postpartum hyperthyroidism is a destructive process, radioiodine uptake will be very low at early and late times after isotope administration. TSH receptor antibodies are not seen unless there is co-existing Graves' disease. Thyrotoxicosis due to postpartum thyroiditis is diagnosed by a suppressed TSH together with an elevated free T_4 or free triiodothyronine (T_3), or elevation of free T_4 and free T_3, with either criterion occurring on more than one occasion. In addition Graves' disease should have been excluded, for instance by ^{99m}Tc scanning or measurement of TSH receptor antibodies. If possible a normal range of thyroid hormone concentrations should be derived in the postpartum period as they fall into a narrower range than the general population. Antibodies to T_4 and T_3 may cause confusion in diagnosis but are infrequent and modern assays are less susceptible to such interference [20].

Hypothyroidism in the postpartum period occurs at a median of 19 weeks, but has been observed as late as 36–40 weeks after the birth. The symptoms are often dramatic and may develop before the decrease in thyroid function is noted.

The most frequent symptoms are lack of energy, aches and pains, poor memory, dry skin and cold intolerance. In the authors' series, hypothyroidism is defined as either TSH >3.6 mU/L, together with free T_4 <8 pmol/L or free $T_3 < 4.2$ pmol/L, or TSH 10 mU/L on one or more occasion. The use of thyroid ultrasonography has demonstrated diffuse or multifocal echogenicity, reflecting the abnormal thyroid morphology and consistent with the known lymphocytic infiltration of the thyroid [21] (see Figure 5.2). The destructive nature of the thyroiditis is also shown by the increase in urinary iodine excretion in the thyrotoxic as well as the hypothyroid phase of the syndrome [22]. There is also evidence that an early rise in serum TG (a further indicator of thyroid destruction) may help in the identification of those women at risk of PPT [23].

Follow up and course of the syndrome

While the thyrotoxicosis of PPT always resolves, several long term studies of the hypothyroid phase have documented persistence in 20–30% of cases [24]. The immunological associations of this are discussed below but a recently completed 9-year follow-up assessment of TPO antibody-positive women (at 16 weeks

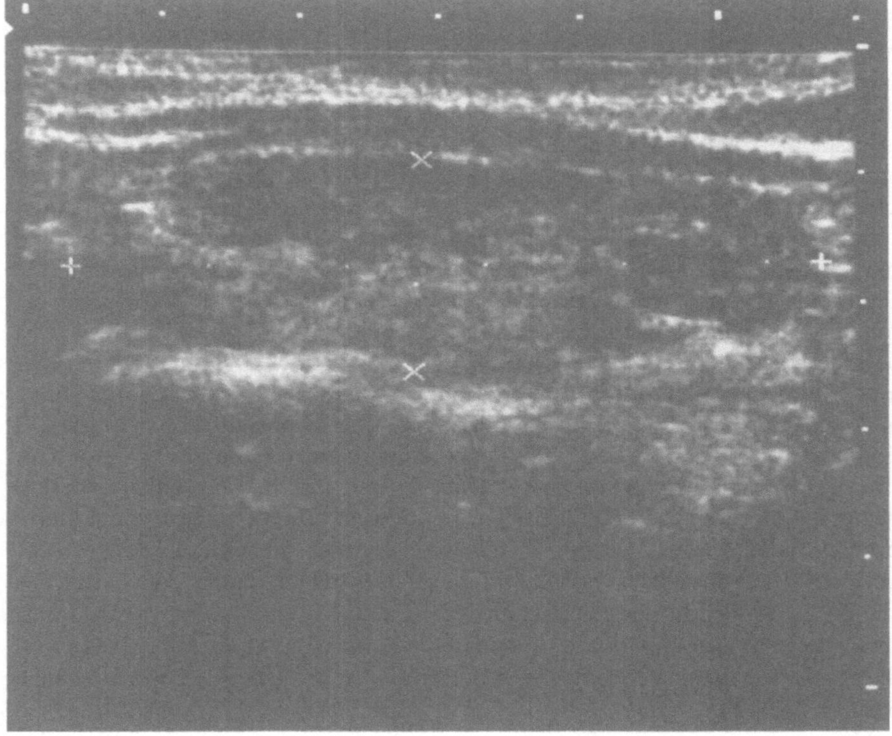

Figure 5.2 Ultrasound of thyroid gland from a patient with postpartum thyroid dysfunction showing hypoechogenicity, consistent with destructive thyroiditis

gestation) showed that the rate of development of hypothyroidism was significantly greater (48% versus 8%) in those who had had PPT than in those who were euthyroid but TPO antibody-positive [25]. Recurrence of transient PPT has been observed in small numbers of patients [26], while a recurrence rate of 30–40% was noted in larger series [27]. In one large group of women, extensively studied in two pregnancies, there was a 70% chance of developing recurrent PPT after a first attack and a 25% risk even if the woman was only TPO antibody-positive without thyroid dysfunction during the first postpartum period [28].

IMMUNOLOGY OF PPT

There is abundant evidence that PPT is an immunologically mediated disease [29]. Biopsy of the thyroid in this syndrome shows lymphocytic infiltration similar to that seen in Hashimoto's thyroiditis [30]. Other aspects of the autoimmune nature of the condition are considered below.

Thyroid antibodies

Amino *et al.* [2] first documented the association of postpartum thyroiditis with high titres of thyroid antibodies, and the dramatic rise of microsomal (TPO) antibody titre after delivery was clearly shown in the study of Fung *et al.* [11] (Figure 5.3). Furthermore, gestation and the postpartum period are characterized by fluctuations in the immune response, and the postpartum increase in thyroid antibodies appears to be a reflection of a general enhancement of immunoglobulin synthesis. Interestingly, the pattern of transient antibody increase in microsomal antibody levels was also observed for serum total IgG and IgG isotype levels but not for IgM, IgA or IgE, or indeed for antibodies against viral and bacterial antigens [31]. Analysis of the IgG subclass distribution in postpartum thyroiditis showed that microsomal antibodies were associated with IgG_1 or IgG_4 subclass, with only minor contributions from IgG_2 and IgG_3 [32]. However, Hall *et al.* [33] showed a significant elevation in the levels of IgG_2 and IgG_3 subclass microsomal antibodies in women who developed biphasic thyroid dysfunction, the elevation of IgG_3 coinciding with the period of thyrotoxicosis. More recently, a study using an ELISA for IgG subclass-associated microsomal antibody activity calibrated against an external reference standard [34] showed a four-fold increase in IgG_1 activity in the PPT group over 12 months postpartum, IgG_3 being low during this time and IgG_4 constant. IgG_2 was also elevated. In contrast, no variation in IgG subclass-associated microsomal antibody activity was found between TPO antibody-positive euthyroid women and women with PPT, during the postpartum year in another study [35].

Clearly the application of varying methodologies to the measurement of IgG subclass distribution has contributed to these results. The rapid perturbation of the immune system in the postpartum year contrasts with the relatively stable

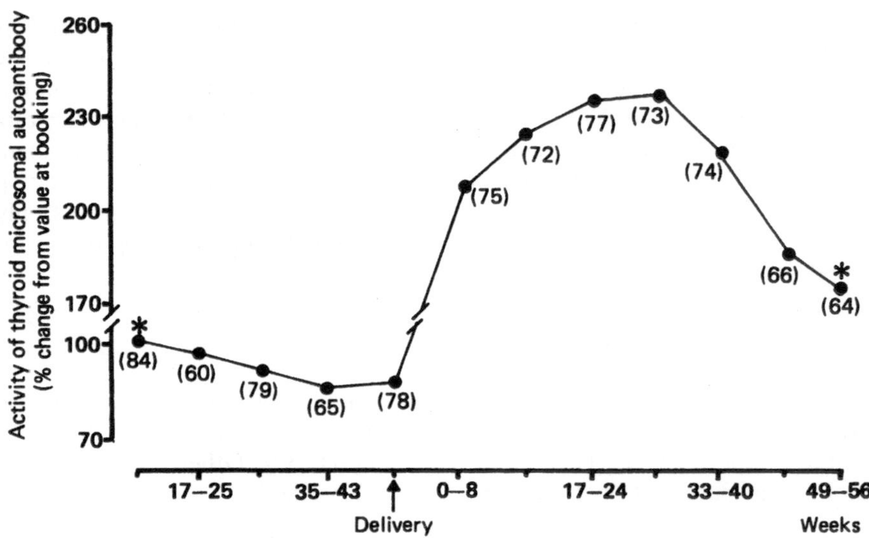

Figure 5.3 Mean titres of microsomal (TPO) antibody during pregnancy and during the postpartum period in a group of women studied prospectively from 16 weeks gestation. Number of women in brackets. Antibody titres are compared to the initial ones set at 100%. (From Fung *et al.*, 1988 with permission.)

situation seen in chronic Hashimoto's thyroiditis (see Chapter 3). It is therefore noteworthy that, using a technique of epitopic profiling of TPO antibodies (epitopic fingerprinting), fingerprint constancy occurred regardless of fluctuations in antibody levels [36] (Figure 5.4). Thus, despite marked variations in TPO epitopic profiles among different individuals, the temporal constancy suggests inheritance of the fingerprint of this antibody. Although the antibody response is dramatic, its precise role in the immunopathogenesis of the condition remains to be determined. Most probably, the antibody titre is merely a marker of disease and the immunological damage is mediated by lymphocyte- and complement-mediated mechanisms, discussed below.

Complement

The strong association between thyroid antibodies and the development of PPT is clear [8,9,11,13,37,38] and, in our experience, PPT does not occur in women in the absence of elevated thyroid antibodies at any time during the postpartum year. However, only around 50% of TPO antibody-positive women become symptomatic. Studies on antibody functional affinity [35] and IgG subclass distribution [34] in PPT suggest that, as in other autoimmune diseases, activation of the complement system may have a role in pathogenesis.

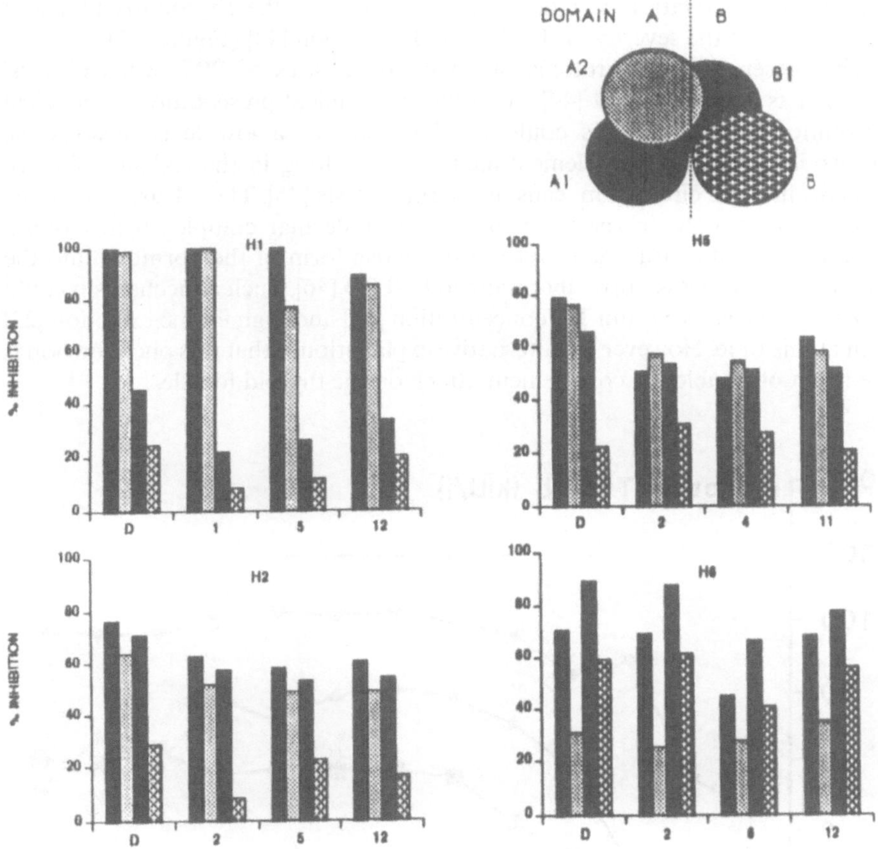

Figure 5.4 TPO antibody epitopic profiles (fingerprints) in four women (H1, H2, H5, H6) who developed postpartum thyroid dysfunction. Sera were characterized at delivery (D) and at the indicated months after delivery. Four immunoglobulin Fab fragments, reactive with the A1, A2, B1 and B2 domains in the immunodominant region as TPO (shown on the right), were used to compete for serum TPO antibody binding to [^{125}I]TPO. Percentage inhibition by each Fab fragment is shown by a bar with shading corresponding to the diagram of the TPO domains on the right. (Adapted from Jaume *et al.*, 1995 with permission.)

To quantify the interaction of the complement system with thyroid antigen/autoantibody complexes, we have developed two assay techniques, one based on the haemolysis of sheep erythrocytes in the presence of excess complement [39] and, the other an ELISA for the quantitation of complement C3b, immobilized as a result of classical complement pathway activation [40]. Applying these techniques to the study of PPT, we have shown that not only is there activation of the complement system by thyroid-directed autoantibodies [41], but also that complement activation is related to the extent of the thyroiditis [42] and correlates with the severity of the thyroid dysfunction [43] (Figure 5.5).

The presence of a thyrotoxic phase in some cases of PPT, when Graves' disease has been ruled out [44], is an unusual clinical presentation of classical Hashimoto's disease. This could be the result of a low level, destructive mechanism, possibly complement-mediated, resulting in the leakage of iodoproteins into the circulation, causing thyrotoxicosis [45]. The released hormone would, however, be in the form of a macromolecular complex which would require enzymatic cleavage to release the active form of the hormone into the circulation, a process normally catalysed by TPO [46]. Such a mechanism could explain the elevated serum TG concentration [23] and high iodine excretion [22] seen at this time. However, an alternative explanation is that this phenomenon is the result of a sublethal complement attack on the thyroid follicle.

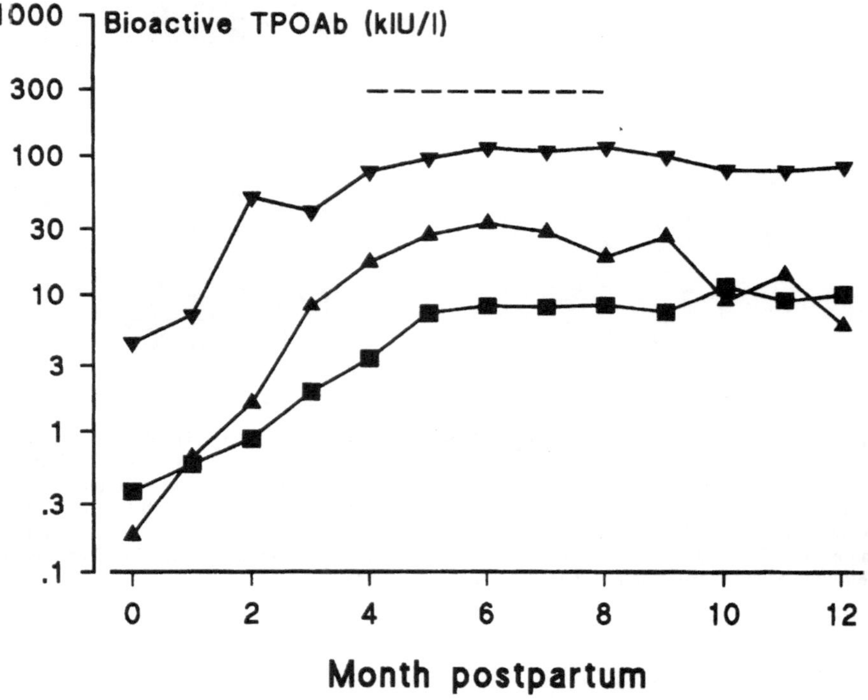

Figure 5.5 Mean serum bioactive TPO antibody activity in TPO antibody-positive postpartum women. ■, 75 women, euthyroid for whole period; ▲, 44 women with transient thyroid dysfunction during the year; ▼, 29 women with persistent thyroid dysfunction. The dotted line at the top shows the time period during which antibody levels in the transient dysfunction group were significantly higher ($p < 0.05$) than euthyroid group. In the persistent dysfunction group, significantly higher TPO antibody levels were observed at all time points. (Adapted from Parkes *et al.* [41] with permission.)

Antibody-directed complement attack on nucleated cells can result in two quite distinct pathophysiological mechanisms [47]. Under the influence of a sublethal complement attack the metabolic activity of cells is increased via a number of mechanisms, including a rapid rise in both intracellular Ca^{2+} ions [48] and cAMP [49]. In the thyroid cell these metabolic changes would mimic the action of TSH [50] leading to the up-regulation of TPO [51] and secretion of thyroid hormones into the circulation with a consequent thyrotoxicosis. However, in this situation one might expect to see an increase in radioiodine uptake (i.e. true hyperthyroidism) which is not seen in PPT. Should the complement-mediated attack be more severe, destruction of thyroid follicular architecture would ensue with a resulting loss of thyroid function, leading eventually to hypothyroidism. As the degree of complement activation increases the transient hyperthyroid phase of the PPT could be missing altogether, the resulting PPT being characterized by hypothyroidism alone. In the most severe cases, damage to thyroid follicular architecture could be extensive and terminal, resulting in a persistent Hashimoto-like hypothyroidism.

In other forms of autoimmune thyroid disease where complement activation has been suspected, it has been possible to measure elevated levels of the C5–C9 membrane attack complex (MAC) in patient serum [52]. However, despite an exhaustive search, we have been unable to detect elevated MAC levels in serum samples from postpartum women who subsequently developed PPT [53].

T cell function

During pregnancy, maternal immune reactions are regulated to prevent rejection of the fetal allograft [54]. Both humoral and cell-mediated immunity have been reported to be depressed during pregnancy. Specifically, the $CD4^+$ T cell population was found to be decreased during pregnancy by some workers [55–57], but these data were not replicated by others [58–60]. More recently, a prospective study of lymphocyte subpopulations in TPO antibody-positive pregnant women and antibody-negative controls showed a significant fall in the $CD4^+/CD8^+$ ratio in late pregnancy and into the postpartum period in the controls [61]. In contrast, women who subsequently developed PPT had a significantly higher $CD4^+/CD8^+$ ratio and T cell activtion than in normal TPO antibody-negative women. In addition, $CD45RA^+$ T cells were also significantly elevated in those women destined to develop PPT, and it is possible that this subset serves as a marker in this respect. Thus, both humoral and cellular immune reactions are involved in the development of PPT but the exact role of the alterations in different T cell subsets requires further clarification.

Immunogenetics

A possible role for HLA antigens in the pathology of autoimmune thyroid disease, and PPT in particular, has been postulated for some time (see Chapters 3 and 4). Initially, no association between HLA-A or -B phenotypes and PPT could be found [62]. However, Tachi *et al.* [63] reported a higher frequency of HLA-A26, -Bw46 and -Bw67, together with a significantly lower frequency of HLA-Bw62 and -Cw7 in women with postpartum hypothyroidism. Later, an increased frequency of HLA-A1 and -B8 in women with this condition was reported [64].

Several HLA class II specificities have also been associated with PPT, in particular HLA-DR3, DR4 and DR5 [65]. Farid *et al.* [66] reported an increased frequency of HLA-DR3 and DR5, and later, DR4 [67] in women with transient hypothyroid PPT. Higher frequencies of DR4 in women with PPT have also been observed [68,69]. Other groups [70,71] have shown a relatively strong association with DR5, confirmed by our own studies [72]. However, an earlier study in Wales [64] identified an association between PPT and DR3. Both studies, however, found a negative association between PPT and HLA-DR2. Tachi *et al.* [63] also reported a negative association between PPT and HLA-DR2, together with an increased frequency of DR3. The frequency of HLA-DQ7 is also raised in PPT and this is likely to be a consequence of the increase in DR5, since both DR11 and DR12 are in linkage disequilibrium with DQ7 [72].

Based on an interpretation of these HLA-DR frequencies, it was suggested that PPT is an early manifestation of Hashimoto's thyroiditis [70]. This seems plausible as Hashimoto's thyroiditis has variously been associated with an increased frequency of HLA-DR3, DR4 and/or DR5, an increased frequency of HLA-DQ7 and a negative association with HLA-DR2 [66,73–78] and is in accord with our own hypothesis, based on clinical and laboratory findings, that PPT and Hashimoto's thyroiditis share a common aetiology [24]. A positive association between an HLA specificity and disease pathology is generally interpreted in one of two ways. Firstly, it may indicate that the disease locus is in linkage disequilibrium with the HLA locus. When interpreted in this way, the data reported by ourselves [72] and others [63,64,66–71] are relatively weak but do not exclude this possibility. Alternatively, the HLA specificity itself may have a direct role in disease process. A complex antigen will produce a number of epitopes when processed within antigen-presenting cells and not all these will be physically compatible with the peptide groove of particular HLA molecules. Thus, the polymorphic forms of the HLA molecules may be one factor influencing the ability of an antigen-presenting cell to present a particular species of antigenic peptide and so modulate disease susceptibility. This may be of particular importance in autoimmune thyroid disease where, despite the large number of potentially antigenic peptide sequences within the three known protein antigens, only a very restricted set of antigenic epitopes are known to exist [80,81].

The class III area of the HLA complex encodes several proteins which are important in the pathogenesis of autoimmune disease (especially tumour necrosis factor-α, heat shock protein 70 and complement). We have measured the allotype frequency of three complement proteins, Bf, C4A and C4B, and found significant differences in their overall frequency distribution in women with PPT. These findings are similar to those reported by Ratanachaiavong *et al.*

[82] in Graves' disease, an autoimmune thyroid disease which is also associated with an increased frequency of HLA-DR3. This may indicate linkage disequilibrium with candidate genes in the class III region, bue could equally be interpreted on a functional basis, as the pathogenesis of PPT is known to be linked to activtaion of the complement system [41,43].

RECENT DEVELOPMENTS

An intriguing study reported by Pop *et al.* [83] compared a number of developmental variables in a group of children born to mothers with TPO antibodies measured at 32 weeks of pregnancy and compared these with a large number of children whose mothers had no thyroid antibodies during gestation. A significant decrement in IQ (10 points) was found at age 9 in the children of antibody-positive mothers, after allowing for confounding factors. The reason why maternal antibodies may be related to subsequent mental impairment is not clear and these important findings require confirmation. A possible explanation may be the existence of low or low/normal maternal T_4 concentrations in early pregnancy.

These data add strength to previous suggestions by ourselves [16] and others [6,84,85] that there is a strong case for routine screening for thyroid antibodies in early pregnancy in all women.

References

1. Roberton HEW. Lassitude, coldness, and hair changes following pregnancy, and their response to treatment with thyroid extract. Br Med J. 1948;2:93–4.
2. Amino N, Miyai KJ, Onishi T et al. Transient hypothyroidism after delivery in autoimmune thyroiditis. J Clin Endocrinol Metab. 1976;42:296–301.
3. Ginsberg J, Walfish PG. Postpartum transient thyrotoxicosis with painless thyroiditis. Lancet. 1977;1:1125–8.
4. Amino N, Iwatani Y, Tamaki H, Mori H, Aozasa M, Miyai K. Postpartum autoimmune thyroid syndromes. In: Walfish PG, Wall JR, Volpé R, eds. Autoimmunity and the Thyroid. London: Academic Press; 1985:289–314.
5. Stagnaro-Green A. Postpartum thyroiditis: prevalence, etiology and clinical implications. Thyroid Today. 1993;16:1–11.
6. Hall R. Pregnancy and autoimmune endocrine disease. Baillière's Clin Endocrinol Metab. 1995;9:137–55.
7. Smallridge RC. Postpartum thyroid dysfunction: a frequently undiagnosed endocrine disorder. Endocrinologist. 1996;6:44–50.
8. Amino N, Mori H, Iwantani Y et al. High prevalence of transient post-partum thyrotoxicosis and hypothyroidism. N Engl J Med. 1982;306:849–52.
9. Jansson R, Bernander S, Karlsson A, Levin KK, Nilsson G. Autoimmune thyroid dysfunction in the postpartum period. J Clin Endocrinol Metab. 1984;58:681-7.
10. Nikolai TF, Turney SL, Roberts RC. Postpartum lymphocytic thyroiditis. Arch Intern Med. 1987;147:221–4.
11. Fung HYM, Kologlu M, Collison K et al. Postpartum thyroid dysfunction in Mid Glamorgan. Br Med J. 1988;296:241–4.
12. Rajatanavin R, La-or C, Tirarungsikul K, Chalayondeja W, Jittivanich U, Puapradit W. Postpartum thyroid dysfunction in Bangkok: a geographical variation in the prevalence. Acta Endocrinol. 1990;122:283–7.

13. Walfish PG, Meyerson J, Provias JP, Vargas MT, Papsin FR. Prevalence and characteristics of post-partum thyroid dysfunction: results of a survey from Toronto, Canada. J Endocrinol Invest. 1992;15:265–72.
14. Gerstein HC. How common is postpartum thyroiditis? A methodologic overview of the literature. Arch Intern Med. 1990;150:1397–400.
15. Weetman AP. Insulin-dependent diabetes mellitus and postpartum thyroiditis: an important association. J Clin Endocrinol Metab. 1994;79:7–9.
16. Lazarus JH, Hall R, Othman S et al. The clinical spectrum of postpartum thyroid disease. Q J Med. 1996;89:429–35.
17. Harris B, Othman S, Davies J et al. Association between postpartum thyroid dysfunction and thyroid antibodies and depression. Br Med J. 1992;305:152–6.
18. Cunningham ET, Souza EB. Interleukin 1 receptors in the brain and endocrine tissues. Immunol Today. 1993;14:171–6.
19. Lazarus JH, Harris B, Parkes AB. Depression and postpartum thyroid disease [PPTD] – A clinical enigma. Proceedings of the First National Congress of Neuroendocrinology, Sept 27–28, 1996, Bucharest. Bucharest: Romanian Psychoneuroendocrine Society, in press.
20. John R, Othman S, Parkes AB, Lazarus JH, Hall R. Interference in thyroid function tests in postpartum thyroiditis. Clin Chem. 1991;37:1397-400.
21. Adams H, Jones MC, Othman S et al. The sonographic appearances in postpartum thyroiditis. Clin Radiol. 1992;45:311–18.
22. Othman S, Phillips DIW, Lazarus JH, Parkes AB, Richards C, Hall R. Iodine metabolism in postpartum thyroiditis. Thyroid. 1992;2:107–11.
23. Parkes AB, Black EG, Adams H et al. Serum thyroglobulin – an early indicator of autoimmune postpartum thyroid disease. Clin Endocrinol. 1994;41:9–14.
24. Othman S, Phillips DIW, Parkes AB et al. A long-term follow-up of postpartum thyroiditis. Clin Endocrinol. 1990;32:559–64.
25. Premawardhana LDKE, Lazarus JH, Adams H, Parkes AB. Abnormalities of thyroid function and morphology 7–10 years after postpartum thyroid dysfunction [PPTD]. J Endocrinol Invest. 1996;19:74.
26. Amino N, Miyai K, Kuro P et al. Transient postpartum hypothyroidism: fourteen cases with autoimmune thyroiditis. Ann Intern Med. 1977;87:155–9.
27. Dahlberg PA, Jansson R. Different aetiologies in post-partum thyroiditis. Acta Endocrinol. 1983;104:195–200.
28. Lazarus JH, Ammari F, Oretti R, Parkes AB, Richards CJ, Harris B. Clinical aspects of recurrent postpartum thyroiditis. J Roy Coll Gen Pract. 1997;47:305–8.
29. Weetman AP, McGregor AM. Autoimmune thyroid disease: further developments in our understanding. Endocr Rev. 1994;15:788–830.
30. Mizukami Y, Michigishi T, Nonomura A et al. Postpartum thyroiditis – a clinical, histologic and immunologic study of 15 cases. Am J Clin Pathol. 1993;100:200–5.
31. Jansson R, Karlsson FA, Linde A, Sjoberg O. Postpartum activation of autoimmunity: transient increase of total IgG levels in normal women and in women with autoimmune thyroiditis. Clin Exp Immunol. 1987;70:68–73.
32. Jansson R, Thompson PM, Clark F, McLachlan SM. Association between thyroid microsomal antibodies of subclass IgG-1 and hypothyroidism in autoimmune postpartum thyroiditis. Clin Exp Immunol. 1986;63:80–6.
33. Hall R, Fung M, Kologlu M et al. Postpartum thyroid dysfunction. In: Pinchera A, Ingbar SH, McKenzie JM, Fenzi GF, eds. Thyroid Autoimmunity. New York: Plenum Press; 1987: 211–19.
34. Briones-Urbina R, Parkes AB, Bogner U, Mariotti S, Walfish PG. Increase in antimicrosomal antibody related IgG1, IgG2 and IgG3 and titres of antithyroid peroxidase antibodies, but not antibody dependent cell mediated cytotoxicity in post-partum thyroiditis with transient hyperthyroidism. J Endocrinol Invest. 1990;13:879–86.
35. Weetman AP, Fung HYM, Richards CJ, McGregor AM. IgG subclass distribution and relative functional affinity of thyroid microsomal antibodies in postpartum thyroiditis. Eur J Clin Invest. 1990;20:133–6.
36. Jaume JC, Parkes AB, Lazarus JH et al. Thyroid peroxidase autoantibody fingerprints. II. A longitudinal study in postpartum thyroiditis. J Clin Endocrinol Metab. 1995;80:1000–5.
37. Lervang HH, Pryds O, Kristensen HPO. Thyroid dysfunction after delivery: incidence and clinical course. Acta Med Scand. 1987;222:369–74.

38. Bech K, Hertel J, Rasmussen NG et al. Effect of maternal thyroid autoantibodies and postpartum thyroiditis on the fetus and neonate. Acta Endocrinol. 1991;125:146–9.
39. Parkes AB, Williams S, Howells RD et al. The measurement of complement fixation by autoantibodies directed against thyroid membrane antigens. J Clin Lab Immunol. 1991;35:1–7.
40. Parkes AB, Harris R, Williams S, Lazarus JH, Waters JS. An ELISA for the measurement of complement C3 activation by autoantibodies directed against thyroid membrane antigens. J Clin Lab Immunol. 1991;35:139–45.
41. Parkes AB, Othman S, Hall R, John R, Richards CJ, Lazarus JH. The role of complement in the pathogenesis of postpartum thyroiditis. J Clin Endocrinol Metab. 1994;79:395–400.
42. Parkes AB, Adams H, Othman S, Hall R, John R, Lazarus JH. The role of complement in the pathogenesis of postpartum thyroiditis. Ultrasound echogenicity and the degree of complement induced thyroid damage. Thyroid. 1996;6:169–74.
43. Parkes AB, Othman S, Hall R, John R, Lazarus JH. The role of complement in the pathogenesis of postpartum thyroiditis: relationship between complement activation and disease presentation and progression. Eur J Endocrinol. 1995;133:210–15.
44. Hidaka Y, Tamaki H, Iwatani Y, Tada H, Mitsuda N, Amino N. Prediction of post-partum Graves' thyrotoxicosis by measurement of thyroid stimulating antibody in early pregnancy. Clin Endocrinol. 1994;41:15–20.
45. LiVolsi VA. Postpartum thyroiditis – the pathology slowly unravels. Am J Clin Pathol. 1993; 100:193–5.
46. Nunez J, Pommier J. Formation of thyroid hormones. Vit Horm. 1982;39:175–229.
47. Morgan BP. Complement membrane attack on nucleated cells: resistance, recovery and non-lethal effects. Biochem J. 1989;264:1–14.
48. Morgan BP, Campbell AK. The recovery of human polymorphonuclear leucocytes from sublytic complement attack is mediated by intracellular calcium. Biochem J. 1985;231:205–8.
49. Carney DF, Shin ML. Multiple signals are generated by terminal complement complexes (TCC) to stimulate the elimination of TCC from the surface of nucleated cells (NC). Complement. 1987;4:140.
50. Bastomsky CH, McKenzie JM. Cyclic AMP: a mediator of thyroid stimulation by thyrotropin. Am J Physiol. 1967;213:753–8.
51. Mower J, Rickards CR, Parkes AB, Wynford Thomas D. Thyroid peroxidase expression in the transformed thyroid cell line 'HTORI3' is TSH and cyclic AMP dependent. J Endocrinol Invest. 1992;15:101.
52. Watts M, Dankest JR, Morgan BP. Isolation and characterisation of a membrane-attack complex-inhibiting protein present in human serum and other biological fluids. Biochem J. 1990;265:471–7.
53. McCullough B, Hall R, Morgan BP, Parkes AB, Lazarus JH. Lack of terminal complement component in postpartum thyroiditis (PPT) – a possible explanation for transient disease. J Endocrinol. 1994;140:251.
54. Gleicher N, Deppe G, Cohen CJ. Common aspects of immunologic tolerance in pregnancy and malignancy. Obstet Gynecol. 1979;54:335–42.
55. Sridama V, Pacini F, Yang SL, Moawad A, Reilly M, DeGroot LJ. Decreased levels of helper T-cells: a possible cause of immunodeficiency in pregnancy. N Engl J Med. 1982;307:352–6.
56. Barnett MA, Learmonth RP, Pihl E, Wood EC. T helper lymphocyte depression in early pregnancy. J Reprod Immunol. 1983;5:55–7.
57. Iwatani Y, Amino N, Tachi J et al. Changes of lymphocyte subsets in normal pregnant and postpartum women: postpartum increase of NK/K (Leu 7) cells. Am J Reprod Immunol. 1988;18:52–5.
58. Moore MP, Carter NP, Redman CWG. Lymphocyte subsets defined by monoclonal antibodies in human pregnancy. Am J Reprod Immunol. 1983;3:161–4.
59. Luciuero G, Seluaggi L, Dell'Osso A. Mononuclear cell subpopulations during normal pregnancy: analysis of cell surface markers using conventional techniques and monoclonal antibodies. Am J Reprod Immunol. 1993;4:142–5.
60. Cheney RT, Tomaszewski JE, Raab SJ, Zmijewski C, Rowlands DT. Subpopulations of lymphocytes in maternal peripheral blood during pregnancy. J Reprod Immunol. 1984;6: 111–20.
61. Stagnaro-Green A, Roman H, Cobin RH, El-Harazy E, Wallenstein S, Davies TF. Prospective study of lymphocyte-initiated immunosuppression in normal pregnancy: evi-

dence of a T-cell etiology for postpartum thyroid dysfunction. J Clin Endocrinol Metab. 1992;74:645–53.
62. Jenkins H, Farid NR. Subacute thyroiditis like syndromes in relation to HLA. Tissue Antigens. 1979;13:167–9.
63. Tachi J, Amino N, Tamaki H, Aozaso M, Iwatani Y, Miyai K. Long term follow-up and HLA association in patients with postpartum hypothyroidism. J Clin Endocrinol Metab. 1988;66: 480–4.
64. Kologlu M, Fung H, Darke C, Richards CJ, Hall R, McGregor AM. Postpartum thyroid dysfunction and HLA status. Eur J Clin Invest. 1990;20:56–60.
65. Roman SH, Greenberg D, Rubenstein P, Wallenstein S, Davies TF. Genetics of autoimmune thyroid disease: lack of evidence for linkage to HLA within families. J Clin Endocrinol Metab. 1992;74:496–503.
66. Farid NR, Hawe BS, Walfish PG. Increased frequency of HLA-DR3 and 5 in the syndromes of painless thyroiditis with transient thyrotoxicosis: evidence for an autoimmune etiology. Clin Endocrinol. 1983;19:699–704.
67. Thompson P, Farid NR. Post-partum thyroiditis and goitrous (Hashimoto's) thyroiditis are associated with HLA-DR4. Immunol Lett. 1985;11:301–3.
68. Lervang HH, Pryds O, Kristensen HPO, Jakobsen BK, Svejgaard A. Post-partum autoimmune thyroid disorder associated with HLA-DR4? Tissue Antigens. 1984;23:2500–2.
69. Jansson R, Safwenberg J, Dahlberg PA. Influence of the HLA-DR4 antigen and iodine status on the development of autoimmune postpartum thyroiditis. J Clin Endocrinol Metab. 1985; 60:168–73.
70. Pryds O, Lervang H-H, Ostergaard Kristensen HP, Jakobsen BK, Svejgaard A. HLA-DR factors associated with postpartum hypothyroidism: an early manifestation of Hashimoto's thyroiditis? Tissue Antigens. 1987;30:34–7.
71. Vargas MT, Briones-Urbina R, Gladman D, Papsin FR, Walfish PG. Antithyroid microsomal autoantibodies and HLA-DR5 are associated with postpartum thyroid dysfunction: evidence supporting an autoimmune pathogenesis. J Clin Endocrinol Metab. 1988;67:327–33.
72. Parkes AB, Darke C, Othman S et al. MHC class II and complement polymorphism in postpartum thyroiditis. Eur J Endocrinol. 1996;134:449–53.
73. Weissel M, Hofer R, Zasmeta H, Mayr WR. HLA-DR and Hashimoto's thyroiditis. Tissue Antigens. 1980;16:256–7.
74. Farid NR, Sampson I, Moens H, Barnard LM. The association of goitrous autoimmune thyroiditis with HLA-DR5. Tissue Antigens. 1981;17:265–8.
75. Sakurami T, Ueno Y, Iwaki Y et al. HLA-DR specificities among Japanese with several autoimmune diseases. Tissue Antigens. 1982;19:129–33.
76. Svejgaard A, Platz P, Ryder LP. HLA and disease susceptibility: clinical implications. Clin Immunol Rev. 1994;4:567–80.
77. Stenszky V, Balazs C, Kraszits E et al. Association of goitrous autoimmune thyroiditis with HLA-DR3 in eastern Hungary. J Immunogen. 1987;14:143–8.
78. Badenhoop K, Schwarz G, Walfish PG, Drummond V, Usadel KH, Bottazzo GF. Susceptibility to thyroid autoimmune disease: molecular markers for goitrous Hashimoto's thyroiditis. J Clin Endocrinol Metab. 1990;71:1131–7.
79. Tandon N, Zhang L, Weetman AP. HLA associations with Hashimoto's thyroiditis. Clin Endocrinol. 1991;34:383–6.
80. Fukuma N, McLachlan SM, Petersen VB et al. Human thyroglobulin autoantibodies of subclass IgG2 and IgG4 bind to different epitopes on thyroglobulin. Immunology. 1989;67: 129–31.
81. Chazenbalk GD, Portolano S, Russo D, Hutchinson JS, Rapoport B, McLachlan S. Human organ-specific autoimmune disease. Molecular cloning and expression of an autoantibody gene repertoire for a major autoantigen reveals an antigenic immunodominant region and restricted immunoglobulin gene usage in the target organ. J Clin Invest. 1993;92:62–74.
82. Ratanachaiavong S, Demaine AG, Campbell RD, McGregor AM. Heat shock protein 70 (HSP70) and complement C4 genotypes in patients with hyperthyroid Graves' disease. Clin Exp Immunol. 1991;84:48–52.
83. Pop VJ, de Vries E, van Baar AL et al. Maternal thyroid peroxidase antibodies during pregnancy: a marker of impaired child development. J Clin Endocrinol Metab. 1995;80: 3561–6.

84. Hayslip CC, Fein HG, O'Donnell VM, Friedman DS, Klein TA, Smallridge RC. The value of serum antimicrosomal antibody testing in screening for symptomatic postpartum thyroid dysfunction. Am J Obstet Gynecol. 1988;159:203–9.
85. Solomon BL, Fein HG, Smallridge RC. Usefulness of antimicrosomal antibody titers in the diagnosis and treatment of postpartum thyroiditis. J Fam Pract. 1993;36:177–82.

[illegible]

[illegible]

6
Thyroid-associated ophthalmopathy

R. M. CUDDIHY AND R. S. BAHN

CLINICAL FEATURES

Graves' disease (GD) is an autoimmune disease in which autoantibodies directed against the thyrotropin receptor (TSHR) are produced. Interaction of these stimulatory antibodies with the TSHR on thyrocytes results in hyperthyroidism (Chapter 4). Thyroid-associated ophthalmopathy (TAO) is the eye disease that commonly accompanies GD. Approximately 20–25% of patients with Graves' hyperthyroidism have clinically evident TAO [1]. However, subtle ocular involvement can be demonstrated in the vast majority of patients when sensitive imaging techniques such as orbital ultrasonography are used [2]. Conversely, although approximately 10% of patients with TAO have the characteristic eye changes without current or past evidence of hyperthyroidism ('euthyroid ophthalmopathy'), the vast majority of these patients have laboratory evidence of autoimmune thyroid disease, including antibodies to thyroid peroxidase or to the TSHR [3]. Finally, there is a close temporal relationship between the onset of hyperthyroidism in GD and the development of clinically significant TAO; eye involvement precedes or follows the onset of TAO by 18 months in 85% of affected individuals [1].

Patients with TAO may describe a 'gritty' sensation in the eyes, sensitivity to light, double vision, increased tearing, visual blurring and an orbital pressure-type discomfort. Physical examination may reveal proptosis (forward protrusion of the eyes), extraocular muscle dysfunction, periorbital and eyelid oedema, conjunctival chemosis (swelling) and injection (redness), lid lag and retraction (or 'stare'), and exposure keratitis (corneal injury due to corneal drying) [4] (Figure 6.1). The majority of clinically affected patients experience only minor signs and symptoms of TAO, including mild chemosis, injection and

A.P. Weetman (ed.), Endocrine Autoimmunity and Associated Conditions. 99–111.

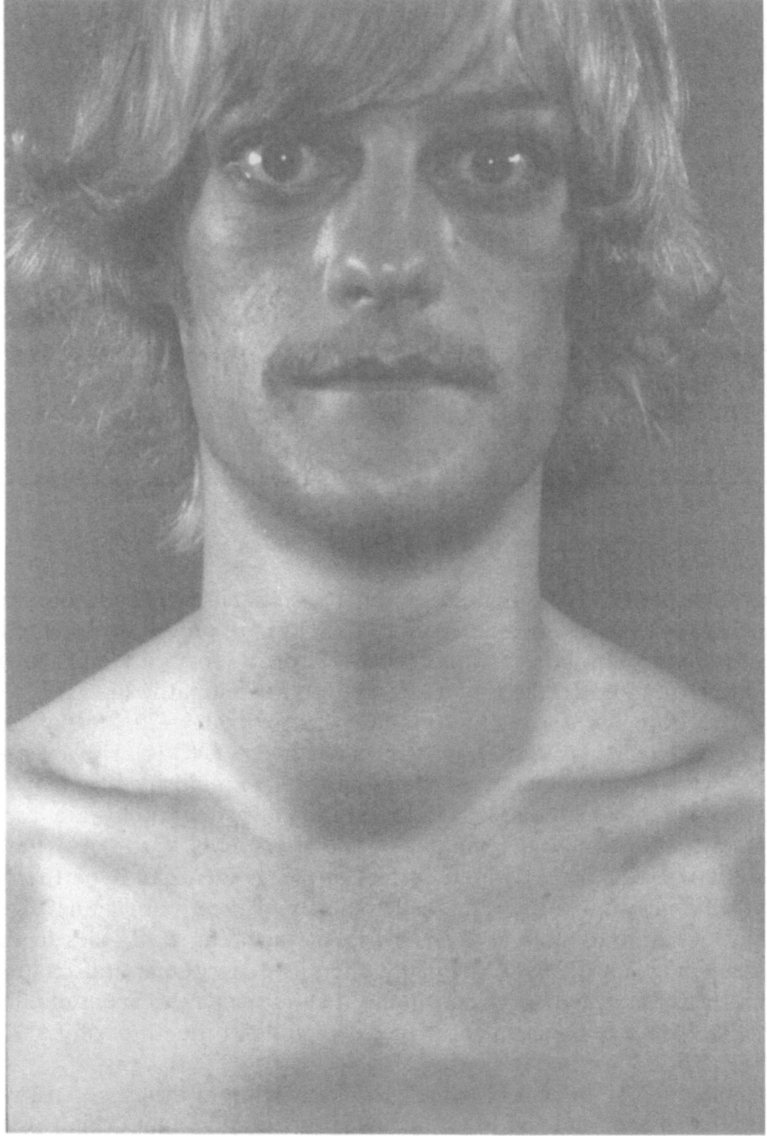

Figure 6.1 Patient with goiter, proptosis and moist, hyperaemic skin

lid oedema, that improve spontaneously within approximately 6–24 months [5]. However, in 10% of patients, the disease progresses for several years from onset and one or more of the symptoms becomes severe. Progression is generally followed by a plateau phase of approximately 1–3 years. Subsequent resolution is gradual and generally incomplete.

Treatment options for symptomatically severe TAO include corticosteroids, orbital radiotherapy and orbital decompression surgery [4]. Double vision may be improved with prisms in spectacle lenses or extraocular muscle surgery may be indicated. Controversy exists concerning whether the form of treatment chosen for Graves' hyperthyroidism (thyroid ablation with radioiodine, anti-thyroid drugs or thyroidectomy) affects the development or worsening of TAO [6]. A well-accepted exacerbating factor for TAO is smoking; there are more smokers among GD patients with TAO than among those without TAO or normal controls [7]. Further, TAO patients who smoke are more likely to have severe eye disease than are non-smokers with TAO. The incidence of GO is highest in women under 50. However, the disease tends to be more severe in men and in patients older than 50 [8], perhaps reflecting the historically higher rate of smoking in men than in women.

Pretibial dermopathy (PTD) is a diffuse or nodular thickening of the skin of the anterior lower leg that is associated with Graves' hyperthyroidism and TAO (Figure 6.2). The characteristic dermal changes occur only rarely on other parts of the body, often following local trauma. PTD is clinically evident in only a small proportion of patients with GD. It occurs primarily in patients with significant TAO, and is preceded in onset by TAO in 78% of cases [9]. Thyroid acropachy is a condition that is seen essentially only in patients who have both TAO and PTD [10]. It is characterized by soft tissue swelling and clubbing of the terminal phalanges with periosteal new bone formation in the hands and feet (Figure 6.3).

HISTOPATHOLOGY

Histological examination of orbital tissues from patients with TAO reveals an accumulation of hydrophilic glycosaminoglycans (GAGs) and oedema within the perimysial connective tissues investing the extraocular muscle cells and within the connective tissue compartments of the orbit [11]. This process produces gross enlargement of the extraocular muscle bodies and swelling of the orbital fatty connective tissue. As a result, the globe is displaced anteriorly (proptosis) and periorbital oedema may arise due to venous obstruction. Histological examination of the extraocular muscle fibres during the acute phase of the disease shows them to be intact; in later stages, the muscles may become fibrotic and atrophic due to chronic inflammation and compression by the surrounding swollen connective tissues [12]. Histological examination of dermal tissues affected by PTD, and of the distal digits in patients with acropachy, reveals a similar pattern of GAG accumulation, oedema and fibrosis [10). In addition to an accumulation of GAGs, orbital tissues from patients with TAO contain an infiltration of activated mononuclear cells. Both $CD4^{+}$ and $CD8^{+}$ T lymphocytes are present, with a slight predominance of the latter [13].

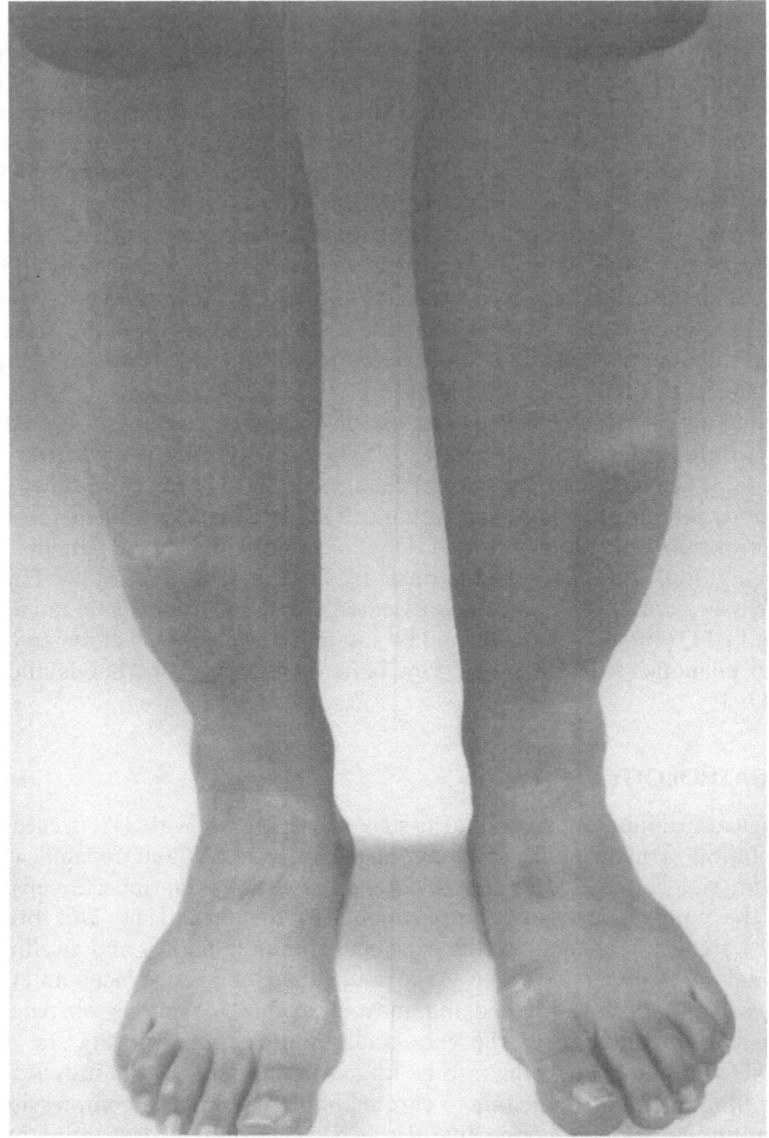

Figure 6.2 Patient with the plaque-like variety of pretibial dermopathy

ROLE OF CYTOKINES

Particular cytokines, including interferon-γ (IFN-γ), tumour necrosis factor-β (TNF-β), and interleukin-1α (IL-1α), are present adjacent to T cell aggregates in

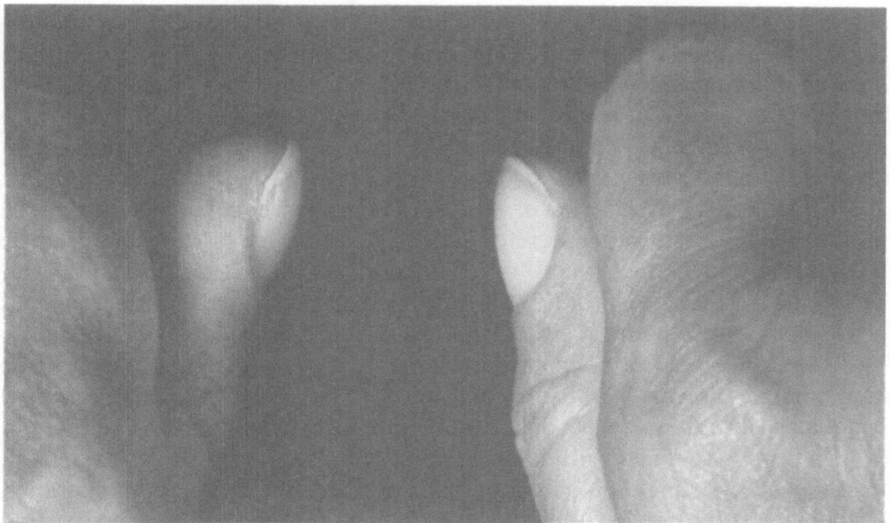

Figure 6.3 Patient with acropachy of the distal phalanges

orbital connective tissues in TAO [14]. These cytokines are produced primarily by the activated lymphocytes and macrophages in the orbit. IFN-γ and IL-1α are potent enhancers of GAG production by cultured orbital fibroblasts and are likely involved in stimulating the accumulation of this substance in affected orbital tissues [15].

Other paracrine effects of cytokines in TAO include stimulation of the expression of certain immunomodulatory proteins on orbital fibroblasts. Among these proteins is a 72 kDa heat shock protein (HSP) that has been shown to be present on the cell surface [16,17]. This protein aids in the protection of cells under stress, but may also play a role in intercellular antigen processing [18]. In addition, human leukocyte antigen (HLA)-DR expression has been demonstrated in endomysial fibroblasts surrounding extraocular muscle fibres and in fibroblasts residing in the orbital fatty connective tissues in TAO [19]. This antigen is normally present on activated cells (including T cells, monocytes, B cells, macrophages and endothelial cells) that are capable of presenting antigens to $CD4^+$ lymphocytes. HLA-DR expression on orbital fibroblasts in TAO is probably stimulated by IFN-γ produced locally by infiltrating lymphocytes. It is possible that orbital fibroblasts are thus able to participate directly in the autoimmune process by functioning as antigen-presenting cells. Adhesion molecules are important receptors for a variety of interactions between immunocompetent cells, connective tissue cells and extra-cellular matrix [20]. Strong immunoreactivity for intercellular adhesion molecule-1 (ICAM-1] is demonstrable on endomysial fibroblasts and throughout the connective tissue in the orbit [21]. ICAM-1 expression can be stimulated *in vitro* on orbital fibroblasts by treatment with IFN-γ, IL-1α or TNF-α [22]. It is likely that these cytokines function similarly *in vivo* and that the resulting ICAM-1 expressed on orbital lymphocytes in TAO acts to aid in the recruitment of activated lymphocytes into the orbit.

The functional classification of helper (CD4$^+$) T lymphocytes is based on the profile of cytokines that are secreted [23]. In general, type I (T_H1] cells produce IFN-γ, IL-2 and TNF-α; type II (T_H2] cells secrete IL-4, IL-5, IL-6 and IL-13. T_H1 cells are involved primarily in cell-mediated responses, while T_H2 cells provide efficient help for B-cell activation and antibody production. In addition, T_H2 cells and their secreted cytokines may play a protective role in some autoimmune diseases [24]. It is of interest that the T_H1 cytokine IFN-γ stimulates fibroblasts to produce GAG and to express immunomodulatory proteins, processes likely to be important in early disease pathology. In contrast, IL-4 (a T_H2 cytokine) is a potent stimulator of orbital fibroblast proliferation [25], a process that may result in the fibrosis of extraocular muscles seen in late-stage disease. It may be that T_H1 cells infiltrate the orbit at the onset of the disease and that the advent of T_H2 cell clones signals the phase of resolution. IL-1, a macrophage product that is also produced by orbital fibroblasts in TAO [14], may be an important mediator throughout the course of the disease (Table 6.1).

Table 6.1 Role of cytokines in thyroid-associated ophthalmopathy

Disease stage	*Early*	*Progressive/plateau*	*Late/resolution*
Clinical signs and symptoms	Chemosis Periorbital oedema Eye discomfort	Proptosis	Fixed diplopia
Cytokines involved	IFN-γ TNF-α IL-1	IFN-γ TGF-β IL-1	IL-4 IL-1
Effect of cytokines on orbital fibroblasts	Stimulation of ICAM, HLA-DR, and HSP-72 surface expression	Stimulation of glycosaminoglycan synthesis	Stimulation of proliferation

TARGET CELL AND AUTOANTIGEN

Controversy exists concerning whether orbital fibroblasts, adipocytes or extraocular muscle cells are the autoimmune targets in TAO [1,26]. Gross pathological examination of orbital tissues from patients with TAO reveals extraocular muscles that are oedematous and may be enlarged several-fold [11]. This striking observation led investigators to believe that the extraocular muscle cell was the autoimmune target in TAO. As a result, early studies using enzyme-linked immunosorbent assays were aimed at the identification of autoantibodies that recognized soluble preparations of eye muscle [27,28]. Tissue preparations used in these studies contained a mixture of components, including eye muscle, connective tissue and circulating blood cells, that did not allow specific identification of the cell type or protein against which sera were reactive. Later immunoblotting studies using cultured human extraocular muscle cells or orbital fibroblasts allowed for the examination of single cell types and early characterization of potential autoantigens [29,30]. These studies, however, yielded no consensus concerning which cell (or antigen) serves as the relevant target in TAO.

As discussed above, orbital fibroblasts in TAO show surface expression of several immunomodulatory proteins, including a 72 kDa HSP, HLA-DR and ICAM-1. Similarly, expression of HLA-DR and HSP-72 by extraocular muscle fibres in TAO has been reported [26]. Expression of these proteins on the two cell types suggests that both may be involved in the autoimmune process in TAO. However, these observations do not clarify whether either one functions as the primary target cell. It may be that inflammatory cytokines within the involved orbit affect nearby cells in a paracrine manner. In an attempt to identify the target cell in TAO, Grubeck-Loebenstein and colleagues examined the proliferation of T cell lines established from the orbital tissues of patients with TAO in response to orbital tissue preparations [31]. These investigators documented HLA class I-restricted proliferation of orbital lymphocytes in response to autologous orbital and skin fibroblasts. However, T cells did not proliferate when exposed to crude eye muscle extract, autologous peripheral blood mononuclear cells, allogeneic cells or purified protein derivative of *Mycobacterium tuberculosis*. These data strongly support the concept that fibroblasts in the orbit and skin, recognized by activated T cells, are the target cells in TAO and PTD.

An extraocular muscle protein of 64 kDa has been studied extensively as a potential target antigen in TAO [29]. Immunoreactivity against this protein was found to be present in thyroid and extraocular muscles, but absent in other skeletal muscle. The corresponding autoantibodies are detectable in sera from 75% of patients with severe, active, orbital inflammation of short duration and in 50% of patients having lid lag, without other signs of progressive ophthalmopathy [32,33]. Normal individuals who possess anti-64 kDa antibodies tend to have low-titre reactivity. Similarly, circulating autoantibodies directed against orbital fibroblasts have been detected in patients with GD and TAO. These autoantibodies recognize a 23 kDa fibroblast protein and are present in the sera of 56% of GD patients and in 15% of normal individuals [34]. Because these eye muscle and fibroblast autoantibodies are present in normal sera and are detectable inconsistently in TAO sera, they are unlikely to play a primary role in pathogenesis. They may arise secondarily as a result of the local inflammatory process in the orbit, and may be directed against cytoskeletal components that are common to many cells [35].

The TSHR is known to be the autoantigen involved in the hyperthyroidism of GD. The relevant autoantigen(s) involved in TAO and PTD has not been identified. It has been suggested that a shared autoantigen present in thyroid, ocular and dermal tissues serves as a common target against which the autoimmune process is directed in GD. If this were proven to be the case, the close clinical association between Graves' hyperthyroidism, TAO and PTD could be explained. The TSHR, or a closely related protein, would seem to be a likely candidate for such a cross-reactive antigen. As a result, several groups of investigators have sought its presence in orbital and dermal tissues. Our laboratory has demonstrated the presence of RNA corresponding to a 705 bp fragment of the extracellular domain of the human TSHR in orbital fibroblasts obtained from patients with TAO [36]. Other investigators, using somewhat different primers and PCR systems, have also identified full-length or variant TSHR transcripts in orbital connective tissues [37–39]. Similarly, cultured human pretibial skin fibroblasts have been shown to produce transcripts encoding the TSHR extracellular domain [40]. Immunoblotting studies with human TSHR antibody and TAO sera demonstrated several specific bands in fibroblast preparations, suggesting that a protein species antigenically related to the TSHR is present in these cells [41]. No TSHR RNA or protein has been detected in eye muscle cells. Whether the TSHR (or a related protein) is a target antigen common to thyroid, orbital and dermal tissues is unknown at present and awaits further study.

IMMUNOGENETICS OF TAO

It is a well known clinical axiom that autoimmune thyroid disorders tend to cluster in families [42]. It is not uncommon to find families with many affected individuals, some of whom have GD with or without TAO, while others have Hashimoto's thyroiditis or postpartum thyroiditis [43]. Even in the same individual, the clinical course of autoimmune thyroid disease may begin as hypothyroidism due to Hashimoto's thyroiditis and evolve into Graves' hyperthyroidism (hashitoxicosis). Thus it appears that these disorders have a genetic basis, and that many autoimmune thyroid disorders (including GD with or without TAO, Hashimoto's thyroiditis, atrophic thyroiditis, silent thyroiditis, and postpartum thyroiditis) may be closely related from a genetic standpoint. It is also likely that these conditions are not determined solely by genetic inheritance, but depend on other non-genetic or environmental factors (see Chapters 3, 4 and 5). This concept is supported by the relatively low concordance rates (between 20 and 50%) for these disorders in genetically identical monozygotic twins [44,45]. However, regardless of the other factors involved, population studies and analyses of affected family members have shown that genetic factors exert the primary influence on predisposition to autoimmune thyroid diseases.

Specific HLA loci have been reported to be increased in frequency in patients with GD who have clinically apparent TAO. Several investigators have noted that GD patients possessing the HLA-B8 allele, or the tightly linked HLA-DR3 specificity, are at high risk for the development of TAO [46,50]; others have not reproduced these findings [51,52]. A closer association between TAO and HLA-B8 than between TAO and HLA-DR3 has been reported, and it has been suggested that HLA-DR7 may increase the risk for TAO in the presence of B8 [46]. Associations between TAO and DQA1*0501 [53] or TAO and DRB3*0202/*0202 heterozygosity [54] have also been noted. In addition, HLA-DR4 was reported to be increased in frequency in Caucasians with GD and TAO [47]. Both HLA-DR4 and HLA-DR13 (DRw6] are increased in American blacks with GD and TAO, while the frequency of HLA-DR5 is increased in blacks having GD without clinical evidence of TAO [55]. In the Japanese population, euthyroid TAO was found to be associated with increased frequencies of HLA-B40, -DR9, -DQw3, -Dw15, -B12 and -Cw1 [56]. Finally, certain HLA specificities (e.g. Dqw3.1, B12 and DR2] have been reported to be negatively associated with the occurrence of TAO, presumably providing protection [46,57]. Despite these reported genetic associations, family studies using lod scores have failed to demonstrate linkage between the DR3 locus [58] or the HLA-DQ beta locus [59] and GD or TAO. Thus, while it is clear that particular HLA loci confer some degree of susceptibility to GD or TAO, they do not appear to be the major genetic determinants of these disorders [60]. More extensive family studies, perhaps using microsatellite-based large-scale screening methods, will be needed in order to identify the gene(s) conferring highest risk for GD and TAO.

It has been suggested that certain non-HLA alleles, rather than functioning primarily as genes influencing susceptibility to disease, may act to modify the course of an existing autoimmune disease. The interleukin-1 receptor antagonist (IL-1ra) A2 allele has been shown to be associated with increased severity of several autoimmune diseases, including alopecia areata [61], systemic lupus erythematosus [62] and nephropathy in insulin-dependent diabetes mellitus [63]. Our studies, while finding no association between the IL-1ra A2 allele and GD itself, have suggested that the IL-1ra A2 allele may be associated with increased disease severity as defined by the presence of extrathyroidal manifestations of GD (i.e. TAO, PTD and acropachy) [64]. We found a carriage rate for this allele of 29% in 28 patients with GD who did not have TAO, PTD or acropachy. However, the carriage rate was 42% in 98 patients with GD and TAO, 57% in seven patients with GD, TAO and PTD, and 63% eight in patients having GD, GO, PTD and acropachy. Clearly, the number of patients studied with the extrathyroidal manifestations is too small (and thus prone to type II statistical error) to reach a definite conclusion. However, studies of the IL-1ra A2 allele in larger populations of patients with TAO, PTD and acropachy are warranted in order to further explore its potential association with the severity of GD.

Our understanding of the mechanisms by which particular genes may function as susceptibility genes is based on the concept that autoimmunity results from an abnormal immune response to a normal self-antigen [65]. Thus, it seems unlikely that a polymorphic self-antigen would confer risk for an autoimmune disorder. We have, however, documented an association between the occurrence of GD and the presence of a polymorphic form of the TSHR in a Caucasian female population [66,67]. In contrast, study of a population in the UK by another group of investigators failed to reproduce these findings [68]. In further analyses of our population, we found that three of five patients having GD with TAO, PTD and acropachy carried the TSHR polymorphism (60%), and that four of 10 GD patients who had TAO and PTD (but not acropachy) possessed this polymorphism (40%). However, only seven of 55 GD patients with TAO, who did not have clinically evident PTD or acropachy, carried the TSHR polymorphism (13%) [66]. Because of the small number of affected individuals within these each of these subgroups, and the multiple comparisons made between groups, no statistical significance can be attached to these observations. However, these findings suggest that the codon 52 TSHR polymorphism is another genetic factor (in addition to the IL-1ra A2 allele) that may act to modify the course of GD towards greater clinical severity.

CONCLUSION

Graves' hyperthyroidism, TAO and PTD (and likely acropachy) are autoimmune conditions that are clinically closely associated. That these conditions are manifestations of a single autoimmune disease is suggested by (i) their close temporal profiles in presentation; (ii) the evidence of thyroid autoimmune disease common to affected individuals; (iii) the similarities in histopathology seen in the diverse regions involved; and (iv) the sharing of particular susceptibility genes among individuals who manifest several of these conditions. Controversy exists concerning whether extraocular muscle cells or orbital fibroblasts are the autoimmune targets in TAO. However, if TAO, PTD and acropachy are indeed manifestations of a single autoimmune disease, it seems likely that a cell common to the orbit, pretibial skin and distal digits (i.e. the fibroblast) would be involved. Further, TAO and PTD are characterized histologically by an accumulation of GAG and the presence of particular cytokines in affected tissues. Certain of these cytokines are potent stimulators of GAG synthesis *in vitro* by orbital and pretibial fibroblasts. It is likely that this same process occurs in the orbit and pretibial skin in TAO and PTD. The resulting accumulation of GAG, oedema and inflammation in orbital and dermal tissues leads to development of the characteristic clinical signs and symptoms of these conditions. Further insight into the pathogenesis and treatment of TAO and PTD awaits information concerning the specific autoantigen(s) involved. The link between these conditions and thyroid autoimmunity may be explained in the future by the identification of an autoantigen common to fibroblasts and thyrocytes.

References

1. Bahn RS, Heufelder AE. Mechanisms of disease: pathogenesis of Graves' ophthalmopathy. N Engl J Med. 1993;329:1468–75.
2. Werner S, Coleman DJ, Franzen LA. Ultrasonic evidence of a consistent orbital involvement in Graves' disease. N Engl J Med. 1974;29:1447–50.
3. Salvi M, Zhang Z-G, Haegert D et al. Patients with endocrine ophthalmopathy not associated with overt thyroid disease have multiple thyroid immunological abnormalities. J Endocrinol Metab. 1990;70:89–94.
4. Bahn RS. Assessment and management of the patient with Graves' ophthalmopathy. Endocr Pract. 1995;1:172–8.
5. Hales IB, Rundle FF. Ocular changes in Graves' disease. A long-term follow-up study. Q J Med. 1960;29:113–25.
6. DeGroot LJ, Gorman CA, Pinchera A et al. Therapeutic controversies: radiation and Graves' ophthalmopathy. J. Clin Endocrinol Metab. 1995;80:339–49.
7. Shine B, Fells P, Edwards OM, Weetman AP. Association between Graves' ophthalmopathy and smoking. Lancet. 1990;335:1261–3.
8. Kendler DL, Lippa J, Rootman J. The initial clinical characteristics of Graves' orbitopathy vary with age and sex. Arch Ophthalmol. 1993;111:197–201.
9. Fatourechi V, Pajouhi M, Fransway AF. Dermopathy of Graves' disease (pretibial myxedema). Review of 150 cases. Medicine. 1994;73:1–7.
10. Smith TJ, Bahn RS, Gorman CA. Connective tissue, glycosaminoglycans, and diseases of the thyroid. Endocr Rev. 1989;10:366–91.
11. Campbell RJ. Pathology of Graves' ophthalmopathy. In: Gorman CA, Waller RA, Dyer JA, eds. The Eye and Orbit in Thyroid Disease. New York: Raven Press; 1984:25–31.
12. Tallstedt L, Norberg R. Immunohistochemical staining of normal and Graves' extraocular muscle. Invest Ophthalmol Vis Sci. 1988;29:175–84.
13. Weetman AP, Cohen S, Gatter KC et al. Immunohistochemical analysis of the retrobulbar tissues in Graves' ophthalmopathy. Clin Exp Immunol. 1989;75:222–7.
14. Heufelder AE, Bahn RS. Detection and localization of cytokine immunoreactivity in retroocular connective tissue in Graves' ophthalmopathy. Eur J Clin Invest. 1993;23:10–8.
15. Korducki JM, Loftus SJ, Bahn RS. Glycosaminoglycan production in retroocular fibroblasts. Invest Ophthalmol Vis Sci. 1992;33:2037–42.
16. Heufelder AE, Wenzel BE, Gorman CA, Bahn RS. Detection, cellular localization, and modulation of heat shock proteins in cultured fibroblasts from patients with extrathyroidal manifestations of Graves' disease. J Clin Endocrinol Metab. 1991;73:739–45.
17. Heufelder AE, Wenzel BE, Bahn RS. Cell surface localization of a 72 kilodalton heat shock protein in retroocular fibroblasts from patients with Graves' ophthalmopathy. J Clin Endocrinol Metab. 1992;74:732–6.
18. Lindquist S. The heat-shock response. Annu Rev Biochem. 1986;55:1151–91.
19. Heufelder AE, Smith TJ, Gorman CA, Bahn RS. Increased induction of HLA-DR by interferon-gamma in cultured fibroblasts derived from patients with Graves' ophthalmopathy and pretibial dermopathy. J Clin Endocrinol Metab. 1991;73-307–13.
20. Shimizu Y, Shaw S. Lymphocyte interaction with extracellular matrix. FASEB J. 1991;5: 2292–9.
21. Heufelder AE, Bahn RS. Elevated expression in situ of selectin and immunoglobulin superfamily type adhesion molecules in retroocular connective tissues from patients with Graves' ophthalmopathy. Clin Exp Immunol. 1993;91:381–9.
22. Heufelder AE, Bahn RS. Graves' immunoglobulins and cytokines stimulate the expression of intercellular adhesion molecule-1 (ICAM-1) in cultured Graves' orbital fibroblasts. Eur J Clin Invest. 1992;22:529–37.
23. Mosmann TR, Sad S. The expanding universe of T-cell subsets: Th1, Th2 and more. Immunol Today. 1996;17:138–46.

24. Fowell D, Powrie F, Saoudi A et al. The role of subjects of CD4 and T cells in autoimmunity. Aba Foundation Symposium. 1995;195:173–82.
25. Heufelder AE, Bahn RS. Modulation of orbital fibroblast proliferation by cytokines and glucocorticoid receptor agonistsl. Invest Ophthalmol Vis Sci. 1994;35:120–7.
26. Kiljanski JI, Nebes V, Wall JR. The ocular muscle cell is a target of the immune system in endocrine ophthalmopathy. Int Arch Allergy Immunol. 1995;106:204–12.
27. Atkinson S, Holcombe M, Kendall-Taylor P. Ophthalmic immunoglobulins in patients with Graves' ophthalmopathy. Lancet. 1984;2:374–6.
28. Miller A, Sikorska H, Salvi M, et al. Evaluation of an enzyme-linked immunosorbent assay for the measurement of autoantibodies against eye muscle membrane antigens in Graves' ophthalmopathy. Acta Endocrinol (Copenh) 1986;113:514-22.
29. Salvi M, Muller A, Wall JR. Human orbital tissue and thyroid membranes express a 64 kDa protein which is recognized by autoantibodies in the serum of patients with thyroid-associated ophthalmopathy. FEBS Lett. 1988;232:135–9.
30. Bahn RS, Gorman CA, Johnson CM, Smith TJ. Presence of autoantibodies in the sera of patients with Graves' disease recognizing a 23 kilodalton fibroblast protein. J Clin Endocrinol Metab. 1989;69:622–8
31. Grubeck-Loebenstein B, Trieb K, Sztankay A, Holter W, Anderl H, Wick G. Retrobulbar T cells from patients with Graves' ophthalmopathy are $CD8^+$ and specifically recognize autologous fibroblasts. J Clin Invest. 1994;93:2738–43.
32. Salvi M, Bernard N. Muller A, Ahang ZG, Gardini E, Wall JR. Prevalence of antibodies reactive with a 64 kDa eye muscle membrane antigen in thyroid associated ophthalmopathy. Thyroid. 1991;1:207–13.
33. Wall JR, Hayes M, Scalise D et al. Native gel electrophoresis and isoelectric focusing of a 64-kilodalton eye muscle protein shows that it is an important target for serum autoantibodies in patients with thyroid-associated ophthalmopathy and not expressed in other skeletal muscles. J Clin Endocrinol Metab. 1995;80:1226–32.
34. Bahn RS, Gorman CA, Johnson CM, Smith TJ. The presence of antibodies in the sera of patients with Graves' disease recognizing a 23 kilodalton fibroblast protein. J Clin Endocrinol Metab. 1989;69:622–8.
35. Weetman AP. Thyroid-associated ophthalmopathy. Autoimmunity 1992;12:215–21.
36. Heufelder AE, Dutton CM, Sarkar G, Donovan KA, Bahn RS. Detection of TSH receptor RNA in cultured retroocular fibroblasts from patients with Graves' ophthalmopathy and pretibial dermopathy. Thyroid. 1993;3:297–300.
37. Mengistu M, Lukes YG, Nagy EV et al. TSH receptor gene expression in fibroblasts. J Clin Endocrinol Invest. 1994;17:437–41.
38. Feliciello A, Porcellini A, Ciullo I et al. Expression of thyrotropin-receptor mRNA in healthy and Graves' disease retro-orbital tissue. Lancet. 1993;342:337–8.
39. Paschke R, Metcalfe A, Alcalde L, Vassart G, Weetman, Ludgate M. Presence of nonfunctional thyrotropin receptor variant transcripts in retroocular and other tissues. J Clin Endocrinol Metab. 1994;79:1232–3.
40. Chang T-C, Wu S-L, Hsiao Y-L. TSH and TSH receptor antibody binding sites in fibroblasts of pretibial myxedema are related to the entire extracellular domain of the TSH receptor. Clin Immunol Immunopathol. 1994;71:113–20.
41. Burch HB, Sellitti D, Barnes SG, Nagy EV, Bahn RS, Burman KD. Thyrotropin receptor antisera for the detection of immunoreactive protein species in retroocular fibroblasts obtained from patients with Graves' ophthalmopathy. J Clin Endocrinol Metab. 1994;78: 1384–91.
42. Stenszky V, Kozma L, Balazs C, Rochlitz S, Bear JC, Farid NR. The genetics of Graves' disease: HLA and disease susceptibility. J Clin Endocrinol Metab. 1986;61:735–40.
43. Schleusener H, Bogner U, Peters H et al.The relevance of genetic susceptibility in Graves' disease and immune thyroiditis. Exp Clin Endocrinol. 1991;97:127–32.
44. Farid NR. Graves' disease. In: Farid NR, eds. HLA in Endocrine and Metabolic Disorders. New York: Academic Press; 1981:85.
45. Irvine WJ, MacGregor AG, Stuart AE, Hall GH. Hashimoto's disease in uniovular twins. Lancet. 1961;2:850–3.
46. Frecker MF, Preus M, Kozma L et al.Heterogeneity by cluster analysis techniques of Graves' patients typed for HLA DR and IgG heavy chain markers. Mol Biol Med. 1986;3:63–71.
47. van der Gaag R, Wiersinga WM, Koornneef L et al. HLA-DR4 associated response to corticosteroids in Graves' ophthalmopathy patients. J Endocrinol Invest. 1990;13:489–92.

48. Frecker M, Stenszky V, Balazs C, Kozma L, Kraszits E, Farid NR. Genetic factors in Graves' ophthalmopathy. Clin Endocrinol (Oxford). 1986;25:479–85.
49. Stenszky V, Balazs C, Kozma L, Rochlitz S, Bear JC, Farid NR. Identification of subsets of patients with Graves' disease by cluster analysis. Clin Endocrinol (Oxford). 1983;18:335–45.
50. Sergott RC, Felberg NT, Savino PJ, Blizzard JJ, Schatz NJ, Sanford CA. Association of HLA antigen Bw35 with severe Graves' ophthalmopathy. Invest Ophthalmol Vis Sci. 1983;24:124–7.
51. Kendall-Taylor P, Stephenson A, Stratton A, Papiha SS, Perros P, Roberts DF. Differentiation of autoimmune ophthalmopathy from Graves' hyperthyroidism by analysis of genetic markers. Clin Endocrinol (Oxford). 1988;28:601–10.
52. Weetman AP, So AK, Warner CA, Foroni L, Fells P, Shine B. Immunogenetics of Graves' ophthalmopathy. Clin Endocrinol (Oxford). 1988;28:619–28.
53. Badenhoop K, Schleusener H, Usadel KH. Immunogenetics of endocrine ophthalmopathy and Graves' disease. In: Kahaly G, ed. Endocrine Ophthalmopathy: Molecular, Immunological and Clinical Aspects. Basel: Karger; 1993:11–9.
54. Boehm BO, Kuhnl P, Manfras BJ et al. HLA-DRB3 gene alleles in Caucasian patients with Graves' disease. Clin Invest. 1992;70:956–60.
55. Sridama V, Hara Y, Fauchet R, DeGroot LJ. HLA immunogenetic heterogeneity in black American patients with Graves' disease. Arch Intern Med. 1987;147:229–31.
56. Inoue D, Sato K, Meada M et al. Genetic differences shown by HLA typing among Japanese patients with euthyroid Graves' ophthalmopathy, Graves' disease and Hashimoto's thyroiditis: genetic characteristics of euthyroid ophthalmopathy. Clin Endocrinol (Oxford). 1991;34: 57–62.
57. Weetman AP, Zhang L, Webb S, Shine B. Analysis of HLA-DQB and HLA-DPB alleles in Graves' disease by oligonucleotide probing of enzymatically amplified DNA. Clin Endocrinol (Oxford). 1990;33:65–71.
58. Roman SH, Greenberg D, Rubinstein P, Wallenstein S, Davies T. Genetics of autoimmune thyroid disease: lack of evidence for linkage to HLA within families. J Clin Endocrinol Metab. 1992;74:496–503.
59. O'Connor G, Neufeld DS, Greenberg DA, Concepcion ES, Roman S. Lack of disease associated HLA-DQ restriction fragment length polymorphisms in families with autoimmune thyroid disease. Autoimmunity. 1993;14:237–41.
60. McLachlan SM. The genetic basis of autoimmune thyroid disease: time to focus on chromosomal loci other than the major histocompatibility complex (HLA in man). J Clin Endocrinol Metab. 1993;77:605A–605C.
61. Tarlow JK, Clay FE, Cork MJ et al.Severity of alopecia areata is associated with a polymorphism in the interleukin-1 receptor antagonist gene. J Invest Dermatol. 1994;103: 387–90.
62. Blakemore AI, Tarlow JK, Cork MJ, Gordon C, Emery P, Duff GW. Interleukin-1 receptor antagonist gene polymorphism as a disease severity factor in systemic lupus erythematosus. Arthritis Rheum. 1994;37:1380–5.
63. Blakemore AIF, Cox A, Gonzalez A et al. Interleukin-1 receptor antagonist allele (IL1RN*2) associated with nephropathy in diabetes mellitus. Hum Genet. 1996;97:369–74.
64. Cuddihy RM, Bahn RS. Lack of an association between alleles of interleukin-1α and interleukin-1 receptor antagonist genes and Graves' disease in a North American Caucasian population. J Clin Endocrinol Metab. 1996;81:4476–8.
65. Volpé R. A perspective on human autoimmune thyroid disease: is there an abnormality of the target cell which predisposes to the disorder? Autoimmunity. 1992;13:3–9.
66. Cuddihy RM, Dutton CM, Bahn RS. A polymorphism in the extracellular domain of the thyrotropin receptor is highly associated with autoimmune thyroid disease in females. Thyroid. 1995;5:89–95.
67. Cuddihy RM, Schaid DS, Bahn RS. Multivariate analysis of HLA loci in conjunction with a thyrotropin receptor codon 52 polymorphism in conferring risk of Graves' disease. Thyroid. 1996;6:261–5.
68. Watson PF, French A, Pickerill AP, McIntosh RS, Weetman AP. Lack of association between a polymorphism in the coding region of the thyrotropin receptor gene and Graves' disease. J Clin Endocrinol Metab. 1995;80:1032–5.

7
Beta cell antigens

A. PLESNER and Å. LERNMARK

INTRODUCTION

Insulin-dependent (type 1) diabetes mellitus (IDDM) is classified as an autoimmune disorder, since it is associated with specific autoimmunity towards the insulin-producing cells in the islets of Langerhans. The disease process that results in IDDM is not fully understood and whether it is initiated by endogenous or exogenous antigens, or a combination, remains to be clarified. The clinical onset of IDDM is characterized by weight loss and an abrupt or gradual onset of hyperglycaemia; dependence on insulin injections to sustain life; presence of different types of islet cell autoantibodies in more than 90% of patients, although this is not possible to document in the individual patient and lymphocytic infiltration of the islets of Langerhans (insulitis) in about 60% of patients [1,2]. While mononuclear cell infiltration of the pancreatic islets was described in the last century, it was not until 1965 that a systematic study [1] documented the presence of insulinitis in patients with IDDM of short duration. Later it was demonstrated that the β cells were specifically eradicated [3]. Subsequent observations that organ-specific autoimmune diseases are more common among patients with IDDM [4–6] and that IDDM was associated with certain HLA types [7,8] further supported the notion of IDDM as an autoimmune disorder. The demonstration of islet cell antibodies (ICA) using an indirect immunofluorescence test on frozen sections of human blood group pancreas [9,10] was additional evidence of islet autoimmunity. Possible etiologic mechanisms in IDDM are summarized in Table 7.1. ICA reacted, however, not only with the β cells, but with all islet endocrine cells [11]. As indicated above, the β cells are specifically lost in IDDM and it was therefore difficult to envisage a role for ICA in the pathogenetic process. Alternative assays, such as binding of

A.P. Weetman (ed.), Endocrine Autoimmunity and Associated Conditions. 113–144.

Table 7.1 Possible aetiologic mechanisms in insulin dependent (type 1) diabetes

Hypothetical series of events:

Stage I:
- Genetic susceptibility: HLA-DQ2, DQ8 or both
- Environmental factors initiate β cell destruction:
  - Latent virus infection (Coxsackie B)
  - Virus lysis (rubella, mumps)
  - Toxin necrosis (nitrosamines)

Stage II:
- HLA-DQ (A1*0301, B1*0201, B1*0302) restricted peptide presentation to initiate an immune response eventually leading to insulitis

Alternative hypothetical series of events:

Stage I:
- Environmental insults, for example:
  - Gestational infections (congenital rubella)
  - Toxins
- Islet antigen presentation which will occur on all HLA types:
  - GAD65 antibodies formation
- IDDM2, IDDM12 or other susceptibility genetic factors

Stage II:
- HLA-DQ2, DQ8 acceleration of β cell autoreactivity but only to select autoantigens

antibodies to the surface of living β cells were, therefore, tested in the search for a subset of autoantibodies which would reflect the loss of β cells [6,12]. A variety of islet cell preparations [13,14]. and insulin-producing islet tumour cell lines [15,16] was used to demonstrate that many patients with recent onset IDDM, as well as their first degree relatives, had islet cell surface antibodies [14,15,17]. Since immunoglobulin is not thought to permeate cells, IDDM would be associated with at least two types of autoantibodies, one type would be detected by standard immunofluorescence by binding primarily to autoantigens present intracellularly, and another type would recognize autoantigens expressed on the cell surface. The latter type of autoantigens could represent receptor or transport molecules. Interestingly, although further studies are needed, autoantibodies interfering with glucose transport [18], or glucose-stimulated insulin release [19], have been detected in serum from patients with recent onset IDDM.

The diverse set of reactions between IDDM autoantibodies and miscellaneous islet cell preparations suggested that IDDM sera would recognize different autoantigens. It was assumed that the inflammatory process in the islets resulted in the generation of β cell autoantibodies directed against not one but several autoantigens. In addition, it could not be excluded that the autoantibodies would detect different epitopes on the same autoantigen. Finally, the autoantibody profile seemed likely to differ between patients [11].

Novel methods for the identification and study of membrane proteins [20–22] made it possible to use IDDM sera in immunoprecipitation experiments with radioactively labelled islets. The islets were isolated from human or rodent pancreas and used to identify islet autoantigens by analysing the immunoprecipitate by gel electrophoresis [12,23,24]. These experiments showed that about 80% of new onset patients had antibodies which immunoprecipitated a 64 kDa protein from the human islet extracts. In some sera a 38 kDa component was also detected [23]. The demonstration of the 64 kDa protein was followed by about 8 years of research until it was shown that the immunoprecipitated 64 kDa protein had glutamic acid decarboxylase activity [25]. This elegant demonstration came shortly after a report that patients with both stiff man syndrome and diabetes have not only ICA, but also antibodies detecting a band by immunoblotting that was similar to 64 kDa [26].

The human islet 64 kDa protein was identified as a novel isoform (GAD65) of glutamic acid decarboxylase (GAD) [27]. Both 65 kDa and 67 kDa GAD were also present in the brain of humans [28] and rodents [29]. In human islets, GAD65 is unique to the β cells and little, if any, GAD67 is expressed [30]. Numerous subsequent studies confirmed that autoantibodies to GAD65 are strongly associated both with progression to and with the onset of IDDM [for reviews and standardization of GAD65 autoantibodies see References 31–36]. The interest in islet autoreactivity therefore shifted from a mere registration of whether islet cell autoantibodies were present or not, to autoantigen-specific analysis, which is both precise and reproducible and allows the autoantigen specificity to be expressed quantitatively. Although immuno-precipitation was used in initial studies to identify autoantigens, a number of approaches have subsequently been used in attempts to detect additional autoantigens. In one approach, candidate autoantigens were tested: this resulted in the discovery of insulin as an autoantigen [37]. In another approach, islet cell expression libraries were screened with IDDM sera which resulted in the discovery of the ICA512 [38] and IA-2 [39] autoantigens (Table 7.2), as well as others which are discussed below.

Insulin is a truly β cell-specific protein and would seem to be the ultimate autoantigen in IDDM. Using iodinated insulin it was demonstrated that almost 50% of children with new onset IDDM had insulin autoantibodies (IAA) [37]. This observation was followed by a large number of confirming investigations [40,41]. and a demonstration, although still unresolved, that the IAA may primarily be directed towards proinsulin [42,43]. Insulin and proinsulin are uniquely associated with the islet β cells although low levels may be expressed in the thymus are of possible importance for tolerance induction [44].

The ICA512 autoantigen was detected by screening an islet expression library with IDDM serum [45] and the presence of autoantibodies reacting to the product of a full-length cDNA clone, IA-2, was confirmed [39]. In earlier studies, it was demonstrated that trypsin treatment of immunoprecipitated 64 kDa protein generated three major fragments of relative molecular mass 50 kDa, 40 kDa and 37 kDa [46,47]. While the 50 kDa fragment is from GAD65, the 37 kDa is the cytoplasmic tail of the ICA512/IA-2 protein [48] and the 40 kDa from the isoform IA-2β isoform [49]. The presence of ICA512 antibodies is

Table 7.2 Recombinant β cell autoantigens – high sensitivity autoantibodies

Antigen	*Nature, location and autoantibody assay*
Proinsulin/Insulin	Beta cell specific 10 kDa and 6 kDa proteins stored in secretory granules. Less than 10% of proinsulin is secreted. Standardized radioligand ([^{125}I]-insulin) assay detects insulin autoantibodies (IAA) in about 50% of new onset IDDM children. Less in adults.
GAD	Two isoforms of 65 and 67 kDa are expressed in human islet cells. GAD65 (formerly 64 kDa protein) seems β cell-specific. Also expressed in the brain and other non-neuronal locations. Standardized radioligand ([^{35}S]- or [^{3}H]GAD65) assay detect autoantibodies (GAD65 antibodies) in about 80% of new onset IDDM children and adults. GAD67 antibodies are found primarily in GAD65 antibodies positive sera.
ICA 512/IA-2	Beta cell receptor-type protein tyrosine phosphatase (PTPase) first detected as a 40 kDa tryptic fragment of the 64 kDa protein. Expressed as a transmembrane molecule in the secretory granules of the β cells and other secretory cells. The cytoplasmic end has all autoantibody epitopes. Standardized radioligand ([^{35}S]- or [^{3}H]IA-2) assay detects autoantibodies (ICA512 antibodies or IA-2 antibodies) in about 50% of new onset IDDM children and adults. ICA512 antibodies are unique to IDDM, develop after GAD65 antibodies and closer to the clinical IDDM onset.
IA-2β /Phogrin	Beta cell PTPase isoform of IA-2 representing a 37 kDa tryptic fragment of immunoprecipiated 64 kDa protein. IA-2β is 74% homologous to IA-2 and the two molecules share most of the autoantibody epitopes. Radioligand ([^{35}S]- or [^{3}H]IA-2) assay detects autoantibodies (IA-2β antibodies) in about 50% of new onset IDDM children and adults. Not formally standardized.

age dependent and the highest diagnostic sensitivity is observed in young age at onset IDDM patients [50]. It has been suggested that ICA512 antibodies may mark rapid progression to clinical onset among immune marker-positive first degree relatives [51]. It has been suggested that the autoantibody reactivity to the three autoantigens, GAD65, insulin and ICA512, delimit the ICA immunofluorescence reaction [52]. Taken together, IDDM is therefore strongly associated with three autoantigens, GAD65, insulin and ICA512 (IA-2/IA-2β) (Figure 7.1).

Subsequent to the discovery of these three autoantigens, a number of approaches have been used to detect not only autoantibodies, but also T cell reactivity to a growing number of autoantigens [for recent reviews see References 31,53,54]. It is however impossible to distinguish between autoreactivity, which is primary and pathogenic, and autoreactivity which is

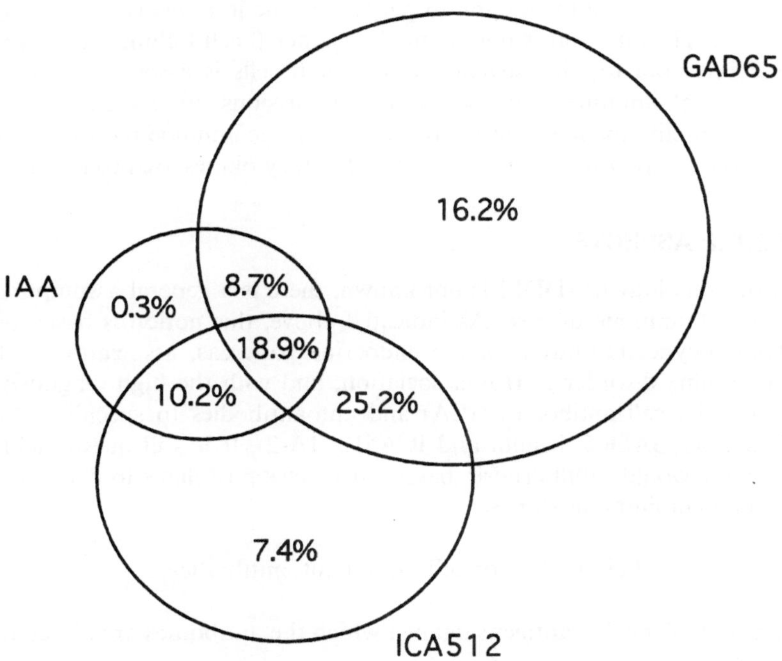

Figure 7.1 Venn diagram of the diagnostic sensitivity (%) of GAD65, ICA512 and insulin (IAA) autoantibodies in IDDM

secondary to a primary β or islet cell destruction (Table 7.1). It cannot be excluded that the autoreactivity which develops after an initial lesion itself adds to the pathogenesis of β cell killing. In this review, we will summarize recent data on β cell antigens detected by different methods. The focus will be on human IDDM, but comparisons will be made to the spontaneously diabetic NOD mouse and the BB rat. The underlying hypothesis, summarized in Table 7.1, is that a specific autoantigen is the target in an immune attack on the β cells. The alternative hypothesis is that autoreactivity to multiple autoantigens is the result of a primary destructive process resulting in autoimmune reactivity to multiple β cell antigens.

IDDM is often referred to as a T cell-mediated disease. This notion is based primarily on adoptive transfer of IDDM in animal experiments (Chapter 8). In man there is no evidence that β cell killing is achieved solely by T cells without the involvement of a full immune response, including a variety of β cell-specific autoantigens. The immune response would include uptake and processing of autoantigen by antigen presenting cells (macrophages, dendritic cells and B lymphocytes), activation and differentiation of $CD4^+$ T cells followed by dual activation of both $CD8^+$ T cells and antibody-producing B lymphocytes. A

B lymphocyte–CD4 T cell interaction to perpetuate the immune response may also be critical. The question is not so much whether β cell killing is achieved solely by T cells, but to what extent the loss of β cells is associated with a particular type of immune response. Recent discussions often focus on the possibility to simplify the mechanisms by describing the immune response as a T_H1 or T_H2 type response dependent on what T cell cytokines are produced.

AUTOIMMUNE ASPECTS

Although the aetiology of IDDM is not known, there is a general assumption that it is an autoimmune disease. As indicated above, this notion is based on specific lymphocytic infiltration of the endocrine pancreas, association with other autoimmune disorders, HLA association, and with the high diagnostic sensitivity of islet cell antibodies (ICA) and autoantibodies to specific autoantigens, such as GAD65, insulin and ICA512 (IA-2). It is still questionable whether IDDM would fulfill criteria based on Koch's postulates to define the aetiology of an autoimmune disease:

(1) demonstration of circulating or cell-bound autoantibodies;

(2) recognition of specific antigens against which the antibodies are directed;

(3) production of antibodies against the antigen in experimental animals;

(4) appearance of pathological changes similar to those in human disease of actively sensitized experimental animals.

So far, IDDM seems to fulfill three of these criteria. Autoantibodies have been demonstrated and specific antigens such as GAD65, insulin and ICA512 have been identified. Antibodies against both GAD65 and insulin have been produced, but, the fourth postulate is not yet convincingly fulfilled.

Early studies with insulin immunizations using crude insulin and complete Freund's adjuvant and major species barriers showed insulitis in immunized animals [55]. Subsequent experiments, however, indicated that the purer the insulin, the less severe the insulitis. It is yet to be determined whether immunization with GAD65 or ICA512 induces insulitis. Koch's postulates transposed to autoimmune disease may however be an oversimplification that will be of little help in our attempts to understand the aetiology and pathogenesis of IDDM. On the other hand, the nature of the initiating or triggering antigen(s) still remains to be determined (Table 7.1). This task is complicated not only by the large variety of autoantibodies, which have been associated with IDDM but also by the difficulty in studying preclinical IDDM, at the time when the disease is initiated. Investigations at the time of clinical onset probably represent late events since in some patients developing IDDM, the autoantibodies have been present for many years. Ascertainment of non-diabetic subjects for longitudinal studies have often used autoantibodies as inclusion criteria. The presence of the antibody marker may signify that the autoimmune response has been established. Once a triggering antigen has been identified, it will be critical to elucidate the mechanisms by which that antigen is able to induce β cell killing and the subsequent development of clinical IDDM. In the following, we will discuss the different autoantigens identified so far. We have divided the autoantigens into recombinant autoantigens with high or low prevalence of autoantibodies, respectively.

RECOMBINANT AUTOANTIGENS – HIGH PREVALENCE OF AUTOANTIBODIES

Based on detection of circulating autoantibodies, several autoantigens have been associated with the pathogenesis of autoimmune IDDM. Serum or plasma is used to detect the autoantigen either by immunoprecipitation or immunoblotting. The highest diagnostic sensitivity and specificity has been achieved when the autoantibody analyses are carried out with serum and recombinant autoantigens in non-solid phase assays. Three autoantigens, GAD65, insulin and ICA512 (IA-2 and IA-2β) will first be discussed (Table 7.2).

Insulin

Insulin has been tested as a candidate autoantigen. Insulin autoantibodies (IAA) were, however, not convincingly demonstrated until [^{125}I]-insulin was used in a radioligand binding assay [37]. In the first study, it was carefully documented that the patients with IAA had not been given insulin before the clinical diagnosis. The prevalence of IAA at clinical diagnosis was about 40%; however, later studies in an assay with prolonged incubation show a higher IAA frequency at onset [41,56]. The overall prevalence is dependent on age: IAA are more common among young children than among adolescents or adults [57,58]. So far, it has not been possible to distinguish IAA from insulin antibodies formed in response to daily subcutaneous insulin injections. IAA have been the subject of several comprehensive reviews [54,59].

It has long been possible to detect insulin antibodies using radiolabelled insulin. Numerous radioimmunoassays for insulin have been developed and there is a large number of methods to separate free from antibody bound ^{125}I-labelled insulin. In an early assay for insulin, free insulin was absorbed to activated charcoal while in other assays, the free insulin is allowed to remain in the supernatant after the antibodies, including the insulin–antibody complexes, are precipitated with a second antibody or polyethylene glycol (PEG) [59]. A combination of these two assay systems was used in the IAA assay that reached the highest diagnostic sensitivity and specificity in several international standardization workshops [60,61]. After the ELISA tests or similar solid phase analyses had failed, [62,63] the IAA radiobinding assay used has two steps. The first is to treat the serum or plasma with acid charcoal to displace antibody-bound insulin and to remove free insulin, which otherwise would compete with the radioactive insulin which is added to the neutralized sample. The samples are then incubated with or without an excess of non-radioactive insulin to demonstrate specific binding. Free and antibody-bound insulin is finally separated by PEG in the presence of carrier immunoglobulin [61]. Prolonged incubation and the use of larger volumes of sera seem to increase the sensitivity of the assay [56,58,64].

The role of insulin as an autoantigen in the pathogenesis of IDDM is still not understood. It remains to be determined when and why insulin is processed and insulin peptides presented. Using insulin analogues and mutated insulin in the IAA assays with serum from primarily first degree relatives who later developed IDDM, an IAA epitope was tentatively located to the B chain [65]. The IAA epitope is different from that detected by insulin antibodies in the hypoglycaemic insulin antibody syndrome (Hirata's disease). The association between IAA and HLA may help to define epitope restriction. Among first degree relatives to IDDM patients, IAA was reported to be associated with DR4 [66] (the DR4 subtype is still unclear) as well as with linked DQA1 alleles [67]. Further studies are required to clarify the IAA epitopes, their possible HLA restriction and compare them with the epitopes for the insulin antibodies which develop after the initiation of insulin therapy. Insulin antibodies are more frequent and develop to higher titres among $DR4^+$ IDDM patients [68]. Many more B lymphocytes are committed to production of IgG anti-insulin among recent onset IDDM patients than in controls [69]. It cannot be excluded that the immune response to human insulin injected subcutaneously may be different from that to endogenous insulin or proinsulin.

The diagnostic sensitivity and specificity of IAA for IDDM have been assessed in numerous studies of selected patients [56,64,0], population- and Diabetes Registry-based studies of consecutively diagnosed patients and matched controls [57,71,72], as well as among first degree relatives progressing [41,73,74] or not [75,76] to IDDM. While the diagnostic specificity is high (99%), there are major differences in sensitivity (40–80%) depending on the type of assay used and whether recent onset patients have been studied [57,58,71,77]. Although IDDM primarily develops among children and young adults with no family history of IDDM, there are more studies on select first degree relatives followed to diagnosis than on individuals in the general population. In contrast to the view that IAA predicts IDDM among autoantibody-positive first degree relatives who have been followed to onset of IDDM, it may be argued that IAA have low predictive value (3%) in children and young adults in the general population [57]. Large follow-up studies of marker-positive individuals detected by screening the general population [78,79]. will be required to define the predictive values of IAA for IDDM alone, or in combination with other autoantibodies (GAD65 and ICA512) and genetic markers.

It is a common theme in IDDM research that T cells with specific T cell receptors (TCR) to autoantigen peptides or epitopes, have been difficult to identify and clone. The T cell epitopes of interest are those which are detected on either HLA class II molecules by TCR on $CD4^+$ (autoreactive helper cells), or HLA class I molecules on $CD8^+$ (autoreactive cytotoxic T cells) T cells. Such T cell clones have been produced in the spontaneously diabetic NOD mouse [80]. In summary, insulin and perhaps proinsulin [42,81] are significant autoantigens in insulin dependent diabetes. The positive predictive value of IAA for IDDM is still not fully established, but current data indicate that IAA in combination with GAD65, ICA512 or both autoantibodies may have predictive values as high as 50–70%. The mechanisms of insulin autoantigen processing, HLA class II presentation and susceptibility in DR4-DQ8 positive individuals need to be established.

Glutamic acid decarboxylase (GAD)

Before their identification, GAD65 autoantibodies (GAD65 antibodies) were known as 64 kDa autoantibodies, detectable in serum samples from children with newly diagnosed IDDM by immunoprecipitation of detergent extracts of radiolabelled human islets [23]. The 64 kDa protein was linked to GAD based on the observation of unusually high 64 kDa autoantibody titres in patients with stiff-man syndrome, a rare neurological disorder which has a 25% coincidence with IDDM [25,26,82,83]. Cloning GAD in a human islets showed the 64 kDa protein to be a novel isoform of GAD, GAD65 [27] also present in human brain [28]. The two isoforms of GAD, GAD65 and GAD67 are both expressed in neurons and both catalyse the formation of the main neuroinhibitor γ-aminobutyric acid (GABA) from L-glutamate [84,85]. In contrast, the role of GAD65 and GABA in the islets of Langerhans remains elusive [86–88]. However, following the demonstration of GAD65 as the major autoantigen in IDDM [27,83,89–91], special interest has been focused on this autoantigen since administration of GAD65 to spontaneously diabetic NOD mice prevents or delays the onset of IDDM [92,93]. Following intervention, GAD65 not only prevents overt IDDM, but also reduces the degree of T cell proliferation to other implicated autoantigens [93]. Therefore, it has been speculated that GAD65 plays a primary role in the initial stages of IDDM pathogenesis.

Studies of the GAD gene have demonstrated at least two human non-allelic isoforms of 65 kDa (GAD65) and 67 kDa (GAD67) (Table 7.3) encoded by separate genes presumably derived from a common ancestral GAD gene [27,28,94,95]. Sib-pair analysis suggest that the *GAD2* but not the *GAD1* gene is linked to IDDM susceptibility [96]. Different biochemical features and the differential expression patterns found between man, mouse and rat are summarized in Table 7.3.

In contrast to man, several biochemical isoforms have been detected in porcine brain, and four isoforms with distinct properties have been identified in rat brain [97–99]. Cloning and characterization of the 67 kDa isoform from rat islets proved complete identity with rat brain GAD67 [29,100]. The overall deduced amino acid sequence homology between human islet and brain GAD65 or GAD67 is near 100%, whereas the two isoforms are approximately

Table 7.3 Biochemical features of GAD65 and GAD67, and their respective differential expression pattern in man, mouse and rat

Feature	*GAD65*	*GAD67*
Chromosome, gene	10, GAD2 (5.6 kb transcript)	2, GAD1 (3.7 kb transcript)
Molecular weight	65 kDa	67 kDa
Hydropathy	Amphiphilic, membrane-bound	Hydrophilic
Location	Synaptic-like microvesicles	Cytosolic
Regulation	PLP/ATP activity	GABA biosynthesis
Half-life	20 to 30 h	2–3 h
pI	About 6.7	6.9 to 7.1
Expression	Human, mouse and rat brain Human β cells	Human, mouse and rat brain Low levels in human islets

65% identical. The N-terminal region has only 40% amino acid identity between the two isoforms compared to 80% in the remaining sequence [27,28,100,101]. There are major homologies between mammalian e.g. human, murine and feline, sequences.

Both isoforms associate into dimers of approximately 120 kDa, but differ in their interaction with the GAD cofactor, pyridoxal L-phosphate (PLP). The activity of GAD65 is regulated by the holo-apoenzyme cycle whereas GAD67 is primarily regulated at the level of expression [87,98,99,102,103]. Furthermore, it has been demonstrated that GAD65 consists of two subunits, an α and a β subunit [104,105] whereas GAD67 is recognized as a single entity following immunoprecipitation or Western blotting [30,89].

An early attempt to determine the function of pancreatic GAD was assessed by incubating rat islets with ^{14}C-labelled glucose, which showed specific incorporation into both GAD and GABA, but at 2–4 times higher in GABA, suggesting an apparent intracellular compartmentation of GAD [106]. It was later shown that GAD65 is co-localized with synaptophysin which is found in synaptic-like microvesicles also in the islet β cells [107–110]. GAD65 is most often found membrane bound to these microvesicles whereas GAD67 is usually cytosolic, but both isoforms can exist in both forms (Table 7.3). Both isoforms of GAD have, to a lesser degree, been detected in testis, ovary and colon [84,88,111].

Although high GAD activity and high concentrations of GABA have been detected in islets, at levels comparable with those encountered in the CNS, the physiological function of GAD and GABA in the pancreas remains an enigma [112,113]. Neural and endocrine systems of vertebrates utilize GABA for regulatory and trophic roles, and both paracrine and metabolic effects of islet GABA have been proposed [113,114]. In contrast to serotonin, which is co-localized with insulin to the β cell secretory granules [115], GABA is found in small neurosecretory vesicles. Co-secretion with insulin does not seem to occur

[112] and insulin secretagogues do not affect GABA secretion [116]. It was proposed that inhibition of arginine stimulated glucagon secretion by GABA would be explained by the binding of GABA to $GABA_A$ receptors present on α cells [117]. However, inhibiting the binding of GABA to its receptor with bicuculline, which specifically interferes with the post-synaptic $GABA_A$ receptors, did not influence glucose-induced inhibition of glucagon release [116]. No alteration in the secretion of insulin by β cells or somatostatin by delta cells has been found following treatment with GABA [112]. If GABA serves as a fuel generated by a pathway alternative to glycolysis, GABA could play a role in β cell energy metabolism by generating NADH and ATP in the 'GABA shunt', i.e. the cycle of reactions which include GAD and GABA transaminase [53,113].

The autoantibody response to GAD in IDDM seems to be heterogeneous since immunoprecipitation assays have demonstrated the combined precipitation of both GAD65 and GAD67 in metabolically labelled rat but not human islets of Langerhans [89,118,119]. Comparison of GAD65 and GAD67 expressed after transfection to a fibroblast cell line [89] or expressed by *in vitro* transcription and translation [90,120] revealed that 70–80% of IDDM sera recognized GAD65 whereas only 10–20% recognize GAD67 [120–122]. Shortly after the report that the 64 kDa protein had GAD activity, several assays to detect GAD autoantibodies were developed, including ELISA [123], immunoprecipitated GAD activity [124,125] and radioimmunoassays [126] with GAD from brain homogenates. The availability of recombinant human GAD65 cDNA made it possible to label GAD65 with either ^{35}S, ^{3}H or ^{14}C by coupled *in vitro* transcription and translation [90,91,127]. This approach allowed the development of precise and reproducible radioligand binding assays to detect GAD65 antibodies, as demonstrated in two international standardization workshops [35,36]. This assay system is now widely employed to detect a variety of autoantibodies including ICA512, [52,128,129], ICA69 [130] or 21-hydroxylase in Addison's disease [131]. The advantage of the *in vitro* generated labelled autoantigen seems to be the direct labelling during biosynthesis, which may not harm critical conformational epitopes which may be affected by iodination or biotinylation and perhaps lost when recombinant GAD is absorbed to plastic in an ELISA test.

The highest diagnostic sensitivity of GAD65 antibodies has been found at the onset of IDDM [120,124,130,132] when about 80% of patients have GAD65 antibodies. The sensitivity is lower in young boys [120,124] but does not seem to decrease with increasing age, as is the case for IAA and ICA512 antibodies [50,132]. The frequency of GAD65 antibodies is increased among first degree relatives and predicts IDDM [83,128,130,133]. The positive predictive value for IDDM of GAD65 antibodies alone or in combination with other islet autoantibodies is probably 50–60%. However, prospective studies in which all first degree relatives, and not only those identified because of ICA positivity and loss of β cell function, are needed. Investigations of antibody-positive individuals following screening in the general population are also needed. The diagnostic specificity is about 99% [90,121]. The frequency (1%) is the same as that of all newborns who will develop diabetes over a lifetime [53]. Although newborn children may have GAD65 antibodies [134,135], it is unclear to what extent they predict IDDM and how frequent they are temporary. When do GAD65 antibodies appear if they are not present at birth? The presence of GAD65 autoantibodies at diagnosis has been suggested to be associated with a more rapid loss of β cell function, i.e. indirectly indicating a short remission period [91,136]. Within 2 years after diagnosis, levels of GAD65 antibodies decrease somewhat, but the prevalence of GAD65 antibodies in long-term patients is surprisingly high [83,137].

The availability of simple, precise and reproducible assays has resulted in GAD65 antibodies, as well as GAD67 antibodies analyses in a large variety of disorders to better understand the diagnostic sensitivity of this IDDM marker. The presence of GAD65 antibodies is very high among patients with the autoimmune polyendocrine syndrome-1 (APS-1; Chapter 9), whether or not the patients develop diabetes [138,139]. Both GAD65- and GAD67-specific autoantibodies were detected in Swedish non-diabetic patients with Graves' disease [140], and also in Japanese, who more often have both diseases. [136,141]. GAD65 antibodies were not increased in frequency among patients with idiopathic Addison's disease without diabetes [131].

The availability of GAD65 and GAD67 cDNA has made it possible to mutate GAD65 to study the autoantibody epitopes [142–145]. It is important in this respect that IDDM-associated GAD65 antibodies do not recognize linear GAD65 epitopes, for example when the antigen is blotted onto nitrocellulose, since conformational epitopes are lost [142,146]. Deletion mutants, which for example, can be used with sera from stiff man syndrome [146–148], may not yield interpretable results with IDDM sera. Using 10 different human monoclonal ICA (MICA 1-10) [149–151] several GAD65 epitopes have been identified: N-terminal region (starting at position 39 for MICA 8/9); middle region (amino acid position 245–449 for MICA 4/6 and 10), and C-terminal region (amino acid position 450–570 for MICA 1/3 and 7). The results of these MICA isolated from three IDDM patients were supported in a study with GAD65/67 chimeric molecules using sera from consecutively diagnosed IDDM children [143] demonstrating that the middle (E1) and C-terminal (E2) region antibodies dominate. In addition, it was observed that an increase in antibody levels to the C terminal (E2) region was associated with conversion to IDDM [143]. In these studies, the GAD65 autoantibody epitopes are detected by IgG anti-GAD65; however, the epitope specificity, as well as HLA association for IgM, IgA and IgE anti-GAD65, as well as for IgG 1-4 subclasses need to be determined. Since somatic mutations of the GAD65 antibody molecules most likely are antigen driven by $CD4^+$ T cell-dependent mechanisms [150,152]. it is critical to determine GAD65 T cell receptor epitopes.

Peripheral blood mononuclear cell (PBMC) reactivity to GAD65 at onset of IDDM and in high-risk relatives have been reported [153–155]. Significant proliferation expressed as a stimulation index was reported in 47–67% of newly diagnosed IDDM patients, and was higher among ICA-positive (63–68%) than in ICA-negative relatives (11%) with no effect of ICA titre, HLA-type or gender [153]. GAD67-reactive PBMC have also been demonstrated in both prediabetic (40%) and diabetic patients (38%) [156]. The relevance of cell proliferation in response to GAD67 is unclear and GAD67 immunodominant epitopes have not been identified [157].

Overlapping GAD65 peptides were used to study binding to HLA-DQ [158,159] and DR [160]. GAD65 peptides with strong homology to the PC-2 Coxsackie virus antigen bound strongly to DQ8 but not to DQ7 and DQ9 [159,161]. Mutagenesis of anchor residues of the peptide identified the importance of hydrophobic residues for pocket 4 binding. However, no DQ-restricted T cell proliferative responses have been detected so far to this epitope [162,163]. DRB1*0401-restricted GAD epitopes have been defined by two cloned T cell hybridomas detecting the sequences 115–126 and 254–262 [160]. One of these T cell epitopes was also detected with T cells isolated from three adult IDDM patients [163]. In the latter study, a number of other T cell peptide epitopes were identified (Figure 7.2). However none of the T cell lines proliferated in response to the Coxsackie B4 PCV-2 antigen peptide [163]. It is possible that the binding is not strong enough to induce tolerance by positive selection in the thymus.

The mechanisms by which the GAD65 (and other islet cell autoantigens) autoantigen is processed and presented on HLA-DR or DQ molecules remains to be elucidated. The possible role of molecular mimicry is still unclear. Based on experiments in spontaneously diabetic NOD mice, it has been proposed that immunization with peptides from either insulin or GAD65 would be capable in preventing human Type 1 diabetes [92,93,164]. Peptides have been eluted and

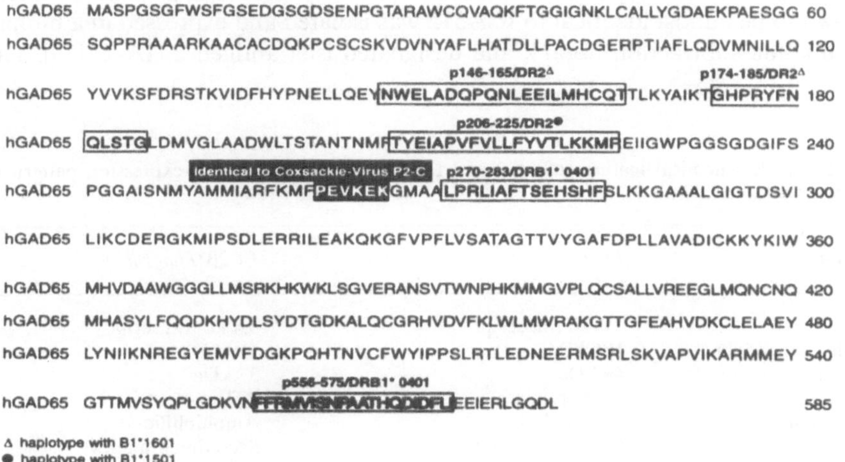

Figure 7.2 GAD65 epitopes reconized by T cell lines from three recent onset adult patients with insulin-dependent diabetes mellitus. [Reproduced from Endl *et al*, J Clin Invest. 1997;99:2405–15, by copyright permission of the American Society for Clinical Investigation]

sequenced from both DQ8 and DQ2 molecules to define peptide binding motifs of these IDDM-associated HLA class II molecules [165]. Such motifs may be useful to identify GAD peptides which may be involved in IDDM pathogenesis or perhaps of aetiological importance. Similar approaches will be needed to determine GAD65 peptide binding to HLA class I molecules to define GAD65-dependent cytotoxic T cells (CTL). A recent study has demonstrated the presence of MHC class I restricted $CD8^+$ CTL specific for a naturally processed GAD65 peptide in peripheral blood of newly diagnosed IDDM patients [166]. $CD8^+$ T cells have been observed in insulitis but their peptide-dependence and HLA class I restriction, i.e. their target, has yet to be elucidated.

IA-2/ICA512

Antibodies to islet proteins distinct from the 64 kDa protein were identified in human diabetic sera by trypsin treatment of immunoprecipitation products [46] with radiolabelled rat insulinoma cell which lack expression of both GAD65 and GAD67 [47,167]. The limited proteolytic cleavage of the immunoprecipitate revealed three different antibody specificities binding fragments of molecular mass (Mr) 37 kDa, 40 kDa and 50 kDa (Table 7.2). The 50 kDa immunoprecipitation moiety could be bound by GAD65 antibodies whereas the 37 kDa and 40 kDa fragments appeared to be derived from a different protein since neither recombinant GAD65 or GAD67 competed for autoantibody binding to their 64 kDa precursor [168]. Subsequently, islet cell antigen 512 (ICA512) was identified from an islet cDNA expression library by screening with sera from IDDM patients [38,45]. (Table 7.4). Simultaneously, the 37 kDa/40 kDa protein shown to be almost identical to ICA512 was isolated and expressed in a human insulinoma subtraction library, and designated islet antigen 2 (IA-2) [39]. The

Table 7.4 Biochemical features of IA-2 and IA-2β, and their respective expression pattern in man, mouse and rat.

Feature	*IA-2*	*IA-2β/Phogrin*
Gene	3.6 kb transcript	5.4 kb transcript
Molecular weight	106 kDa	110 kDa
Tryptic fragment Mr	40 kDa	37 kDa
Protein	PTP protein	PTP protein
Hydropathy	Amphiphilic	Amphiphilic
Location	Secretion granules	Secretion granules
pI	7.09	Predicted 5.66
Expression	Human brain, pituitary, pancreas and tumour cell lines	Human brain and islets
	Mouse CNS and neuroendocrine	Rat islets

3.6 kb cDNA of IA2/ICA512 revealed a 979 amino acid protein (106 kDa) with sequence homology to receptor-type protein tyrosine phosphatases (PTP), which catalyse the removal of phosphate groups from tyrosine residues by protein tyrosine kinase [39,169]. In contrast to most other identified transmembrane PTP, which contain two tandem copies of the PTP domain, the intracellular segment of IA-2 only contains one copy. Apart from being present in various insulinoma cell lines, the IA-2 gene has also been found in normal human brain, pituitary, pancreas and brain tumour cell lines [170]. This suggests that IA-2 is a tissue-restricted PTP which is part of the PTP family, which includes leukocyte CD45 and neural tissue PTP. The function of IA-2 in the islet β cells remains unknown, but transmembrane PTP regulate cell growth and proliferation, cell cycle and cytoskeletal integrity in response to external stimuli [171]. Since IA-2 is an integral membrane protein in the insulin secretion vesicle it is possible that it is of importance to signal internalization of vesicular membrane components [170].

Further analysis of the association between IA-2 and the 37 kDa and 40 kDa tryptic fragments of immunoprecipitated 64 kDa revealed that only the 40 kDa moiety is a product of the intracellular domain of IA-2 [48,169]. The 37 kDa fragment was identified as derived from a different, although related protein, IA-2b (described below). However, both fragments share common epitopes which has complicated their identification as distinct proteins, as well as having specific sites unique to either fragment.

The availability of recombinant IA-2 enables studies of the importance of IA-2 in the pathogenesis of IDDM by assaying for specific autoantibody and T cell reactivity and possibly establishing IA-2-specific immunotherapy. Initially, autoantibodies against islet tryptic fragments of 37 kDa/40 kDa protein were detected in 50% of new onset IDDM patients and 67% of prediabetic twins [47,51]. These data have been further supported by several recent data demonstrating a diagnostic sensitivity of about 50–60% and specificity of 98–99% [48,172,173]. Several investigators believe that the combined GAD65 antibodies, IAA and IA-2 antibodies tests may replace ICA testing [52, 128,173] (Figure 7.1).

In vitro transcribed and translated IA-2 cDNA has been used to determine autoantibody epitopes. First, although the cytoplasmic PTP-like domain is homologous to other tyrosine phosphatases, phosphatase activity has not been detected [45,48]. The ectodomain is unique and does not show homology to known proteins. Second, similar to GAD65, the autoantibody reactivity is directed to the cytoplasmic domain. Sera from patients with recent onset IDDM contain antibodies which react to at least four cytoplasmic domains [174]. Two were mapped to the juxtamembrane domain (amino acid positions 605–620 and 605–682) and an additional two in the PTP-like domain (amino acid positions 777–937 and 687–979). The majority of IDDM sera (83%) reacted at the PTP-like domain followed by the juxtamembrane (56%) and reactivity (39%) with both domains [174]. This heterogeneity is not understood, but may be explained by HLA restriction since IA-2 (ICA512) in IDDM is associated with DQ8

[173,175]. Before a discussion of diagnostic sensitivity, specificity and predictive value of ICA512/IA-2 autoantibodies for IDDM, a novel isoform of IA-2, IA-2β, will be discussed.

IA-2β

A novel transmembrane PTP, IA-2β (Table 7.4), which is closely related but distinct from IA-2, was identified from cDNA libraries of a mouse neonatal brain [169], human colon carcinoma cells [176] and human islets [49]. The intracellular domain of the two β cell IA-2 isoforms show 74% amino acid identity, but the core sequence differs by only one amino acid, whereas part of the extracellular domain only shows 26% identity. Similar to IA-2, IA-2β is primarily expressed in pancreatic islets and brain. The IA-2β (also referred to as IAR or phogrin) cDNA was used in *in vitro* transcription and translation to prepare a radiolabelled autoantigen to demonstrate that about 50% of new onset patients have IA-2β autoantibodies [48,49,176]. Most IA-2 autoantibody-positive sera react with both isoforms. However, some IDDM sera have been found which distinguish between unique epitopes on either IA-2 or IA-2β [49].

The successful cloning of IA-2β also seems to solve the problem of the origin of the 37 kDa fragment which is immunoprecipitated with diabetic sera as it is able to block binding of radiolabelled 37 kDa tryptic fragments prior to immunoprecipitation [48]. Limited proteolysis suggests that IA-2β is the precursor of the 37 kDa fragment [169,176]. The diagnostic sensitivity of IA-2β for IDDM is about 50% and the specificity 99%. IA-2β reactivity is very similar to IA-2 and it is unclear as yet whether IA-2β should be included in the panel of IDDM autoantigens. It is possible to determine the extent IDDM sera may contain autoantibodies detecting epitopes unique to either IA-2 or IA-2β. For example, an IA-2/IA-2β hybrid molecule can be constructed and used as an autoantigen to maximize sensitivity and specificity. Future studies also need to define T cell epitopes and the apparent effect of age at onset on the diagnostic sensitivity, as well as association between HLA and the IA-2/IA-2β autoantibodies. The subcellular distribution and the function of the two IA-2 isoforms also need to be clarified, as well as when and why these two sister molecules are recognized as autoantigens associated with development of IDDM in about 50–60% of the patients.

RECOMBINANT AUTOANTIGENS – LOW PREVALENCE OF AUTOANTIBODIES

The following molecules have all been implicated as tentative autoantigens in IDDM either based on their ability to block the binding of diabetic sera to pancreas sections, or their detection by the use of selected sera from IDDM patients to screen different expression libraries (Table 7.5). Some of the molecules are candidate autoantigens because of observations in experimental animals or in other diseases of autoimmune character. A frequent problem is

Table 7.5 Recombinant β cell autoantigens – low sensitivity or questionable autoantibodies

Antigen	*Nature, location and autoantibody assay*
ICA69	Endocrine and exocrine 69 kDa protein. The rat but not the human ICA69 is homologous to a 17 amino acid peptide (ABBOS) of BSA. Western blotting but not radioligand assay detected ICA69 antibodies in 30% of ICA-positive first degree relatives later developing IDDM. Assay not standardized.
38 kD jun-B	Transcription factor expressed in the nucleus of many cells including islet β cells. T cell responses found in most recent onset IDDM patients. Immunoblotting detected jun-B antibodies in 33% IDDM new onset patients. Assays not standardized.
Carboxypeptidase H	A 52 kDa converting enzyme expressed in islet cell secretory granules. Not β cell specific. Immunoblotting detected CPH antibodies among ICA-positive first degree relatives but a radioligand assay failed to detect an increased frequency of CPH antibodies in new onset patients. Assays not standardized.
Heat shock protein	One of several HSPs inducible under hyperthermic conditions. Sequence homology with GAD65. ELISA test with recombinant murine hsp60 indicate an increased frequency of antibodies in Japanese IDDM and rheumatoid arthritis patients. Assay not standardized.
Aromatic-L-amino decarboxylase	AADC is a cytoplasmic 51 kDa protein expressed in the β cells and other cells synthesizing biogenic amines. Radioligand ([^{35}S]AADC) assay detect AADC autoantibodies in 51% APS 1 patients without and with IDDM but not necessarily in new onset IDDM patients. Assay not standardized.
DNA topoisomerase II	Nuclear 170 kDa enzyme which is expressed in β cells and many other cell types. May be a marker for autoimmunity. Autoantibodies to both full-length and fragments of DNA topoisomerase type II have been detected in 48% IDDM patients. Assay not standardized.

that initial publications appear with, as later realized, too few IDDM and control sera. Currently, the importance of this group of putative autoantigens remains to be determined, since many are only based on a single publications which have not yet been confirmed. However, some of these autoantigens have been cloned which will permit the production of a significant amount of protein for further characterization.

ICA69

Initially an islet cell antigen of 69 kDa (ICA69) (Table 7.5) was identified as a membrane-bound protein in rat insulinoma cells by crossreactivity with antibodies to bovine serum albumin [177]. ICA69 was cloned from a human islet cDNA expression library, the structural gene was designated ICA1, and it was mapped to human chromosome 7p22 [178]. The open reading frame of ICA69 predicts a 482 amino acid protein with some sequence homology to bovine serum albumin, a milk protein that was proposed to be a triggering factor of IDDM [177,179].

The highest expression of ICA69 mRNA was reported in human pancreatic islets and brain, and in rodent islet cell lines, testis, islets and brain [178–180]. These data correlate with Western blot analysis of human and mouse tissue which also revealed high levels of ICA69 in brain, testis, pancreas and islet cell lines. Further analysis detected that ICA69 is not islet cell specific, but is expressed at similar levels in human endocrine and exocrine pancreas [181]. The function of ICA69 currently remains elusive.

Autoantibodies against ICA69 detected by immunoblotting occur in 20–30% of sera from prediabetic individuals, and in recent onset patients and are independent of other islet autoantibodies such as ICA or IAA [178]. However, in a more recent study, less than 5% of newly diagnosed IDDM patients immunoprecipitated *in vitro* prepared ICA69 [130]. ICA69 autoantibodies alone are not adequate markers of the initial stages of IDDM as they have also been found in patients with rheumatoid arthritis [182].

T cell sensitization to ICA69 was reported to be most pronounced in recent onset IDDM patients compared to patients post-disease onset and non-diabetic first-degree relatives [183]. As has been proposed for GAD67 immune reactivity [154], an inverse correlation between T cell and autoantibody responsiveness to ICA69 was observed. Furthermore, whereas DR3 homozygous patients predominantly show T cell but not autoantibody reactivity to ICA69, DR4 homozygous patients showed the reverse reaction pattern (B. Roep, personal communications). Although available as a recombinant protein, the ICA69 autoantibody reactivity has not been easily reproduced and the role of ICA69 in the pathogenesis of IDDM remains controversial.

Glima 38

Glima 38 (Table 7.6) is a 38 kDa amphiphilic membrane glycoprotein expressed in islet cells and neuronal cell lines, and is immunoprecipitated by sera from about 20% of recent onset IDDM children and 14% of prediabetic first degree relatives [184]. A 38 kDa protein was described in the initial study of the 64 kDa autoantigen [23]. Glima 38 shares the neuroendocrine expression pattern characteristic of GAD65 and IA-2 and is distinct from imogen 38 and jun-B, both of which have a molecular mass of 38 kDa. Vigorous detergent extraction of islet cell proteins seems necessary to obtain significant immunoprecipitation

Table 7.6 Putative islet cell antigens and antigen preparations

Antibody reactive: glima 38	Amphiphilic 38 kDa membrane glycoprotein expressed in islet cells and neuroendocrine cells. Glima 38 antibodies were reported among 19% of recent onset IDDM patients
T cell reactive: imogen 38	Mitochondrial 38 kDa protein expressed in β cells and other cells. Imogen 38 was detected in a peptide display library screened with a T cell clone from an IDDM patient. The cDNA was isolated by hybridization to a mouse islet cell tumour cDNA library. T cell and autoantibody determination remains to be determined.
ISG 38 kDa	An insulin granule containing fraction from rat insulinoma cells used to stimulate human T cells in an autologous system. The 38 kDa component thought to be the responsible autoantigen remains to be identified.

of glima 38 with IDDM sera. Deglycosylation with N-glycanase reduced the molecular mass to 22 kDa. The molecular cloning of glima 38 is yet to be performed and the immunoprecipitation assay in Triton X-114 has been used to establish preliminary diagnostic sensitivity and specificity data for glima 38 autoantibodies in IDDM. While the prevalence of glima 38 autoantibodies in new onset IDDM patients was 19%, it is possible that the combination of GAD65 antibodies, IA-2 antibodies and glima 38 will yield a diagnostic sensitivity well above 90%. The specificity needs to be established since in the initial study too few healthy controls were tested [184]. IDDM sera which were glima 38 antibody-positive by immunoprecipitation were negative in a Western blot analysis, indicating that the IDDM autoantibody epitopes are conformational, as is also the case for GAD65 and IA-2 autoantibodies [184]. The presence of autoantibodies to the glima 38 autoantigen has not been confirmed by others.

38 kDa – jun-B

The early response nuclear transcription protein jun-B (38 kDa; Table 7.5) has been shown to be a target of autoreactive T cells in IDDM [185]. Using a 180 N-terminal amino acid recombinant jun-B preparation, peripheral blood T cell reactivity was demonstrated in 71% of recent onset IDDM patients, 50% of ICA-positive first-degree relatives, 25% off other autoimmune disease subjects and in no healthy controls. Autoantibodies against jun-B were reported to co-precipitate in 33% of GAD65 antibodies-positive sera from IDDM patients. The jun-B putative recombinant antigen is probably different from glima 38, since the former is a non-glycosylated nuclear protein and the latter a glycosylated membrane protein. Antibodies against an islet protein of 38 kDa were found in IDDM subjects carrying cytomegalovirus. Sequence comparison indicated that jun-B shares sequences with human cytomegalovirus and also with related herpes viruses antigens [185]. Again, jun-B as an autoantigen has only been reported once and confirmatory studies are needed.

Carboxypeptidase-H (CPH)

CPH, also known as enkephalin convertase, is a 52 kDa enzyme expressed in islet and neuroendocrine cells (Table 7.5). The enzyme is involved in the conversion of certain prohormones to the active hormone. CPH exists both as a membrane bound and a soluble form co-secreted from the islet granules together with insulin [186]. The serum used for screening an islet cell tumour library was from a single ICA-positive first–degree relative. Immunoprecipitation of the *in vitro* transcribed and translated CPH revealed no difference in antibody frequency between recent onset IDDM patients and controls [130]. This autoantigen has not been subjected to standardization.

Heat shock proteins (HSP)

HSP are stress proteins ubiquitously produced by cells in response to stimuli such as an increase in temperature, cytokines or free radicals. HSP are among the most conserved molecules in phylogeny and have been implicated in the pathogenesis of several autoimmune diseases including rheumatoid arthritis and NOD mouse diabetes [187]. Autoreactivity to an epitope of the 65-kDa HSP has been associated with IDDM, based on sequence homology to GAD65 (Table 7.5). Since HSP65 is reported to appear on the cell surface it could direct an immune response against intact β cells [188]. In addition, recombinant murine HSP60 used in ELISA detected antibodies in 16% of 84 IDDM subjects compared with 20% of 25 rheumatoid arthritis patients and 1% of 85 healthy controls [189]. Patients with slowly progressive IDDM, NIDDM and autoimmune thyroid disease were negative. This report warrants further investigations in other ethnic groups to establish the possible role of heat shock proteins as autoantigens in IDDM.

Aromatic-L-amino acid decarboxylase (AADC)

Sera from patients with APS 1 are often positive for autoantibodies against GAD65 and an unrelated 51 kDa β cell protein [190]. No cross-reactivity against the 51 kDa autoantigen was detected in sera from IDDM patients or from patients with other autoimmune diseases. The 51 kDa protein has been identified as AADC (Table 7.5) by screening an expression library derived from a rat insulinoma cell line [191]. AADC catalyses the decarboxylation of aromatic L-amino acids which are intermediates in the synthesis of catecholamines and indolamine neurotransmitters. As a decarboxylase, AADC uses pyridoxal-L-phosphate (PLP) as cofactor, and is a cytosolic enzyme. Apart from the active site, there is little sequence similarity between AADC and

GAD65. AADC is also present in the peripheral and central nervous system, liver, intestine and kidney.

Autoantibodies against AADC were sought in 69 patients with APS 1 and 138 IDDM patients using *in vitro* transcribed and translated AADC [192]. This study seemed to exclude AADC as an autoantigen in IDDM, since AADC antibodies were found in 51% of the APS 1 patients but in none of the IDDM patients or 91 healthy controls. Interestingly, AADC antibodies were more often found in patients with (92%) than without hepatitis (42%). Similarly, 80% of patients with vitiligo compared to 43% without had AADC antibodies. Although AADC is present in β cells and AADC antibodies are present in APS 1 patients who have a high frequency of IDDM [138], IDDM pathogenesis may not involve this cytoplasmic autoantigen.

DNA topoisomerase II

DNA topoisomerase type I and type II have been implicated as autoantigens in patients with autoimmune progressive systemic sclerosis or systemic lupus erythematosus and juvenile rheumatoid arthritis, respectively (Table 7.5). An increased frequency of nucleoprotein antibodies in IDDM patients and their relatives has been reported [193]. Recently, autoantibodies to both full-length and fragments of DNA topoisomerase type II were detected in 48% of 195 IDDM patients [194]. In contrast to ICA and IAA, the frequency of DNA topoisomerase type II antibodies was unaffected by gender, disease duration and age.

Since DNA topoisomerases are never exposed extracellularly, due to their location in the nucleus, it has been suggested that the autoimmune response originates from antigenic mimicry of other autoantigens or pathogens. Comparing the amino acid sequence of DNA topoisomerase type II with insulin, HSP65 and GAD revealed sequences which shared up to 64% homology. DNA topoisomerase type II antibodies may therefore be a result of an immune attack directed at other cytoplasmatic autoantigens after β cell destruction. Finally, it has been speculated that the overall antigenecity to DNA topoisomerase type II is stronger due to its large molecular mass of 170 kDa and complex structure [194]. It will be important to determine the diagnostic sensitivity and specificity of DNA topoisomerase antibodies using the recombinant protein in a standardized assay.

OTHER AUTOANTIGENS: ANTIBODY REACTIVE

Glycolipid/sialic acid

The possibility that the ICA indirect immunofluorescence reaction is explained by non-protein autoantibodies has been the subject of long term investigations. Organic solvents have been used to extract pancreatic tissue to produce glycolipid-containing fractions depleted of protein [195,196]. It was suggested that the target antigen of ICA was a sialoglycoconjugate since the fractions quantitatively blocked the fluorescence of a standard ICA-positive serum to human pancreatic sections. Evidence for the autoantigenic epitopes being glycolipids rather than glycoproteins was provided by the ability to recover blocking activity following treatment with borohydride. Comparing the co-migration of both human whole pancreas and islet extracts with ganglioside markers suggested that islets differentially express monosialoganglioside [196]. A GM2-1 pancreatic islet ganglioside has tentatively been identified as a putative ICA autoantigen [197].

OTHER AUTOANTIGENS: T CELL REACTIVE

Islet mitochondrial antigen 38 kDa (Imogen 38)

A human diabetic T cell clone was used to screen a recombinant antigen epitope library to identify the imogen 38 solely due to its recognition by T cells [198]. The cDNA of imogen 38 (Table 7.6) was isolated using a βTC3 mouse insulinoma cDNA library. It was speculated that imogen 38 is a target for bystander autoimmune attack rather than being a primary autoantigen in IDDM due to its broad tissue distribution [198]. Further studies are required to disclose the possible role of imogen 38 and similar T cell-defined autoantigens in the pathogenesis of IDDM.

Insulin secretory granule (ISG)

Granules extracted from rat insulinoma cell homogenates have been shown to stimulate proliferation of T cell clones isolated from the peripheral blood of a newly diagnosed IDDM patient [199]. The antigenic determinant of the ISG (Table 7.6) membrane proteins was suggested to be a 38 kDa component [183]. T cell reactivity was detected in 74% of 19 newly diagnosed IDDM patients and in 13% of 16 healthy controls. However, the two healthy subjects who produced responsive T cell lines had high titres of ICA autoantibodies. As discussed above, there are now several candidates for a 38 kDa autoantigen and it remains to be determined whether the 38 kDa ISG component may be glima 38, jun-B or imogen 38.

FUTURE DIRECTIONS

The presence of humoral immune markers, often several years before clinical disease, allows early detection and treatment of susceptible relatives of IDDM patients [200] possibly to be extended to the entire population. Antigen-specific immunotherapy, in particular using GAD65 and insulin, is effective in the NOD mouse [92,93] and the BB rat [201]. Importantly, by using the recombinant islet cell autoantigens GAD65, IA-2 and insulin in analyses of disease-associated antibodies, it has been possible to standardize the assays and to establish

Table 7.7 Diagnostic precision in autoantibody assays with recombinant β cell autoantigens

Autoantigen	*Sensitivity*	*Specificity*	*Predictive value*
Insulin	40–80%	99%	30%
GAD65	70–80%	99%	60%
GAD67	10–20%	99%	Very low
IA-2	50–60%	98–99%	30%
IA-2β	50%	99%	30%
ICA69	5–30%	94%	TBD
Glima 38	20%	100%	TBD
jun-B 38 kDa	33%	TBD	TBD
HSP60	16%	99%	TBD
AADC	0%	100%	TBD
DNA topoisomerase II	48%	99%	TBD

TBD = To be determined. The predictive value is estimated from studies of ICA-positive first degree relatives only.

comparable frequencies of sensitivity, specificity, and predictive values (Table 7.7). However, since GAD antibodies also are present in patients with other autoimmune diseases, e.g. stiff man syndrome, autoimmune thyroid disease and APS 1, they cannot be used alone for prediction of IDDM. Although the diagnostic sensitivity is lower for IAA and IA-2, the combination of the three major autoantigens in standardized autoantibody assays predict IDDM (Figure 7.1).

Several autoantibody workshops have taken place in order to standardize the different antibody assays [35–36]. A first attempt has also been made to standardize T cell proliferation tests with ambiguous results. Prior to extensive screening of school children or first degree relatives to identify individuals at risk for IDDM, it is critical to establish assay quality and concordance by proficiency testing. This is of particular importance if immune intervention therapy is considered. Numerous questions regarding autoantigen processing and presentation, as well as $CD4^+$ and $CD8^+$ T cell responses in relation to the temporal appearance of autoantigen immunoglobulin isotypes and subtypes will have to be answered before IDDM aetiology and pathogenesis is fully understood.

Acknowledgement

The research in the authors laboratory was supported by grants from the National Institutes of Health (DK26190, DK42334) and the Juvenile Diabetes Foundation International DIRP as well as the University of Washington Diabetes Research Council and the R H Williams Endowment. AP was supported by a mentor based fellowship from the American Diabetes Association.

References

1. Gepts W. Pathologic anatomy of the pancreas in juvenile diabetes mellitus. Diabetes. 1965; 14:619–33.
2. Foulis AK, Liddle CN, Farquharson MA, Richmond JA, Weir RS. The histopathology of the pancreas in type I (insulin-dependent) diabetes mellitus: a 25-year review of deaths in patients under 20 years of age in the United Kingdom. Diabetologia. 1986;29:267–74.
3. Gepts W, LaCompte PM. The pancreatic islets in diabetes. Am J Med. 1981;70:105–15.
4. Nerup J, Binder C. Thyroid, gastric and adrenal autoimmunity in diabetes mellitus. Acta Endocrinol. 1973;72:279–86.
5. MacCuish AC, Irvine WJ. Autoimmunological aspects of diabetes mellitus. Clin Endocrinol Metab. 1975;4:435–71.
6. Drell DW, Notkins AL. Multiple immunological abnormalities in patients with Type 1 (insulin-dependent) diabetes mellitus. Diabetologia. 1987;30:132–43.
7. Singal DP, Blajchman MA. Histocompatibility (HL-A) antigens, lymphocytotoxic antibodies and tissue antibodies in patients with diabetes mellitus. Diabetes. 1973;22:429–32.
8. Nerup J, Platz P, Anderssen OO. HL-A antigens and diabetes mellitus. Lancet. 1974;2:864–6.
9. Bottazzo GF, Florin-Christensen A, Doniach D. Islet cell antibodies in diabetes mellitus with autoimmune polyendocrine deficiencies. Lancet. 1974;2:1279–83.
10. MacCuish AC, Barnes EW, Irvine WJ, Duncan LJP. Antibodies to pancreatic islet cells in insulin-dependent diabetics with coexistent autoimmune disease. Lancet. 1974;2:1529–31.
11. Lernmark Å. Islet cell antibodies-theoretical and practical implications. Diabetes Med. 1987; 4:285–92.
12. Lernmark Å, Baekkeskov S. Islet cell antibodies-theoretical and practical implications. Diabetologia. 1981;212:431–5.
13. Lernmark Å. The preparation of, and studies on, free cell suspensions from mouse pancreatic islets. Diabetologia. 1974;10:431–8.
14. Dobersen MJ, Scharff JE, Ginsberg-Fellner F, Notkins AL. Cytotoxic autoantibodies to beta cells in the serum of patients with insulin-dependent diabetes mellitus. N Engl J Med. 1980; 303:1493–8.
15. Eisenbarth GS, Morris MA, Scearce RM. Cytotoxic antibodies to cloned rat islet cells in serum of patients with diabetes mellitus. J Clin Invest. 1981;67:403–8.
16. Rabinovitch A, MacKay P, Ludvigsson J, Lernmark Å. A prospective analysis of islet cell cytotoxic antibodies in insulin-dependent diabetic children: transient effects of plasmapheresis. Diabetes. 1984;33:224–8.
17. Lernmark Å, Freedman ZR, Hofmann C et al. IsleT cell-surface antibodies in juvenile diabetes mellitus. N Engl J Med. 1978;299:375–80.
18. Johnson JH, Crider BP, McCorkle K, Alford M, Unger RH. Inhibition of glucose transport into rat islet cells by immunoglobulins from patients with new-onset insulin-dependent diabetes mellitus. N Engl J Med. 1990;322:653–9.
19. Kanatsuna T, Baekkeskov S, Lernmark Å, Ludvigsson J. Immunoglobulin from insulin-dependent diabetic children inhibits glucose-induced insulin release. Diabetes. 1983;32:520–4.
20. Bordier C. Phase separation of integral membrane proteins in Triton X-114 solution. J Biol Chem 1981;256:1604–7.
21. Baekkeskov S, Kanatsuna T, Klareskog L et al. Expression of major histocompatibility antigens on pancreatic islet cells. Proc Nat Acad Sci USA. 1981;78:6456–60.
22. Lernmark Å, Nathan A, Steiner DF. Preparation and characterization of plasma membrane-enriched fractions from rat pancreatis islets. J Cell Biol. 1976;71:606–23.
23. Baekkeskov S, Nielsen JH, Marner B, Bilde T, Ludvigsson J, Lernmark Å. Autoantibodies in newly diagnosed diabetic children immunoprecipitate human pancreatic islet cell proteins. Nature. 1982;298:167–9.
24. Baekkeskov S, Lernmark Å. Rodent islet antigens recognized by antibodies in sera from diabetic patients. Acta Biol Med Germ. 1982;41:1111–15.
25. Baekkeskov S, Aanstoot HJ, Christgau S et al. Identification of the 64 kDa autoantigen in insulin-dependent diabetes as the GABA-synthesizing enzyme glutamic acid decarboxylase. Nature. 1990;347:151–6.

26. Solimena M, Folli F, Denis-Donini S et al. Autoantibodies directed against glutamic acid decarboxylase (GAD) in the cerebrospinal fluid and serum of a patient with stiff-man syndrome, epilepsy and type I diabetes mellitus. N Engl J Med. 1988;318:1012–20.
27. Karlsen AE, Hagopian WA, Grubin CE et al. Cloning and primary structure of a human islet isoform of glutamic acid decarboxylase from chromosome 10. Proc Natl Acad Sci USA. 1991;88:8337–41.
28. Bu D-F, Erlander MG, Hitz BC et al. Two human glutamate decarboxylases, 65-kDa GAD and 67-kDa GAD, are each encoded by a single gene. Proc Natl Acad Sci USA. 1992;89: 2115–19.
29. Erlander MG, Tillakaratne NJK, Feldblum S, Patel N, Tobin AJ. Two genes encode distinct glutamate decarboxylase. Neuron. 1991;7:91–100.
30. Karlsen AE, Hagopian WA, Petersen JS et al. Recombinant glutamic acid decarboxylase representing a single isoform expressed in human islets detects IDDM associated 64 kDa autoantibodies. Diabetes. 1992;41:1355–9.
31. Atkinson MA, Maclaren NK. Islet cell autoantigens in insulin-dependent diabetes. J Clin Invest. 1993;92:1608–16.
32. Colman PG. IDW GAD Antibody Workshop. 13th International Immunology and Diabetes. Workshop. Montvillargenne, France, 1994.
33. Solimena M, Butler MH, De Camilli P. GAD, diabetes, and stiff-man syndrome: some progress and more questions. J Endocrinol Invest. 1994;17:509-20.
34. Sanjeevi CB, Falorni A, Robertson J, Lernmark A. Glutamic acid decarboxylase (GAD) in insulin-dependent diabetes mellitus. Diabetes Nutr Metab. 1996;9:167–82.
35. Schmidli RS, Colman PG, Bonifacio E, Bottazzo GF, Harrison LC. High level of concordance between assays for glutamic acid decarboxylase antibodies. The First International Glutamic Acid Decarboxylase Antibody Workshop. Diabetes. 1994;43:1005–9.
36. Schmidli RS, Colman PG, Bonifacio E. Disease sensitivity and specificity of 52 assays for glutamic acid decarboxylase antibodies. The Second International Glutamic Acid Decarboxylase Workshop. Diabetes. 1995;44:636–40.
37. Palmer JP, Asplin CM, Clemons P et al. Insulin antibodies in insulin-dependent diabetics before insulin treatment. Science. 1983;222:1337–9.
38. Rabin DU, Pleasic SM, Palmer-Crocker R, Shapiro JA. Cloning and expression of IDDM-specific human autoantigens. Diabetes. 1992;41:183–6.
39. Lan MS, Lu J, Goto Y, Notkins AL. Molecular cloning and identification of a receptor-type protein tyrosine phosphatase, IA-2, from human insulinoma. DNA Cell Biol. 1994;13:505–14.
40. Eisenbarth GS, Jackson GS. Insulin autoimmunity: the rate limiting factor of pre-type 1 diabetes. J Autoimmun. 1992;5:214–46.
41. Vardi P, Keller R, Dib S, Eisenbarth GS, Soeldner JS. Log-linear correlation of CIAA with age in new onset type I diabetics. Diabetes. 1988;37:28A.
42. Böhmer K, Keilacker H, Kuglin B et al. Proinsulin autoantibodies are more closely associated with Type 1 (insulin-dependent) diabetes mellitus than insulin autoantibodies. Diabetologia. 1991;34:830–4.
43. Kuglin B, Gries FA, Kolb H. Evidence of IgG autoantibodies against human proinsulin in patients with IDDM before insulin treatment. Diabetes. 1988;37:130–2.
44. Hanahan D. Transgenic mouse models of self-tolerance and autoreactivity by the immune system. Annu Rev Cell Biol. 1990;6:493–537.
45. Rabin DU, Pleasic SM, Shapiro JA et al. Islet cell antigen 512 is a diabetes-specific islet autoantigen related to protein tyrosine phosphatases. J Immunol. 1994;152:3183–7.
46. Christie MR, Vohra G, Champagne P, Daneman D, Delovitch TL. Distinct antibody specificities to a 64-kD islet cell antigen in type 1 diabetes as revealed by trypsin treatment. J Exp Med. 1990;172:789–94.
47. Christie MR, Tun RYM, Lo SSS et al. Antibodies to GAD and tryptic fragments of islet 64 kDa antigen as distinct markers for development of IDDM. Diabetes. 1992;41:782–7.
48. Payton MA, Hawkes CJ, Christie MR. Relationship of the 37,000- and 40,000-Mr tryptic fragments of islet antigens in insulin-dependent diabetes to the protein tyrosine phosphatase-like molecule IA-2 (ICA512). J Clin Invest. 1995;96:1506–11.
49. Wasmeier C, Hutton JC. Molecular cloning of phogrin, a protein-tyrosine phosphatase homologue localized to insulin secretory granule membranes. J Biol Chem. 1996;271: 18161–70.

50. Hagopian WA, Woo W, Kockum I et al. Age-related prediction of autoimmune diabetes by phenotypic and genotypic markers in the general population. Submitted 1996.
51. Christie MR, Genovese S, Cassidy D et al. Antibodies to islet 37k antigen, but not to glutamate decarboxylase, discriminate rapid progression to IDDM in endocrine autoimmunity. Diabetes. 1994;43:1254–9.
52. Wiest-Ladenburger U, Hartmann R, Hartmann U, Berling K, Böhm BO, Richter W. Combined analysis and single-step detection of GAD65 and IA2 autoantibodies in IDDM can replace the histochemical islet cell antibody test. Diabetes. 1997;46:565–71.
53. Lernmark A. Glutamic acid decarboxylase – gene to antigen to disease. J Internal Med. 1996;240:259–77.
54. Greenbaum CJ, Brooks-Worrell BM, Palmer JP, Lernmark Å. Autoimmunity and prediction of insulin dependent diabetes mellitus. Diabetes Annu. 1994;8:21–52.
55. Grodsky GM, Feldman R, Toreson WE, Lee JC. Diabetes. mellitus in rabbits immunized with insulin. J Am Diabetes Assoc. 1966;15:579–85.
56. Srikanta S, Ricker AT, McCulloch DK, Soeldner JS, Eisenbarth GS, Palmer JP. Autoimmunity to insulin, beta cell dysfunction, and development of insulin-dependent diabetes mellitus. Diabetes. 1986;35:139–42.
57. Landin-Olsson M, Palmer JP, Lernmark Å et al. Predictive value of islet cell and insulin autoantibodies for type 1 (insulin-dependent) diabetes mellitus in a population-based study of newly-diagnosed diabetic and matched control children. Diabetologia. 1992;35:1068–73.
58. Vardi P, Ziegler AG, Matthews JH et al. Concentration of insulin autoantibodies at onset of type I diabetes: inverse log-linear correlation with age. Diabetes Care. 1988;9:736–9.
59. Palmer JP. Insulin autoantibodies: their role in the pathogenesis of IDDM. Diabetes Metab. Rev. 1987;3:1005–15.
60. Palmer JP, Wilkin TJ, Kurtz AB, Bonifacio E. The third international workshop on the standardization of insulin antibody measurement. Diabetologia. 1990;33:60–1.
61. Greenbaum CJ, Palmer JP, Kuglin B, Kolb H. Insulin autoantibodies measured by radioimmunoassay methodology are more related to insulin-dependent diabetes mellitus than those measured by enzyme-linked immunosorbent assay. Results of the Fourth International Workshop on the Standardization of Insulin Autoantibody measurement. J Clin Endcrinol Metab. 1992;74:1040–4.
62. Kuglin B, Kolb H, Greenbaum C, Maclaren NK, Lernmark A, Palmer JP. The fourth international workshop on the standardisation of insulin autoantibody measurement. Diabetologia. 1990;33:638–9.
63. Levy-Marchal C, Bridel M-P, Sodoyez-Goffauz F et al. Superiority of radiobinding assay over ELISA for detection of IAAs in newly diagnosed Type 1 diabetic children. Diabetes Care. 1991;14:61–3.
64. Soeldner JS, Tuttleman M, Srikanta S et al. Insulin-dependent diabetes and autoimmunity: islet cell autoantibodies, insulin autoantibodies and beta cell failure. N Engl J Med. 1985;313:893–4.
65. Castano L, Ziegler A, Ziegler R, Shoelson S, Eisenbarth GS. Characterization of insulin autoantibodies in relatives of patients with insulin-dependent diabetes mellitus. Diabetes. 1993;42:1202–9.
66. Ziegler R, Alper CA, Awdeh ZL et al. Specific association of HLA-DR4 with increased prevalence and level of insulin autoantibodies in first-degree relatives of patients with Type 1 diabetes. Diabetes. 1991;40:709–14.
67. Pugliese A, Bugawan R, Moromisato R et al. Two subsets of HLA-DQA1 alleles mark phenotypic variation in levels of insulin autoantibodies in first degree relatives at risk for insulin-dependent diabetes. J Clin Invest. 1994;93:2447–52.
68. Ludvigsson J, Binder C, Mandrup-Poulsen T. Insulin autoantibodies are associated with islet cell antibodies: their relation to insulin autoantibodies and B-cell function in diabetic children. Diabetologia. 1988;31:647–51.
69. Casali P, Nakamura M, Ginsberg-Fellner F, Notkins A. Frequency of Beta cells committed to the production of antibodies to insulin in newly diagnosed patients with insulin-dependent diabetes mellitus and generation of high affinity human monoclonal IgG to insulin. J Immunol. 1990;144:3741–7.
70. Arslanian SA, Becker DJ, Rabin B et al. Correlates of insulin antibodies in newly diagnosed children with insulin-dependent diabetes before insulin therapy. Diabetes. 1985;34:926–30.
71. Gorus FK, Vandewalle CL, Dorchy H et al. Influence of age on the associations among insulin autoantibodies, islet cell antibodies, and HLA DQA1*0301-DQB1*0302 and siblings

of patients with type 1 (insulin-dependent) diabetes mellitus. J Clin Endocrinol. 1994;78: 1172–8.
72. Vandewalle CL, Decraene T, Schuit FC, De-Leeuw IH, Pipeleers DG, Gorus FK. Insulin autoantibodies and high titre islet cell antibodies are preferentially associated with the HLA DQA1*0301-DQB1*0302 haplotype at clinical type 1 (insulin-dependent) diabetes mellitus before age 10 years, but not at onset between age 10 and 40 years. The Belgian Diabetes. Registry. Diabetologia. 1993;36:1155–62.
73. Bingley PJ. Interactions of age, islet cell antibodies, insulin autoantibodies, and first-phase insulin response in predicting risk of progression to IDDM in ICA(+) relatives: The ICARUS data set. Diabetes. 1996;45(12):1720–8.
74. Thivolet C, Beaufrere B, Beutel H et al. Islet cell and insulin autoantibodies in subjects at high risk for the development of type 1 (insulin-dependent) diabetes mellitus: the Lyon family study. Diabetologia. 1988;31:741–6.
75. McCulloch DK, Klaff LJ, Kahn SE et al. Nonprogression of subclinical ß-cell dysfunction among first degree relatives of IDDM patients: 5-yr follow-up of the Seattle family study. Diabetes. 1990;39:549–56.
76. Bärmeier H, McCulloch DK, Neifing JL et al. Risk for developing type 1 (insulin-dependent) diabetes mellitus and the presence of islet 64 kDa antibodies. Diabetologia. 1991;34:727–33.
77. Sochett E, Daneman D. Relationship of insulin autoantibodies to presentation and early course of IDDM in children. Diabetes Care. 1989;12:517–23.
78. Levy-Marchal C, Tichet J, Fajardy I, Gu XF, Dubois F, Czernichow P. Islet cell antibodies in normal French school-children. Diabetologia. 1992;35:577–82.
79. Rowe RE, Leech NJ, Nepom GT, McCulloch DK. High genetic risk for IDDM in the Pacific Northwest. First report from the Washington State Diabetes. Prediction Study. Diabetes. 1994;43:87–94.
80. Daniel D, Gill RG, Schloot N, Wegmann D. Epitope specificity, cytokine production profile and diabetogenic activity of insulin-specific T cell clones isolated from NOD mice. Eur J Immunol. 1995;25:1056–62.
81. Rudy G, Stone N, Harrison LC et al. Similar peptides from two beta cell autoantigens, proinsulin and glutamic acid decarboxylase, stimulate T cells of individuals at risk for insulin-dependent diabetes. Mol Med. 1995;1:625–33.
82. Solimena M, De Camilli P. Autoimmunity to glutamic acid decarboxylase (GAD) in stiff man syndrome and insulin-dependent diabetes mellitus. Trends Neurosci. 1991;14:452–7.
83. Kaufman DJ, Erlander MG, Clare-Salzler M, Atkinson MA, Maclaren NK, Tobin AJ. Autoimmunity to two forms of glutamate decarboxylase in Insulin-dependent diabetes mellitus. J Clin Invest. 1992;89:283–92.
84. Erdö SL, Wolff JR. Gamma-aminobutyric acid outside the mammalian brain. J Neurochem. 1990;54:363–72.
85. Martin DL. Short-term control of GABA synthesis in brain. Prog Biophys molec Biol 1993;60:17–28.
86. Okada Y, Taniguchi H, Shimada C. High concentration of GABA and high glutamate decarboxylase activity in rat pancreatic islets and human insulinoma. Science. 1976;194: 620–2.
87. Okada Y. Localization and function of GABA in the pancreatic islets. In: Erdö SL, Bowery NG, eds. GABAergic Mechanisms in the Mammalian Periphery. New York; Raven Press; 1986:223–40.
88. Persson Å, Pelto-Huikko M, Metsis M et al. Expression of the neurotransmitter-synthesizing enzyme glutamic acid decarboxylase in male germ cells. Mol Cell Biol. 1990;10:4701–11.
89. Hagopian WA, Michelsen B, Karlsen AE et al. Autoantibodies in IDDM primarily recognize the 65,000-Mr rather than the 67,000-Mr isoform of glutamic acid decarboxylase. Diabetes. 1993;42:631–6.
90. Grubin CE, Daniels T, Toivola B et al. A novel radioligand binding assay to determine diagnostic accuracy of isoform-specific glutamic acid decarboxylase antibodies in childhood IDDM. Diabetologia. 1994;37:344–50.
91. Petersen JS, Hejnaes KR, Moody A et al. Detection of GAD65 antibodies in diabetes and other autoimmune diseases using a simple radioligand assay. Diabetes. 1994;43:459–65.
92. Kaufman DL, Clare-Salzler M, Tian J et al. Spontaneous loss of T cell tolerance to glutamic acid decarboxylase in murine insulin-dependent diabetes. Nature. 1993;366:69–72.

93. Tisch R, Yang X-D, Singer SM, Liblau RS, Fugger L, McDevitt HO. Immune response to glutamic acid decarboxylase correlates with insulitis in non-obese diabetic mice. Nature. 1993;366:72–5.
94. Bu DF, Tobin AJ. The exon-intron organization of the genes (GAD1 and GAD2) encoding two human glutamate decarboxylases (GAD67 and GAD65) suggests that they derive from a common ancestral GAD. Genomics. 1994;21:222–8.
95. Edelhoff S, Grubin CE, Karlsen AE et al. Mapping of glutamic acid decarboxylase (GAD) genes. Genomics. 1993;17:93–7.
96. Wapelhorst B, Bell GI, Risch N, Spielman RS, Concannon P. Linkage and association studies in insulin-dependent diabetes with a new dinucleotide repeat polymorphism at the GAD65 locus. Autoimmunity. 1995;21:127–30.
97. Martin DL, Wu SJ, Martin SB. Glutamate-dependent active-site labeling of brain glutamate decarboxylase. J Neurochem. 1990;55:524–32.
98. Martin DL, Rimvall K. The regulation of GABA synthesis in the brain. J Neurochem. 1993; 60:395–407.
99. Sheikh S, Martin DL. Heteromers of glutamate decarboxylase isoforms occur in cerebellum. J Neurochem. 1996;66:2082–90.
100. Michelsen BK, Petersen JS, Boel E, Møldrup A, Dyrberg T, Madsen OD. Cloning, characterization, and autoimmune recognition of rat islet glutamic acid decarboxylase in insulin-dependent mellitus. Proc Natl Acad Sci USA. 1991;88:8754–8.
101. Erlander MG, Tobin AJ. The structural and functional heterogeneity of glutamic acid decarboxylase: a review. Neurochem Res. 1991;16:215–26.
102. Martin DL, Martin SB, Wu S, Espina N. Regulatory properties of brain glutamate decarboxylase: the apoenzyme of GAD is present principally as one of two molecular forms of GAD in brain. J Neurosci. 1991;11:2725–31.
103. Rimvall K, Martin DL. The level of GAD_{67} protein is highly sensitive to small increases in intraneuronal gamma-aminobutyric acid levels. J Neurochem. 1994;62:1375–81.
104. Baekkeskov S, Warnock G, Christie M, Rajotte RV, Larsen PM, Fey S. Revelation of specificity of 64 kDa autoantibodies in IDDM serums by high-resolution 2-D gel electrophoresis. Diabetes. 1990;38:1133–41.
105. Christgau S, Schierbeck H, Aanstoot H-J et al. Pancreatic ß cells express two autoantigenic forms of glutamic acid decarboxylase, a 65-kDa hydrophilic form and a 64-kDa amphiphilic form which can be both membrane-bound and soluble. J Biol Chem. 1991;286:21257–64.
106. Briel G, Gylfe E, Hellman B, Neuhoff V. Microdetermination of free amino acids in pancreatic islets isolated from obese-hyperglycemia mice. Acta Physiol Scand. 1972;84:247–53.
107. Reetz A, Solimena M, Matteoli M, Folli F, Takei K, De Camilli P. GABA and pancreatic β-cells: co-localization of glutamic acid decarboxylase (GAD) and GABA with synaptic-like microvesicles suggests their role in GABA storage and secretion. EMBO J. 1991;10: 1275–84.
108. Solimena M, Aggujaro D, Muntzel C et al. Association of GAD-65, but not of GAD-67, with the Golgi complex of transfected Chinese hamster ovary cells mediated by the N-terminal region. Proc Natl Acad Sci USA. 1993;90:3073–7.
109. Solimena M, Dirkx R Jr, Radzynski M, Mudigl O, De Camilli P. A signal located within amino acids 1-27 of GAD65 is required for its targeting to the Golgi complex region. J Cell Biol. 1994;126:331–41.
110. Dirkx R Jr, Thomas A, Linsong L et al. Targeting of the 67-kDa isoform of glutamic acid decarboxylase to intracellular organelles is mediated by its interaction with the NH2-terminal region of the 65-kDa isoform of glutamic acid decarboxylase. J Biol Chem. 1995; 270:2241–6.
111. Erdo SL, Joo F, Wolff JR. Immunohistochemical localization of glutamate decarboxylase in the rat oviduct and ovary: further evidence for non-neural GABA system. Cell Tiss Res. 1989;255:431–4.
112. Michalik M, Nelson J, Erecinska M. GABA production in rat islets of Langerhans. Diabetes. 1993;42:1506–13.
113. Vincent ST, Hökfelt T, Wu J-Y, Eide RP, Morgan LM, Kimmel JR. Immunohistochemical studies of the GABA system in the pancreas. Neuroendocrinology. 1983;36:197–204.
114. Tobin AJ, Breecha N, Chiang M-Y et al. Alternative forms of GAD and $GABA_A$ receptors. In: Biggio G, Costa E, eds. GABAergic Synaptic Transmission. New York: Raven Press; 1992:55–66.

115. Gylfe E. Serotonin as marker for the secretory granules in the pancreatic β-cell. Acta Physiol Scand. 1977;452:125–8.
116. Gilon P, Bertrand G, Loubatieres-Mariani MM, Remacle C, Henquin JC. The influence of γ-aminobutyric acid on hormone release by the mouse and rat endocrine pancreas. Endocrinology. 1991;129:2521–9.
117. Rorsman P, Berggren PO, Bokvist K et al. Glucose-inhibition of glucagon secretion involves activation of GABAA-receptor chloride channels. Nature. 1989;341:233–6.
118. Hagopian WA, Karlsen AE, Petersen JS et al. Regulation of glutamic acid decarboxylase diabetes autoantigen expression in highly purified isolated islets from *Macaca nemestrina*. Endocrinology. 1993;132:2674–81.
119. Velloso LA, Kämpe O, Hallberg A, Christmanson L, Betsholtz C, Karlsson FA. Demonstration of GAD-65 as the main immunogenic isoform of glutamate decarboxylase in type 1 diabetes and determination of autoantibodies using a radioligand produced by eukaryotic expression. J Clin Invest. 1993;91:2084-90.
120. Falorni A, Örtqvist E, Persson B, Lernmark Å. Radioimmunoassays for glutamic acid decarboxylase (GAD65) and GAD65 autoantibodies using ^{35}S or ^{3}H recombinant human ligands. J Immunol Meth. 1995;186:89–99.
121. Vandewalle CL, Falorni A, Svanholm S et al. High diagnostic sensitivity of glutamate decarboxylase autoantibodies in IDDM with clinical onset between age 20 and 40 years. J Clin Endocrinol Metab. 1995;80:846–50.
122. Seissler J, Amann J, Mauch L et al. Prevalence of autoantibodies to the 65- and 67-kD isoforms of glutamate decarboxylase in insulin-dependent diabetes mellitus. J Clin Invest. 1993;92:1394–9.
123. DeAizpurua HJ, Harrison LC, Cram DS. An ELISA for antibodies to recombinant glutamic acid decarboxylase in IDDM. Diabetes. 1992;41:1182–7.
124. Schmidli RS, DeAizpurua HJ, Harrison LC, Colman PG. Antibodies to glutamic acid decarboxylase in at-risk and clinical insulin-dependent diabetic subjects: relationship to age, sex and islet cell antibody status, and temporal profile. J Autoimmun. 1994;7:55–66.
125. Genovese S, Bingley PJ, Bonifacio E et al. Combined analysis of IDDM-related autoantibodies in healthy school children. Lancet. 1994;344:756.
126. Rowley MJ, Mackay JR, Chen Q-Y, Knowles WJ, Zimmet PZ. Antibodies to glutamic acid decarboxylase discriminate major types of diabetes mellitus. Diabetes. 1992;41:548–51.
127. Grubin C, Daniels T, Karlsen AE, Boel E, Hagopian WA, Lernmark Å. The cDNA-directed, in vitro-synthesized nascent peptide of glutamic acid decarboxylase (GAD2) is the autoantigen in insulin-dependent diabetes. Clin Res. 1992;40:299A.
128. Verge CF, Gianani R, Kawasaki E et al. Prediction of type I diabetes in first-degree relatives using a combination of insulin, GAD, and ICA512bdc/IA-2 autoantibodies. Diabetes. 1996; 45:926–33.
129. Gianani R, Rabin DU, Verge CF et al. ICA512 autoantibody radioassay. Diabetes. 1995;44: 1340–4.
130. Bonifacio E, Genovese S, Braghi S et al. Islet autoantibody markers in IDDM: risk assessment strategies yielding high sensitivity. Diabetologia. 1995;38:816–22.
131. Falorni A, Nikosjkov A, Laureti S et al. High diagnostic accuracy for idiopathic Addison's disease with a sensitive radiobinding assay for autoantibodies against recombinant human 21-hydroxylase. J Clin Endocrinol. 1995;80:2752–5.
132. Vandewalle CL, Falorni A, Svanholm S, Lernmark A, Pipeleers DG, Gorus FK. High diagnostic sensitivity of glutamate decarboxylase autoantibodies in insulin-dependent diabetes mellitus with clinical onset between age 20 and 40 years. The Belgian Diabetes. Registry. J Clin Endocrinol Metab. 1995;80:846–51.
133. Yu L, Chase HP, Falorni A, Rewers M, Lernmark Å, Eisenbarth GS. Sexual dimorphism in transmission to offspring of expression of islet autoantibodies. Diabetologia. 1995;38:1353–7.
134. Ivarsson SA, Ackefors M, Carlsson A et al. Glutamate decarboxylase antibodies in non-diabetic pregnancies precedes insulin-dependent diabetes in the mother but not necessarily in the offspring. Autoimmunity. 1997;26:261–9.
135. Norris JM, Beaty B, Klingensmith G et al. Lack of association between early exposure to cow's milk protein and beta cell autoimmunity. Diabetes. Autoimmunity Study in the Young (DAISY) [see comments]. J Am Med Assoc. 1996;276:609–14.
136. Kawasaki E, Takino H, Yano M et al. Autoantibodies to glutamic acid decarboxylase in patients with IDDM and autoimmune thyroid disease. Diabetes. 1994;43:80–6.

137. Sundkvist G, Velloso LA, Kämpe O et al. Glutamic acid decarboxylase antibodies, autonomic nerve antibodies and autonomic neuropathy in diabetic patients. Diabetologia. 1994;37:293–9.
138. Tuomi T, Björses P, Falorni A et al. Antibodies to glutamic acid decarboxylase and insulin-dependent diabetes in patients with autoimmune polyendocrine syndrome type I. J Clin Endocrinol Metab. 1996;81:1488–94.
139. Björk E, Velloso LA, Kämpe O, Karlsson FA. GAD autoantibodies in IDDM, stiff-man syndrome, and autoimmune polyendocrine syndrome type I recognize different epitopes. Diabetes. 1994;43:161–5.
140. Hallengren B, Falorni A, Landin-Olsson M, Lernmark Å, Papadopoulos KI, Sundkvist G. Islet cell and glutamic acid decarboxylase antibodies in hyperthyroid patients: at diagnosis and following treatment. J Intern Med. 1996;239:63–8.
141. Tsuruoka A, Matsuba I, Toyota T, Isshiki G, Nagataki S, Ikeda Y. Antibodies to GAD in Japanese diabetic patients: a multicenter study. Diabetes. Res Clin Pract. 1995;28:191–9.
142. Daw K, Powers AC. Two distinct glutamic acid decarboxylase auto-antibody specificities in IDDM target difference epitopes. Diabetes. 1995;44:216–20.
143. Falorni A, Ackefors M, Carlberg C et al. Diagnostic sensitivity of immunodominant epitopes of glutamic acid decarboxylase (GAD65) autoantibodies epitopes in childhood IDDM. Diabetologia. 1996;39:1091–8.
144. Syren K, Lindsay L, Stoehrer B et al. Immune reactivity of diabetes-associated human monoclonal autoantibodies defines multiple epitopes and detects two domain boundaries in glutamate decarboxylase. J Immunol. 1996;157:5208–14.
145. Butler MH, Solimena M, Dirkx J, R., Hayday A, De Camilli P. Identification of a dominant epitope of glutamic acid decarboxylase (GAD-65) recognized by autoantibodies in stiff-man syndrome. J Exp Med. 1993;178:2097–106.
146. Kim J, Namchuck M, Bugawan T et al. Higher autoantibody levels and recognition of a linear NH2-terminal epitope in the autoantigen GAD65, distinguish stiff-man syndrome from insulin-dependent diabetes mellitus. J Exp Med. 1994;180:595–606.
147. Li L, Hagopian WA, Brashear HR, Daniels T, Lernmark Å. Identification of autoantibody epitopes of glutamic acid decarboxylase in stiff-man syndrome patients. J Immunol. 1994; 152:930–4.
148. Daw K, Ujihara N, Atkinson M, Powers AC. Glutamic acid decarboxylase autoantibodies in stiff-man syndrome and insulin-dependent diabetes mellitus exhibit similarities and differences in epitope recognition. J Immunol. 1996;156:818–25.
149. Richter W, Endl J, Eiermann TH et al. Human monoclonal islet cell antibodies from a patient with insulin-dependent diabetes mellitus reveal glutamate decarboxylase as the target antigen. Proc Natl Acad Sci USA. 1992;89:846–7.
150. Richter W, Jury KM, Loeffler D, Manfras BJ, Eiermann TH, Boehm BO. Immunoglobulin variable gene analysis of human autoantibodies reveals antigen-driven immune response to glutamate decarboxylase in type 1 diabetes mellitus. Eur J Immunol. 1995;25:1703–12.
151. Richter W, Northemann W, Müller M, Böhm BO. Mapping of an autoreactive epitope with glutamate decarboxylase using a diabetes-associated monoclonal antibody and an epitope cDNA library. Hybridoma. 1996;15:103–8.
152. Madec AM, Rousset F, Ho S et al. Four IgG anti-islet human monoclonal antibodies isolated from a type 1 diabetes patient recognize distinct epitopes of glutamic acid decarboxylase 65 and are somatically mutated. J Immunol. 1996;156:3541–9.
153. Atkinson MA, Kaufman DL, Campbell L et al. Response of peripheral-blood mononuclear cells to glutamate decarboxylase in insulin-dependent diabetes. Lancet. 1992;339:458–9.
154. Harrison LC, Honeyman MC, Deaizpurua HJ et al. Inverse regulation between humoral and cellular immunity to glutamic acid decarboxylase in subjects at risk of insulin-dependent diabetes. Lancet. 1993;341:1365–9.
155. Worsaae A, Hejnaes K, Moody A et al. T cell proliferative responses to glutamic acid decarboxylase-65 in IDDM are negatively associated with HLA-DR3/4. J Autoimmun. 1995;22:183–9.
156. Honeyman MC, Cram DS, Harrison LC. Glutamic acid decarboxylase 67-reactive T cells: a marker of insulin-dependent diabetes. J Exp Med. 1993;177:535–40.
157. Lohmann T, Leslie RDG, Hawa M, Geysen M, Rodda S, Londei M. Immunodominant epitopes of glutamic acid decarboxylase 65 and 67 in insulin-dependent diabetes mellitus. Lancet. 1994;343:1607–8.

158. Kwok WW, Nepom GT, Raymond FC. HLA-DQ polymorphisms are highly selective for peptide binding interactions. J Immunol. 1995;155:2468–76.
159. Kwok WW, Domeier ML, Raymond FC, Byers P, Nepom GT. Allele-specific motifs characterize HLA-DQ interactions with a diabetes-associated peptide derived from glutamic acid decarboxylase. J Immunol. 1996;156(6):2171–7.
160. Wicker LS, Chen SL, Nepom GT et al. Naturally processed T cell epitopes from human glutamic acid decarboxylase identified using mice transgenic for the type 1 diabetes-associated human MHC class II allele, DRB1*0401. J Clin Invest. 1996;98:2597–603.
161. Nepom BS, Nepom GT, Coleman M, Kwok WW. Critical contribution of beta chain residue 57 in peptide binding ability of both HLA-DR and -DQ molecules. Proc Natl Acad Sci USA. 1996;93:7202–6.
162. Atkinson MA, Bowman MA, Campbell L, Darrow BL, Kaufman DL, Maclaren NK. Cellular immunity to a determinant common to glutamate decarboxylase and coxsackie virus in insulin-dependent diabetes. J Clin Invest. 1994;94:2125–9.
163. Endl J, Otto H, Jung G et al. Identification of naturally processed T cell epitopes from glutamic acid decarboxylase presented in the context of HLA-DR alleles by T lymphocytes of recent onset IDDM patients. J Clin Invest. 1997;99:2405–15.
164. Petersen JS, Karlsen AE, Markholst H, Worsaae A, Dyrberg T, Michelsen B. Neonatal tolerization with glutamic acid decarboxylase but not with bovine serum albumin delays the onset of diabetes in NOD mice. Diabetes. 1994;43:1478–84.
165. Godkin A, Friede T, Davenport M et al. Use of eluted peptide sequence data to identify the binding characteristics of peptides to the insulin-dependent diabetes susceptibility allele HLA-DQ8 (DQ 3.2). Int Immunol. 1997;9:905–11.
166. Panina-Bordignon P, Lang R, van Endert PM et al. Cytotoxic T cells specific for glutamic acid decarboylase in autoimmune diabetes. J Exp Med. 1995;181:1923–7.
167. Christie MR, Brown TJ, Cassidy D. Binding of antibodies in sera from Type 1 (insulin-dependent) diabetic patients to glutamate decarboxylase from rat tissues. Evidence for antigenic and non-antigenic forms of the enzyme. Diabetologia. 1992;35:380–4.
168. Christie MR, Hollands JA, Brown TJ, Michelsen BM, Delovitch TL. Detection of pancreatic islet 64,000 Mr autoantigens in insulin-dependent diabetes distinct from glutamate decarboxylase. J Clin Invest. 1993;92:240–8.
169. Lu J, Notkins AL, Lan MS. Isolation, sequence and expression of a novel mouse brain cDNA, mIA-2, and its relatedness to members of the protein tyrosine phosphatase family. Biochem Biophys Res Commun. 1994;204:930–6.
170. Solimena M, Dirkx R, Jr., Hermel JM et al. ICA 512, an autoantigen of type I diabetes, is an intrinsic membrane protein of neurosecretory granules. EMBO J 1996;15:2102–14.
171. Stone RL, Dixon JE. Protein-tyrosine phosphatases. J Biol Chem. 1994;269:31323–6.
172. Bonifacio E, Lampasona V, Genovese S, Ferrari M, Bosi E. Identification of protein tyrosine phosphatase-like IA2 (islet cell antigen 512) as the insulin-dependent diabetes-related 37/40 kDa autoantigen and a target of islet cell antibodies. J Immunol. 1995;155:5419–26.
173. Gorus FK, Goubert P, Semakula C et al. IA-2-autoantibodies complement GAD(65)-autoantibodies in new-onset IDDM patients and help predict impending diabetes in their siblings. Diabetologia. 1997;40:95–9.
174. Lampasona V, Bearzatto M, Genovese S, Bosi E, Ferrari M, Bonifacio E. Autoantibodies in insulin-dependent diabetes recognize distinct cytoplasmic domains of the protein tyrosine phosphatase-like IA-2 autoantigen. J Immunol. 1996;157:2707–11.
175. Sanjeevi CB, Falorni A, Kockum I, Hagopian WA, Lernmark Å. HLA and glutamic acid decarboxylase in human insulin-dependent diabetes mellitus. Diabetic Med. 1996;13:209–17.
176. Cui L, Yu W-P, DeAizpurua HJ, Schmidli RS, Pallen CJ. Cloning and characterization of islet cell antigen-related protein-tyrosine phosphatase (PTP), a novel receptor-like PTP and autoantigen in insulin-dependent diabetes. J Biol Chem. 1996;271:24817–13.
177. Martin JM, Trink B, Daneman D, Dosch H-M, Robinson B. Milk proteins in the etiology of insulin-dependent diabetes mellitus (IDDM). Ann Med. 1991;23:447–52.
178. Pietropaolo M, Castano L, Babu S et al. Islet cell autoantigen 69 KDa (ICA69): Molecular cloning and characterization of a novel diabetes-associated autoantigen. J Clin Invest. 1993; 92:359–71.
179. Karjalainen J, Martin JM, Knip M et al. A bovine albumin peptide as a possible trigger of insulin-dependent diabetes mellitus. N Engl J Med. 1992;327:302–7.
180. Karges W, Pietropaolo M, Ackerley CA, Dosch HM. Gene expression of islet cell antigen p69 in human, mouse and rat. Diabetes. 1996;45:513–21.

181. Mally MI, Cirulli V, Otonkoski T, Soto G, Hayek A. Ontogeny and tissue distribution of human GAD expression. Diabetes. 1996;45:496–501.
182. Martin S, Kardorf J, Schulte B et al. Autoantibodies to the islet antigen ICA 69 occur in IDDM and in rheumatoid arthritis. Diabetologia. 1995;38:351–5.
183. Roep BO, Duinkerken G, Schreuder GM, Kolb H, deVries RR, Martin S. HLA-associated inverse correlation between T cell and antibody responsiveness to islet autoantigen in recent-onset insulin-dependent diabetes mellitus. Eur J Immunol. 1996;26:1285–9.
184. Aanstot HJ, Kang SM, Kim J et al. Identification and characterization of glima 38, a glycosylated islet cell membrane antigen, which together with GAD(65) and IA2 marks the early phases of autoimmune response in type 1 diabetes. J Clin Invest. 1996;97:2772–83.
185. Honeyman MC, Cram DS, Harrison LC. Transcription factor jun-B is target of autoreactive T cells in IDDM. Diabetes. 1993;42:626–30.
186. Castano L, Russo E, Zhou L, Lipes M, Eisenbarth G. Identification and cloning of a granule autoantigen (carboxypeptidase-H) associated with type 1 diabetes. J Clin Endocrinol Metab. 1991;73:1197–201.
187. Elias D, Reshef T, Birk OS, van der Zee R, Cohen IR. Vaccination against autoimmune mouse diabetes with a T cell epitope of human 65-kDa heat shock protein. Proc Natl Acad Sci USA. 1991;88:3088–91.
188. Jones DB, Hunter NR, Duff GW. Heat-shock protein 65 as a ß cell antigen of insulin-dependent diabetes. Lancet. 1990;336:583–598.
189. Ozawa Y, Kasuga A, Nomaguchi H et al. Detection of autoantibodies to the pancreatic islet heat shock protein 60 in insulin-dependent diabetes mellitus. J Autoimmun. 1996;9:517–24.
190. Velloso LA, Winqvist O, Gustafsson J, Kämpe O, Karlsson FA. Autoantibodies against a novel 51 kDa islet antigen and glutamate decarboxylase isoforms in autoimmune polyendocrine syndrome type I. Diabetologia. 1994;37:61–9.
191. Rorsman F, Husebye ES, Winqvist O, Björk E, Karlsson FA, Kämpe O. Aromatic L-amino acid decarboxylase, a pyridoxalphosphate-dependent enzyme, is a beta cell autoantigen. Proc Natl Acad Sci USA. 1995;92:8626–9.
192. Husebye ES, Gebre-Medhin G, Tuomi T et al. Autoantibodies against aromatic L-amino acid decarboxylase in autoimmune polyendocrine syndrome Type I. J Clin Endocrinol Metab. 1997;82:147–50.
193. Huang SW, Hallquist Haedt L, Rich S, Barbosa J. Prevalence of antibodies to nucleic acids in insulin-dependent diabetes and their relatives. Diabetes. 1981;30:873–4.
194. Chang YH, Hwang J, Shang HF, Tsai ST. Characterization of human topoisomerase II as an autoantigen recognized by patients with IDDM. Diabetes. 1996;45:408–14.
195. Nayak RC, Omar MAK, Rabizadeh A, Srikanta S, Eisenbarth GS. 'Cytoplasmic' islet cell antibodies. Evidence that the target antigen is a sialoglycoconjugate. Diabetes. 1985;34:617–19.
196. Colman PG, Nayak RC, Campbell IL, Eisenbarth GS. Binding of cytoplasmic islet cell antibodies is blocked by human pancreatic glycolipid extracts. Diabetes. 1988;37:645–52.
197. Dotta F, Previti M, Lenti L et al. GM2-1 pancreatic islet ganglioside: identification and characterization of a novel islet-specific molecule. Diabetologia. 1995;38:1117–21.
198. Arden SD, Roep BO, Neophytou PI et al. Imogen 38: A novel 38-kD islet mitochondrial autoantigen recognized by T cells from a newly diagnosed type 1 diabetic patient. J Clin Invest. 1996;97:551–61.
199. Roep BO, Arden SD, de Vries RRP, Hutton JC. T cell clones from a type-1 diabetes patient respond to insulin secretory granule proteins. Nature. 1990;345:632–4.
200. Group D-S. The diabetes prevention trial – type 1 diabetes (DPT-1): implementation of screening and staging of relatives. Transplant Proc. 1995;27:3377.
201. Bieg S, Möller C, Olsson T, Lernmark Å. The lymphopenia (lyp) gene controls the intrathymic cytokine ratio in congenic BioBreeding rats. Diabetalogia. 1997;40:786–92.

8
Aetiology and pathogenesis of insulin-dependent diabetes mellitus (IDDM)

J.-F. BACH

It was only in the late 1970s that the autoimmune origin of IDDM appeared as the most plausible hypothesis. The consistent finding of islet cell antibodies (ICA) [1] provided a firm basis for the existence of selective β cell directed autoimmune response. Approximately at the same time, *in vitro* evidence for cell-mediated immunity to islet cells was presented [2]. In the following years, two exceptionally informative spontaneous models of the disease, the bio breeding (BB) rat and the non-obese diabetic (NOD) mouse provided direct evidence for the role of autoimmunity. A considerable bulk of data has been collected since on the immunology and on the genetics of murine and human IDDM allowing a clear understanding of major aspects of the disease pathogenesis and to a lesser degree of its aetiology [3]. Many pending questions persist though. It is the aim of this chapter to review the main prevailing concepts of the immunology of IDDM and discuss the yet unsettled questions.

IDDM IS A T_H1 CELL-MEDIATED AUTOIMMUNE DISEASE

Autoimmune origin of the disease

The role of autoimmunity and more precisely of autoreactive T cells in the pathogenesis of IDDM is now clearly established based on four types of evidence.

A.P. Weetman (ed.), Endocrine Autoimmunity and Associated Conditions. 145–161.

The disease is associated with β cell-specific autoimmune reactivity

In addition to the ICAs mentioned above that are detected by indirect immunofluorescence on human pancreas sections [1], several well defined anti-β cell autoantibodies have now been described (see Chapter 7). The most important of these antibodies react with insulin [4], glutamic acid decarboxylase (GAD) [5] and IA-2, a tyrosine phosphatase [6]. They are found in the vast majority of patients at the onset of the disease and can be detected several years before such onset. They are also found in the NOD mouse and the BB rat although at lower titres [7]. Additionally, autoreactive T lymphocytes specific to islet cells [8,9] or GAD [10–12] are found in a large percentage of patients [9,12] as well as in the animal models [8,10,11].

The islets are consistently infiltrated with mononuclear cells (insulitis) [13]

Insulitis comprises T and at a lesser degree B cells, macrophages and eosinophils. It appears early in the disease history, as early as 3 weeks of age in the NOD mouse [7]. It presents initially as periinsulitis, then peripheral insulitis before becoming fully invading and destructive.

The disease can be transferred by lymphoid cells

The clearest data have been obtained in animal models. Thus, in the NOD mouse, IDDM can be transferred to prediabetic neonatal [14], irradiated [15] or severe combined immune deficiency (SCID) [16] adults by infusing spleen cells from overtly diabetic mice. In man, transfer has been reported after bone marrow transplantation from a diabetic donor [17].

The disease can be prevented or even reversed by T cell blockade

This has been achieved in animal models by a variety of methods including cyclosporin A [18], anti-T cell monoclonals [19,20], neonatal thymectomy [21] or backcrosses to the nude background [22]. The observation has been confirmed in man using cyclosporin A [23,24].

The direct role of T cells is further illustrated by diabetes transfer obtained in SCID mice by injecting β cell-specific T cell clones derived from overtly diabetic mice [25] and by the rapid appearance of diabetes in transgenic NOD mice expressing T cell receptor genes from one of such clones [26].

The precise nature of the T cell subsets involved in this process remains the matter of hot debate, for both the respective role of CD4 versus CD8 T cells and that of T_H1 vs T_H2 cells.

CD4 versus CD8 T cells

Mature T cells are classified into two major subsets, CD4 and CD8, that are for the most part respectively restricted by major histocompatibility complex (MHC) class II and class I molecules. $CD4^+$ T cells, commonly designated as 'helper T cells', act by producing a wide array of cytokines that effectively 'help' the differentiation of B cells and of $CD8^+$ T cells. These cytokines can also exert effector functions notably through macrophage activation or the direct toxic effect of some cytokines such as TNF. $CD8^+$ T cells are essentially known for their killer function. They destroy their target cells in a totally antigen-specific fashion.

Both $CD4^+$ and $CD8^+$ T cells are involved in diabetes pathogenesis as exemplified by the requirement for both cell subsets for rapid disease transfer in neonates [14], irradiated [27] or SCID [28] adults using spleen cells from overtly diabetic mice.

Evidence in favour of a predominant (if not exclusive) role of $CD4^+$ T cells in the induction of the β cell lesion is brought by the possibility to transfer diabetes in SCID recipients by $CD4^+$ T cell clones [25] and by the appearance of diabetes in NOD transgenic mice expressing a T cell receptor (TCR) derived from a $CD4^+$ T cell clone expressed in the majority of $CD4^+$ T cells [26]. These data demonstrate that β cell-specific $CD4^+$ T cells, when present in a very large number, can induce the β cell lesion alone, in the absence of $CD8^+$ T cells (if one admits that SCID mice are not leaky), but this does not prove that $CD4^+$ T cells have this exclusive role in the spontaneous disease occurring in unmanipulated mice or in patients, where the size of the β cell-reactive $CD4^+$ T cell pool is probably not as large as in mice exposed to monoclonal β cell-reactive T cells.

In fact, diabetes transfer has also been obtained with cytotoxic T cell lines derived from NOD mice [29] and $CD8^+$ T cell clones have been obtained in transgenic NOD mice expressing the B7 co-stimulatory molecule on β cells [30]. Diabetes does not develop in MHC class I deficient mice [31] and these mice are resistant to diabetes transfer after infusion of polyclonal diabetogenic T cells [32]. Transfer is only seen in such mice when MHC class I molecules are expressed in β cells (after transgene administration coupled to the insulin gene promoter (RIP)).

The problem is complicated by the fact that $CD8^+$ T cells do not home to the β cells in the absence of $CD4^+$ T cells whereas $CD4^+$ T cells can invade islets when injected alone [33].

Taken together these data might suggest that:

(1) both $CD4^+$ and $CD8^+$ β cell-specific T cells can induce destructive insulitis when reaching the islets in sufficient number;

(2) in the spontaneous disease, $CD8^+$ T cells are probably needed to induce the lesion even if $CD4^+$ T cells are required for their homing to the islets and their diffentiation and expansion, and if $CD4^+$ T cells can by themselves contribute to the lesion induction.

T_H1 vs T_H2 cells

$CD4^+$ T cells have recently been divided into two major functional subsets distinguished by their cytokine pattern. T helper 1 (T_H1) cells produce interleukin-2 (IL-2), interferon gamma (IFN-γ) and tumour necrosis factor (TNF). T helper 2 (T_H2) cells produce interleukin 4 (IL-4), (IL-5), (IL-10) and (IL-13).

Converging evidence indicates that IDDM is a T_H1-dependent autoimmune disease.

(1) Insulitis comprises a majority of IFN-γ-containing $CD4^+$ T cells as shown by immunofluorescence [34] and immunoenzymatic [35] studies with very few IL-4 producing cells.

(2) This pattern is drastically altered after various manoeuvres leading to diabetes prevention such as administration of oral insulin [35] or of complete Freund's adjuvant [34]. IL-4 producing cells are then the predominant T cell type over IFN-γ–producing cells; the cytokine content of β islet-infiltrating cells has also been examined at the mRNA level by RT-PCR but data are still controversial, probably due to the insufficient quantitation of the technique.

(3) Blockade of T_H1 cells by anti-IFN-γ [36,37] or anti-IL-2 receptor [38] monoclonal antibodies prevents diabetes onset or transfer whereas IL-12, a T_H1 differentiating agent, precipitates diabetes onset [39].

The β cell lesion

The intimate mechanisms of the β cell lesion remain uncertain. There is first the already mentioned debate about $CD4^+$ and $CD8^+$ T cells which intervene through totally distinct mechanisms: $CD4^+$ T cell-produced lymphokines induce inflammatory lesions with involvement of nitric oxide (NO) and probably IL-1; $CD8^+$ T cells act through a Fas-mediated apoptosis killing mechanism.

In any case, it is important to stress that the β cell-selective atrophic phase which characterizes IDDM is preceded by a phase of T cell-mediated reversible inflammation as assessed by the recovery of insulin production by islet cells of overtly diabetic NOD mice after *in vitro* culture [40] and by the spectacular normalization of glycaemia observed in recently diagnosed diabetic NOD mice 24 h after administration of an anti-TCR monoclonal antibody [41].

LOSS OF ISLET SELF TOLERANCE IS DRIVEN BY β CELL AUTOANTIGEN(S)

The role of β cell antigen(s)

Autoreactive T cells and natural autoantibodies are found in normal healthy subjects. The question has been raised whether the pathogenic autoimmunity which characterizes autoimmune diseases such as IDDM is due to the non-antigen specific polyclonal activation of these autoreactive clones or whether it is more conventionally due to an autoantigen-driven autoimmune response. This latter hypothesis is illustrated but not demonstrated by the induction of a wide variety of autoimmune diseases after immunization with autoantigen incorporated in Freund's complete adjuvant. The question is particularly pertinent in IDDM inasmuch as no good model of experimental autoantigen-induced animal model is available.

Several pieces of indirect evidence argue in favor of an autoantigen-driven autoimmune response:

(1) There is some evidence for restriction of TCR gene usage among T cells contributing to insulitis in both the NOD mouse [42,43] and human IDDM [44]. Positive mouse data that have been obtained in very young NOD mice are submitted to the criticism of artificial amplification of the very small number of cells infiltrating the islets at the very early stages of insulitis. In fact, restriction is no longer found after 6 weeks of age in NOD mice [45]. Human data showing Vβ7 preferential usage [44] have not yet been confirmed by other authors and could be explained by technical considerations.

(2) IDDM is highly associated with MHC class II genes in both human disease and animal models. Although it may receive other explanations (see below), this association is usually taken as a strong argument for particular predisposition of the patient to present antigenic peptides binding to the HLA molecule in question.

(3) Induction of tolerance to several β cell autoantigens prevents diabetes onset (see below). This argument is weakened by the fact that several unrelated β cell autoantigens can achieve such protection.

Direct evidence in favour of the driving role of β cell autoantigens has been brought by experiments showing the exhaustion of diabetogenic T cells in β cell-depleted NOD mice [46]. Such mice, in whom β cells were destroyed by alloxan treatment, were irradiated and injected with diabetogenic T cells. Their spleen cells showed no capacity to transfer diabetes, unlike spleen cells from non alloxan-treated mice. These results indicate that the presence of β cells is necessary to maintain diabetogenic T cells.

The requirement for autoantigen stimulation poses two central questions: what is the nature of the autoantigen(s) triggering the β cell targeted autoimmune response?, and what are the cellular and molecular events that render these autoantigens immunogenic, i.e. capable of triggering an autoimmune response?

Several candidate autoantigens

Autoantibodies and autoreactive T cells are found against a large number of β cell autoantigens in diabetic patients and in NOD mice (Table 8.1). A number of criteria should be fulfilled, though, before accepting these as plausible candidate autoantigens:

Table 8.1 Candidate autoantigens in IDDM

1.	(Pro-) insulin
2.	Glutamic acid decarboxylase (GAD 65)
3.	IA-2/ICA512/40 kDa antigen (tyrosine phosphatase)
4.	Heat shock protein 65 (hsp 65)/p277
5.	p69 (cross-reaction with BSA)
6.	IA-5 (37 kDa antigen)
7.	GLIMA (38 kDa)
8.	Imogen (mitochondria)
9.	Gangliosides, sulphatide, etc.
10.	Peripherin
11.	Carboxypeptidase H
12.	β granule-associated protein (β GAP)

(1) Their tissue distribution should be reasonably restricted to β cells (only β cells are affected by the autoimmune process).

(2) Intraislet and, to a lesser degree, circulating T cells should react to the antigen.

(3) The disease should be prevented by tolerance induction against the said antigen in NOD mice or BB rats and induce diabetes in non-autoimmune mice (with the adequate genetic background) after immunization.

None of the antigens listed in Table 8.1 fulfil all these criteria. It is fair to recognize, however, that four major antigens fulfil most of them (Table 8.2). The problem is that none clearly emerges over the others, opening the intriguing possibility of the concomitant existence of several diabetes autoantigens.

One logical way to identify the diabetes autoantigen among several candidate molecules is to determine whether induction of tolerance to that antigen prevents disease onset. This has been achieved in NOD mice with three of the major candidate autoantigens, using a variety of procedures.

Table 8.2 Requirements for candidate β cell autoantigens

	GAD	*Insulin*	*hsp 60*	*IA-2*
β cell exclusive distribution	β cells/brain	β cells	Ubiquitous (β cells+)	β cells
Autoreactivity in human IDDM T cells	+ (80%)	+ (30%)	+	+ (50%)
	+	±	+	?
Protective tolerance in NOD mice				
Peripheral	+	+	+	?
Central (transgenic mice)	–	+	+	?
Reactivity with pathogenic T cell clones	+	+	+	?
De novo induction of IDDM	–	–	+	?

Tolerance to GAD was obtained by injecting GAD intravenously [10] or intrathymically [11] at the age of 3 weeks. Diabetes onset was delayed and even prevented in some animals. Similarly administration of insulin by various routes (oral [47], nasal [48], sc [49]) induced tolerance and diabetes prevention. Finally, sensitization against the p277 peptide of heat shock protein 60 (hsp 60) protected NOD mice from becoming diabetic [50]. The fact that these three unrelated antigens all provide protection is incompatible with a mechanism of central tolerance since one would not understand then why the deletion of T cells reacting to any of these three antigens protects from disease onset. A more plausible hypothesis to explain these results is active peripheral tolerance. This is corroborated by the observation of the presence of T_H2-dependent autoantibody isotypes in mice rendered tolerant to GAD and hsp 60 [51].

An attractive way to induce central tolerance is to provoke negative intrathymic deletion by transgenic expression of the autoantigen in the thymus. This has been achieved with GAD using an Ig promoter (A. Lehuen, in preparation), proinsulin [52] and hsp 60 using a MHC class II promoter [53]. Diabetes was prevented in the two latter cases. It is not clear however whether the prevention was associated with central tolerance.

We are thus presently faced with the unexpected conclusion that several autoantigens may be concomitantly operating in the triggering of the pathogenic β cell lesion.

Rupture of β cell ignorance: the triggering of the β cell specific response

Normal individuals do not present with lesions of the various organs against which they show naturally occurring autoreactive T cells. This state of ignorance is well illustrated by a double transgenic mice experiment performed in the lymphochoromeningitis virus (LCMV) model [54]. A first set of transgenic mice expresses the LCMV glycoprotein in the β cells after administration of RIP-coupled transgene. A second set of transgenic mice expresses the TCR of anti-

LCMV gp T cell clone. The F1 hybrids derived from these two sets of transgenic mice do not develop diabetes although they coexpress an external antigen in their β cells and the corresponding TCR in large amounts. This state of ignorance is overcome after infection with LCMV which activates the LCMV gp-specific T cell clones. Interestingly, in some mouse strains, ignorance was not observed in the double transgenic mice which became diabetic without T cell activation [55].

The question is then to determine the factors in diabetics that have overcome the ignorance observed in normal individuals. Several hypotheses have been proposed:

(1) Increased expression of molecules contributing to antigen presentation: MHC class I or class II molecules, B7 and adhesins. Increased expression of MHC class I and class II molecules has been reported on β cells in both human IDDM [56] and animal models [57,58] but the data are controversial and it is difficult to exclude that such abnormal expression is not secondary to the T cell-mediated autoimmune attack, notably through the production of IFN-γ, a cytokine known to exert such effects.

(2) Cross reactivity between a β cell autoantigen and an infectious agent as in the case of GAD and Coxsackie B4 [59]. T cells react then against the unignored viral epitope and provide help to the silent autoreactive T cell clones.

(3) Modification of the autoantigen conformation by a chemical or a virus protein which renders it immunogenic according to a mechanism close to that of autoantigen mimicry just described.

Taken together, these data open the possibility that whether or not it is initially triggered by a single autoantigen, the autoimmune response rapidly spreads to other specificities secondary to the local inflammation induced by the initial aggression (which may or may not be immunological) (Figure 8.1). The possibility of preventing disease onset by inducing tolerance to β cell antigens suggests that a similar spreading occurs at the level of suppressor cytokines. Regulatory T cells are guided to the β cell and their target autoantigen but exert then a suppressor effect which extends to T_H1 cells with other specificities present on the spot.

THE ANTI-β CELL AUTOIMMUNE RESPONSE IS EXACERBATED AND PERPETUATED BY A FAILURE OF IMMUNOREGULATION

Regulatory cells in young prediabetic NOD mice.

Young adult prediabetic NOD mice do not become diabetic after infusion of spleen cells from overtly diabetic mice. The transfer is only obtained when the recipient mice are irradiated [15] or given anti-CD4 monoclonal antibody (+ adult thymectomy) [60]. The transfer is also readily obtained when using

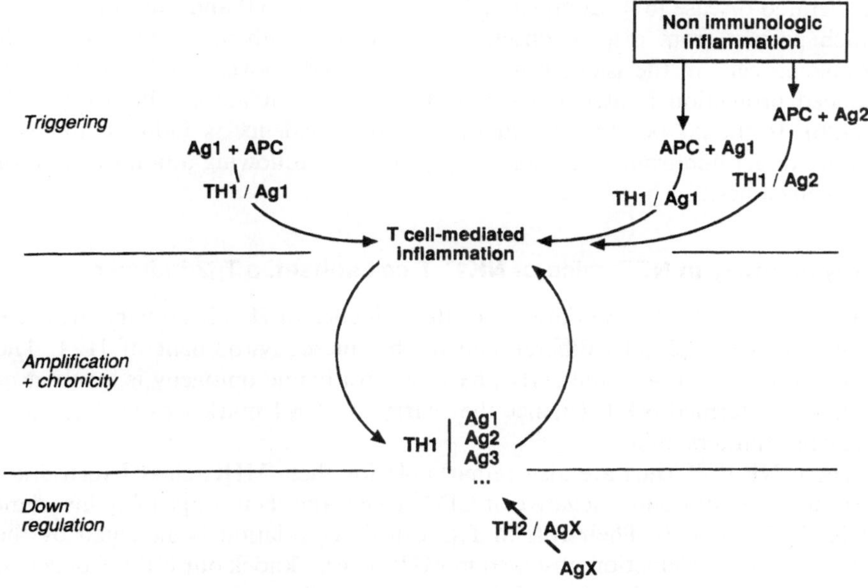

Figure 8.1 Immunoregulatory circuits controlling autoimmune responses

immunoincompetent recipients, such as neonates (up to 3 weeks of age) [14] or SCID/NOD mice [16].

The absence of diabetes before the age of 15–20 weeks in such mice is under the control of regulatory T cells, as exemplified by the acceleration of diabetes onset observed after thymectomy performed at 3 weeks of age [61] and cyclophosphamide therapy [62]. In both cases, the accelerating effect is specific since it is abrogated by infusion of T cells from untreated prediabetic animals.

The existence of the regulatory T cells has been directly demonstrated in cotransfer experiments where the simultaneous transfer of $CD4^+$ cells from prediabetic mice prevents diabetes transfer afforded by spleen cells from overtly diabetic mice [63]. It will be important to determine whether the few T cell clones shown to protect from diabetes onset in similar settings are related to the $CD4^+$ protector subset.

Indirect evidence for the regulatory role of T_H2 cells

Converging but still indirect evidence suggests that the $CD4^+$ regulatory cells just described are of the T_H2 type. Diabetes onset in NOD mice is prevented by systemic IL-4 administration [64] or β cell IL-4 transgenic expression [65]. Diabetes onset is also prevented by IL-10 treatment [66] but, unexpectedly, transgenic NOD mice expression of large amounts of IL-10 in the islets induces accelerated disease [67]. Complete Freund's adjuvant [34] and oral insulin [35], which protect from disease onset, are associated with appearance of IL-4-producing cells in the islets. Finally, as mentioned above, GAD and hsp 60-induced protection is associated with T_H2 dependent autoantibodies (IgG1, IgG2b). It should be emphasized that all this evidence is indirect and will require direct confirmation, notably by protection following administration of T_H2 cell clones.

Early anomaly in NOD mice of $NK1^+$ T cell subset, a T_H2 inducer

Whereas T_H1 cells differentiate under the influence of IL-12, growing evidence indicates that T_H2 cells differentiate in the microenvironment of IL-4. The major source of IL-4 in the early phase of intrathymic ontogeny is a subset of thymocytes termed NK1 T (since they carry the NK1 marker as well as other NK cells markers) [68].

These $NK1^+$ T cells are also remarkable for their MHC class I restriction (very unusual for double negative or $CD4^+$ cells), and their usage of an invariant TCR (Vα14, Vβ8.2). Their role in T_H2 cell differentiation is indicated by the absence of IgE production observed in MHC class I knock out NK1 T-deficient mice. We have recently reported that $NK1^+$ T cells present a major defect in NOD mice both numerically and functionally (IL-4 production) [69]. This deficiency is observed in both the thymus and the periphery (the precocious production of IL-4 following *in vivo* administration of anti-CD3 antibody which is mediated by $NK1^+$ T cells is absent in young NOD mice). This $NK1^+$ T cell deficiency is fully corrected both *in vitro* and *in vivo* by IL-7, a T cell growth factor that has been shown to have a preferential effect on $NK1^+$ T cells [70] .

Conclusions

Taken together, these data tend to indicate that a subset of $CD4^+$ T cells, presumably of the T_H2 type (although the role of TGF-β-producing cells has not been excluded), affords protection from diabetes in young NOD mice for several weeks. However, this protection mechanism progressively wanes between 10 and 20 weeks of age in the NOD mouse, transforming the insulitis from a peripheral pattern to an invading and destructive one. One may hypothesize that the $NK1^+$ T cell deficiency that precedes this failure of protection mechanisms is at its origin, although again this remains to be demonstrated.

AETIOLOGICAL FACTORS ARE BOTH GENETIC AND ENVIRONMENTAL

The hereditary transmission of IDDM is well established: the disease concordance rate varies from 35 % in monozygotic twins to 7 % in siblings (15 % in HLA identical sibs) [3]. The role of genetic factors is also illustrated by the tight genetic control of IDDM onset in the NOD mouse and the BB rat.

Role of the MHC

The central role of the MHC genes is well established in both human disease and animal models. Thus, in the NOD mouse, NOD.H-2^k congenic mice which do not express the NOD I-A genes are protected from diabetes (whereas they still show thyroiditis) [71]. Conversely, however, C57Bl/6 mice congenic for I-A^{NOD} do not become diabetic except if they express an IL-10 transgene in β cells [72]. Note, lastly, that transgenic NOD mice expressing I-A^k or I-A^b are protected from diabetes and that this protection is probably an active one since it is broken down by cyclophosphamide treatment [73,74]. In human IDDM, the HLA association with the predisposing HLA alleles DR3 and DR4 has been extensively documented [3]. Recent data indicate that only some DR4 subtypes may predispose to disease onset. The DR2 DQB1*0602 allele provides strong protection from disease but not from autoantibody appearance.

Three major mechanisms can be put forward to explain the HLA association with IDDM. In the first, predisposing but not protective alleles present crucial autoantigenic peptides. This is in fact the classical immune response gene model based on the central phenomenon of HLA restriction of T cell responses. It is difficult however to accept this hypothesis, at least in an exclusive way, because of the dominance of DR2-associated protection over DR3- or DR4-associated susceptibility. Additionally, DRB5*0101, a probable protective allele, has been shown to present very effectively a GAD65 epitope to T cells from diabetic patients (P. van Endert, personal communication). In the second hypothesis, predisposing and protective alleles compete for autoantigen binding ('determinant capture'). This hypothesis is supported by the observation that autoantigens bind to protective alleles. However, it does not take consideration of the fact that autoantigens possess numerous T cell epitopes located in distinct protein domains. Any individual class II allele is unlikely to bind crucial epitopes of all important antigens. A last and perhaps more attractive hypothesis is that predisposing and protective alleles stimulate different types of T cell subsets (T_H1/T_H2). This hypothesis explains dominance of protection by dominance of T_H2 type lymphokines and the benefit of 'determinant capture' by protective alleles. It is also compatible with the notion of multiple important autoantigens and epitopes. Lastly, it explains protection of transgenic NOD mice expressing I-$A^{non\text{-}NOD}$ [73,74].

Non-MHC genes

The role of non-MHC genes in predisposition to IDDM is illustrated in man by the difference between disease concordance rate in monozygotic twins (35%) and HLA identical siblings (15%). Only a few non-HLA genes have been clearly identified: the insulin gene [75,76] and the CTLA-4 gene [77] have modest linkage and questionable significance. Other chromosomal predisposing regions have also been suggested [78] (Table 8.3).

Table 8.3 Loci linked to IDDM susceptibility

Disease locus	*Chromosome location*
IDDM1	6p21
IDDM2	11p25
IDDM3	15q
IDDM4	11q13
IDDM5	6q25
IDDM6	18q
IDDM7	2q31
IDDM8	6q27
IDDM9	3q21-q25
IDDM10	10cen
IDDM11	Xq
IDDM12	7p

Table 8.4 Idd loci in NOD mice

Locus	*Chromosome location*	*Distance (cm)*
Idd1	17	19
Idd2	9	22
Idd3	3	30
Idd4	11	44
Idd5	1	30
Idd6	6	77
Idd7	7	4
Idd8	14	3
Idd9	4	82
Idd10	3	55
Idd11	4	53
Idd12	14	12
Idd13	2	71
Idd14	13	13
Idd15	15	27
Idd16	1	9

More data have been collected in NOD mice where, thanks to the systematic segregation studies of several laboratories, notably that of John Todd, 16 loci have been localized [79] (Table 8.4). Much work remains to be done to identify the genes in question and their biological significance in relation to disease pathogenesis. The problem is complicated by the existence of protective genes such as the Fcγ receptor II gene, recently shown in our laboratory to be abnormal in NOD mice and to confer paradoxical partial protection, notably in males [80].

Environmental factors

The relatively low penetrance of the human disease, indicated by the 35% concordance rate in monozygotic twins, brings strong evidence in favour of a major role for environmental factors. The nature of these factors is still poorly defined. Viruses and bacteria are probably central but their role is complicated by the fact that they may act in both directions of disease promotion or protection. The protective role of some viral infections has been well demonstrated in NOD mice and BB rats that show the highest incidence of disease in specific pathogen-free colonies [3,81,82]. It could explain the north-south gradient of disease incidence observed in both Europe and North America [82].

CONCLUSIONS

IDDM is a multifactorial and polygenic autoimmune disease. Data presented in this review indicate the potential central role of three orders of aetiologic factors:

(1) abnormal immunogenicity of β cell autoantigens, probably secondary to local inflammation, whether or not this inflammation is of immunological nature;

(2) genetically controlled T cell capacity for recognizing the antigen peptides;

(3) an immune dysregulation perpetuating the autoimmune response.

Interestingly, genetic factors probably intervene at all steps and environmental factors at several levels. One may hope that the dissection of all these mechanisms will provide a better understanding of IDDM pathogenesis and new tracks for immunotherapy and antigen specific disease prevention.

References

1. Bottazzo GF, Florin-Christensen A, Doniach D. Islet-cell antibodies in diabetes mellitus with autoimmune polyendocrine deficiencies. Lancet. 1974;2:1279–83.
2. Nerup J, Andersen OO, Bendixen G, Egeberg J, Poulsen JE. Antipancreatic cellular hypersensitivity in diabetes mellitus. Diabetes. 1971;20:424–7.
3. Bach JF. Insulin-dependent diabetes mellitus as an autoimmune disease. Endocrine Rev. 1994;15:516–42.
4. Palmer JP, Asplin CM, Clemons P et al. Insulin antibodies in insulin-dependent diabetics before insulin treatment. Science. 1983;222:1337–9.
5. Baekkeskov S, Landin M, Kristensen JK et al. Antibodies to a 64,000 Mr human islet cell antigen precede the clinical onset of insulin-dependent diabetes. J Clin Invest. 1987;79:926–34.
6. Lan MS, Wasserfall C, MacLaren NK, Notkins AL. IA-2, a transmembrane protein of the protein tyrosine phosphatase family, is a major autoantigen in insulin- dependent diabetes mellitus. Proc Natl Acad Sci USA. 1996;93:6367–70.
7. Bach JF. The natural history of the islet specific autoimmune response in the NOD mouse. In: Leiter E, Atkinson MA, eds. The NOD Mouse. Austin: R.G. Landes; 1996 [in press].

8. Burtles SS, Trembleau S, Drexler K, Hurtenbach U. Absence of T cell tolerance to pancreatic islet cells. J Immunol. 1992;149:2185–93.
9. Honeyman MC, Cram DS, Harrison LC. Glutamic acid decarboxylase 67-reactive T cells: a marker of insulin-dependent diabetes. J Exp Med. 1993;177:535–40.
10. Kaufman DL, Clare-Salzler M, Tian J et al. Spontaneous loss of T-cell tolerance to glutamic acid decarboxylase in murine insulin-dependent diabetes. Nature. 1993;366:69–72.
11. Tisch R, Yang XD, Singer SM, Liblau RS, Fugger L, McDevitt HO. Immune response to glutamic acid decarboxylase correlates with insulitis in non-obese diabetic mice. Nature. 1993;366:72–5.
12. Atkinson MA, Kaufman DL, Campbell L et al. Response of peripheral-blood mononuclear cells to glutamate decarboxylase in insulin-dependent diabetes. Lancet. 1992;339:458–9.
13. Gepts W, Lecompte PM. The pancreatic islets in diabetes. Am J Med. 1981;70:105–15.
14. Bendelac A, Carnaud C, Boitard C, Bach JF. Syngeneic transfer of autoimmune diabetes from diabetic NOD mice to healthy neonates. Requirement for both $L3T4^+$ and $Lyt\text{-}2^+$ T cells. J Exp Med. 1987;166:823–32.
15. Wicker LS, Miller BJ, Mullen Y. Transfer of autoimmune diabetes mellitus with splenocytes from nonobese diabetic (NOD) mice. Diabetes. 1986;35:855–60.
16. Rohane PW, Shimada A, Kim DT et al. Islet-infiltrating lymphocytes from prediabetic NOD mice rapidly transfer diabetes to NOD-scid/scid mice. Diabetes. 1995;44:550–4.
17. Lampeter EF, Homberg M, Quabeck K et al. Transfer of insulin-dependent diabetes between HLA-identical siblings by bone marrow transplantation. Lancet. 1993;341:1243–4.
18. Mori Y, Suko M, Okudaira H et al. Preventive effects of cyclosporin on diabetes in NOD mice. Diabetologia. 1986;29:244–07.
19. Wang Y, Pontesilli O, Gill RG, La Rosa FG, Lafferty KJ. The role of $CD4^+$ and $CD8^+$ T cells in the destruction of islet grafts by spontaneously diabetic mice. Proc Natl Acad Sci USA. 1991;88:527–31.
20. Hutchings P, O'Reilly L, Parish NM, Waldmann H, Cooke A. The use of a non-depleting anti-CD4 monoclonal antibody to reestablish tolerance to beta cells in NOD mice. Eur J Immunol. 1992;22:1913–18.
21. Like AA, Kislauskis E, Williams RR, Rossini AA. Neonatal thymectomy prevents spontaneous diabetes mellitus in the BB/W rat. Science. 1982;216:644–6.
22. Matsumoto M, Yagi H, Kunimoto K, Kawaguchi J, Makino S, Harada M. Transfer of autoimmune diabetes from diabetic NOD mice to NOD athymic nude mice: the roles of T cell subsets in the pathogenesis. Cell Immunol. 1993;148:189-97.
23. Feutren G, Papoz L, Assan R et al. Cyclosporin increases the rate and length of remissions in insulin-dependent diabetes of recent onset. Results of a multicentre double-blind trial. Lancet. 1986;2:119–24.
24. The Canadian-European Randomized Control Trial Group. Cyclosporin-induced remission of IDDM after early intervention. Association of 1 yr of cyclosporin treatment with enhanced insulin secretion. Diabetes. 1988;37:1574–82.
25. Peterson JD, Haskins K. Transfer of diabetes in the NOD-scid mouse by CD4 T-cell clones. Differential requirement for CD8 T-cells. Diabetes. 1996;45:328–36.
26. Katz JD, Wang B, Haskins K, Benoist C, Mathis D. Following a diabetogenic T cell from genesis through pathogenesis. Cell. 1993;74:1089–100.
27 Miller BJ, Appel MC, O'Neil JJ, Wicker LS. Both the $Lyt\text{-}2^+$ and $L3T4^+$ T cell subsets are required for the transfer of diabetes in nonobese diabetic mice. J Immunol. 1988;140:52–8.
28 Christianson SW, Shultz LD, Leiter EH. Adoptive transfer of diabetes into immunodeficient NOD-scid/scid mice. Relative contributions of $CD4^+$ and $CD8^+$ T-cells from diabetic versus prediabetic NOD.NON-Thy-1a donors. Diabetes. 1993;42:44–55.
29. Nagata M, Santamaria P, Kawamura T, Utsugi T, Yoon JW. Evidence for the role of $CD8^+$ cytotoxic T cells in the destruction of pancreatic beta-cells in nonobese diabetic mice. J Immunol. 1994;152:2042–50.
30. Wong FS, Visintin I, Wen L, Flavell RA, Janeway CA. CD8 T cell clones from young nonobese diabetic (NOD) islets can transfer rapid onset of diabetes in NOD mice in the absence of CD4 cells. J Exp Med. 1996;183:67–76.
31. Katz J, Benoist C, Mathis D. Major histocompatibility complex class I molecules are required for the development of insulitis in non-obese diabetic mice. Eur J Immunol. 1993; 23:3358–60.

32. Kay TW, Parker JL, Stephens LA, Thomas HE, Allison J. RIP-beta2-microglobulin transgene expression restores insulitis, but not diabetes, in beta2-microglobulin-null non-obese diabetic mice. J Immunol. 1996;157:3688–93.
33. Thivolet C, Bendelac A, Bedossa P, Bach JF, Carnaud C. $CD8^+$ T cell homing to the pancreas in the nonobese diabetic mouse is $CD4^+$ T cell-dependent. J Immunol. 1991;146: 85–8.
34. Shehadeh NN, Larosa F, Lafferty KJ. Altered cytokine activity in adjuvant inhibition of autoimmune diabetes. J Autoimmun. 1993;6:291–300.
35. Hancock WW, Polanski M, Zhang J, Blogg N, Weiner HL. Suppression of insulitis in non-obese diabetic (NOD) mice by oral insulin administration is associated with selective expression of interleukin-4 and -10, transforming growth factor-beta, and prostaglandin-E. Am J Pathol. 1995;147:1193–9.
36. Debray-Sachs M, Carnaud C, Boitard C et al. Prevention of diabetes in NOD mice treated with antibody to murine IFN gamma. J Autoimmun. 1991;4:237–48.
37. Campbell IL, Kay TW, Oxbrow L, Harrison LC. Essential role for interferon-gamma and interleukin-6 in autoimmune insulin-dependent diabetes in NOD/Wehi mice. J Clin Invest. 1991;87:739–42.
38. Kelley VE, Gaulton GN, Hattori M, Ikegami H, Eisenbarth G, Strom TB. Anti-interleukin 2 receptor antibody suppresses murine diabetic insulitis and lupus nephritis. J Immunol. 1988; 140:59–61.
39. Trembleau S, Penna G, Bosi E, Mortara A, Gately MK, Adorini L. Interleukin 12 administration induces T helper type 1 cells and accelerates autoimmune diabetes in NOD mice. J Exp Med. 1995;181:817–21.
40. Strandell E, Eizirik DL, Sandler S. Reversal of beta-cell suppression in vitro in pancreatic islets isolated from nonobese diabetic mice during the phase preceding insulin-dependent diabetes mellitus. J Clin Invest. 1990;85:1944–50.
41. Sempe P, Bedossa P, Richard MF, Villa MC, Bach JF, Boitard C. Anti-alpha/beta T cell receptor monoclonal antibody provides an efficient therapy for autoimmune diabetes in nonobese diabetic (NOD) mice. Eur J Immunol. 1991;21:1163–9.
42. Sarukhan A, Bedossa P, Garchon HJ, Bach JF, Carnaud C. Molecular analysis of TCR junctional variability in individual infiltrated islets of non-obese diabetic mice: evidence for the constitution of largely autonomous T cell foci within the same pancreas. Int Immunol. 1995;7:139–46.
43. Yang Y, Charlton B, Shimada A, Dal Canto R, Fathman CG. Monoclonal T cells identified in early NOD islet infiltrates. Immunity. 1996;4:189–94.
44. Conrad B, Weidmann E, Trucco G et al. Evidence for superantigen involvement in insulin-dependent diabetes mellitus aetiology. Nature. 1994;371:351–5.
45. Sarukhan A, Gombert JM, Olivi M, Bach JF, Carnaud C, Garchon HJ. Anchored polymerase chain reaction based analysis of the V-beta repertoire in the non-obese diabetic (NOD) mouse. Eur J Immunol. 1994;24:1750–6.
46. Larger E, Becourt C, Bach JF, Boitard C. Pancreatic islet beta cells drive T cell-immune responses in the nonobese diabetic mouse model. J Exp Med. 1995;181:1635–42.
47. Zhang ZJ, Davidson L, Eisenbarth G, Weiner HL. Suppression of diabetes in nonobese diabetic mice by oral administration of porcine insulin. Proc Natl Acad Sci USA. 1991;88: 10252–6.
48. Daniel D, Wegmann DR. Protection of nonobese diabetic mice from diabetes by intranasal or subcutaneous administration of insulin peptide B-(9-23). Proc Natl Acad Sci USA. 1996; 93:956–60.
49. Muir A, Peck A, Clare-Salzler M et al. Insulin immunization of nonobese diabetic mice induces a protective insulitis characterized by diminished intraislet interferon-gamma transcription. J Clin Invest. 1995;95:628–34.
50. Elias D, Reshef T, Birk OS, Van Der Zee R, Walker MD, Cohen IR. Vaccination against autoimmune mouse diabetes with a T-cell epitope of the human 65-kDa heat shock protein. Proc Natl Acad Sci USA. 1991;88:3088–91.
51. Elias D, Cohen IR. The hsp60 peptide p277 arrests the autoimmune diabetes induced by the toxin Streptozotocin. Diabetes. 1996;45:1168–72.
52. French MB, Allison J, Cram DS et al. Transgenic expression of mouse proinsulin II prevents diabetes in non-obese diabetic mice. Diabetes. 1996;46:34–9.
53. Birk OS, Douek DC, Elias D et al. A role of hsp60 in autoimmune diabetes: analysis in a transgenic model. Proc Natl Acad Sci USA. 1996;93:1032–7.

54. Ohashi PS, Oehen S, Buerki K et al. Ablation of 'tolerance' and induction of diabetes by virus infection in viral antigen transgenic mice. Cell. 1991;65:305–17.
55. Scott B, Liblau R, Degermann S et al. A role for non-MHC genetic polymorphism in susceptibility to spontaneous autoimmunity. Immunity. 1994;1:73–82.
56. Bottazzo GF, Dean BM, McNally JM, MacKay EH, Swift PG, Gamble DR. In situ characterization of autoimmune phenomena and expression of HLA molecules in the pancreas in diabetic insulitis. N Engl J Med. 1985;313:353–60.
57. Kay TW, Campbell IL, Oxbrow L, Harrison LC. Overexpression of class I major histocompatibility complex accompanies insulitis in the non-obese diabetic mouse and is prevented by anti-interferon-gamma antibody. Diabetologia. 1991;34:779–85.
58. Hanafusa T, Fujino-Kurihara H, Miyazaki A et al. Expression of class II major histocompatibility complex antigens on pancreatic B cells in the NOD mouse. Diabetologia. 1987;30:104–8.
59. Kaufman DL, Erlander MG, Clare-Salzler M, Atkinson MA, MacLaren NK, Tobin AJ. Autoimmunity to two forms of glutamate decarboxylase in insulin-dependent diabetes mellitus. J Clin Invest. 1992;89:283–92.
60. Sempe P, Richard MF, Bach JF, Boitard C. Evidence of $CD4^+$ regulatory T cells in the non-obese diabetic male mouse. Diabetologia. 1994;37:337–43.
61. Dardenne M, Lepault F, Bendelac A, Bach JF. Acceleration of the onset of diabetes in NOD mice by thymectomy at weaning. Eur J Immunol. 1989;19:889–95.
62. Yasunami R, Bach JF. Anti-suppressor effect of cyclophosphamide on the development of spontaneous diabetes in NOD mice. Eur J Immunol. 1988;18:481–4.
63. Boitard C, Yasunami R, Dardenne M, Bach JF. T cell-mediated inhibition of the transfer of autoimmune diabetes in NOD mice. J Exp Med. 1989;169:1669–80.
64. Rapoport MJ, Jaramillo A, Zipris D et al. Interleukin 4 reverses T cell proliferative unresponsiveness and prevents the onset of diabetes in nonobese diabetic mice. J Exp Med. 1993;178:87–99.
65. Mueller R, Krahl T, Sarvetnick N. Pancreatic expression of interleukin-4 abrogates insulitis and autoimmune diabetes in nonobese diabetic (NOD) mice. J Exp Med. 1996;184:1093–9.
66. Pennline KJ, Roque-Gaffney E, Monahan M. Recombinant human IL-10 prevents the onset of diabetes in the nonobese diabetic mouse. Clin Immunol Immunopathol. 1994;71:169–75.
67. Wogensen L, Lee MS, Sarvetnick N. Production of interleukin 10 by islet cells accelerates immune-mediated destruction of beta cells in nonobese diabetic mice. J Exp Med. 1994;179: 1379–84.
68. Vicari AP, Zlotnik A. Mouse $NK1.1^+$ T cells: a new family of T cells. Immunol Today. 1996; 17:71–6.
69. Gombert JM, Herbelin A, Tancrede-Bohin E, Dy M, Carnaud C, Bach JF. Early quantitative and functional deficiency of $NK1^+$ like thymocyte in the NOD mouse. Eur J Immunol. 1996;26:2989–98.
70. Gombert JM, Tancrede-Bohin E, Hameg A et al. IL-7 reverses $NK1^+$ T cell defective IL-4 production in the non-obese diabetic mouse. Int Immunol. 1996;9:73–9.
71. Wicker LS, Appel MC, Dotta F et al. Autoimmune syndromes in major histocompatibility complex (MHC) congenic strains of nonobese diabetic (NOD) mice. The NOD MHC is dominant for insulitis and cyclophosphamide-induced diabetes. J Exp Med. 1992;176:67–77.
72. Lee MS, Mueller R, Wicker LS, Peterson LB, Sarvetnick N. IL-10 is necessary and sufficient for autoimmune diabetes in conjunction with NOD MHC homozygosity. J Exp Med. 1996; 183:2663–8.
73. Slattery RM, Kjer-Nielsen L, Allison J, Charlton B, Mandel TE, Miller JF. Prevention of diabetes in non-obese diabetic I-Ak transgenic mice. Nature. 1990;345:724–6.
74. Singer SM, Tisch R, Yang XD, McDevitt HO. An Abd transgene prevents diabetes in nonobese diabetic mice by inducing regulatory T cells. Proc Natl Acad Sci USA. 1993;90: 9566–70.
75. Lucassen AM, Julier C, Beressi JP et al. Susceptibility to insulin dependent diabetes mellitus maps to a 4.1 kb segment of DNA spanning the insulin gene and associated VNTR. Nature Genet. 1993;4:305–10.
76. McGinnis RE, Spielman RS. Linkage disequilibrium in the insulin gene region: size variation at the 5′ flanking polymorphism and bimodality among 'class I' alleles. Am J Hum Genet. 1994;55:526–32.
77. Nistico L, Buzzetti R, Pritchard LE et al. The CTLA-4 gene region of chromosome 2q33 is linked to, and associated with, type 1 diabetes. Hum Mol Genet. 1996;5:1075–80.

78. Merriman TR, Todd JA. Genetics of insulin-dependent diabetes: non-major histocompatibility genes. Horm Metab Res. 1996;28:289–93.
79. Wicker LS, Todd JA, Peterson LB. Genetic control of autoimmune diabetes in the NOD mouse. Annu Rev Immunol. 1995;13:179–200.
80. Luan JJ, Monteiro RC, Sautes C et al. Defective FC gamma RII gene expression in macrophages of NOD mice: genetic linkage with upregulation of IgG1 and IgG2b in serum. J Immunol.1996;157:4707–16.
81. Like AA, Guberski DL, Butler L. Influence of environmental viral agents on frequency and tempo of diabetes mellitus in BB/Wor rats. Diabetes. 1991;40:259–62.
82. Bach JF. Predictive medicine in autoimmune diseases: from the identification of genetic predisposition and environmental influence to precocious immunotherapy. Clin Immunol Immunopathol. 1994;72:156–61.

9
Addison's disease and related polyendocrinopathies

P. PETERSON, R. UIBO and K. J. E. KROHN

INTRODUCTION

The clinical disorder caused by adrenocortical destruction was first described by an English physician, Thomas Addison, almost 150 years ago [1] and has since been known as Addison's disease [2]. The clinical signs and symptoms of the condition are due to the failure of adrenal cortex to produce steroid hormones, notably cortisol and aldosterone. The lack of cortisol results in loss of weight, weakness, vomiting and, as the cortisol production is regulated by adrenocorticotrophic hormone (ACTH), elevated blood level of ACTH. By the time the diagnosis of autoimmune Addison's disease is established, the adrenal cortex is usually completely destroyed by the autoimmune reaction.

Some of the cases described by Addison were due to secondary tuberculosis, affecting the adrenal glands: tuberculosis and fungal infections were the primary cause for Addison's disease at that time, and still are in the developing world. Other non-immunological causes of adrenal insufficiency include HIV or cytomegalovirus infection, amyloidosis, tumours, haemorrhage or adreno-leukodystrophy [3], a rare genetic disease caused by a defective very long chain fatty acid transporter gene [4]. In countries where fungal infections and tuberculosis are less common, the idiopathic or autoimmune form of the disease prevails, accounting for 75–90% of the cases [5].

Addison's disease is rare. Estimates of the prevalence have varied between 40 and 70 cases per million [6–8] but a recent retrospective study from Nottingham reported a calculated prevalence of 110/million, and the cause was attributed to autoimmune destruction of adrenals in 93% of the cases. The annual incidence was found to be 5.6 per million [9]. In the present review, the term Addison's disease is used solely for the autoimmune adrenocortical failure.

A.P. Weetman (ed.), Endocrine Autoimmunity and Associated Conditions. 163–182.

The histological picture of the adrenal cortex in Addison's disease is similar to that seen in the autoimmune diseases of other endocrine glands, especially the thyroid in autoimmune thyroiditis (Chapter 3). In the early phase of the disease, one sees heavy lymphocytic infiltration in the cortex, and destruction of the cortical cells. This finding is in agreement with the hypothesis that the destruction of cortical cells is due to cytotoxic T lymphocytes. In late cases, seen most often at autopsy, the active destructive process has been replaced with fibrosis, again resembling the burn-out process observed in autoimmune thyroid diseases or in atrophic A-type gastritis (Chapter 12).

CLINICAL ASSOCIATIONS

Addison's disease belongs to the group of organ-specific autoimmune diseases. Clinically, the disease can occur alone, as a solitary disease or in association with other organ-specific immune diseases. The age of onset varies and at least three clinical entities exist:

Autoimmune polyglandular syndrome type 1 (APS 1)

Type 1 polyglandular syndrome (APS 1), also known as autoimmune polyendocrinopathy-candidiasis-ectodermal dystrophy (APECED;[10]) or autoimmune polyglandular disease type 1 (APD 1), is a rare disorder, and most of the earlier case reports described only single or a few patients. The first large series was published by Ahonen *et al.* from Finland [11]. The highest incidence of the syndrome has been found among isolated populations, such as Finns and Iranian Jews [13,21]. The patient with APS 1 develops chronic mucocutaneous candidiasis soon after birth; later, several organ-specific autoimmune diseases, mainly hypoparathyroidism and Addison's disease occur (Table 9.1). These are the most consistent disorders, and by definition APS 1 should have at least two

Table 9.1 Addison's disease and associated disorders in APS 1, APS 2 and solitary Addison's disease [adapted from References 11,18,50]

	APS 1 %	*APS 2 %*	*Solitary disease*
Addison's disease	72	100	100
Hypoparathyroidism	79	–	–
Mucocutaneous candidiasis	100	–	–
Autoimmune thyroid disease	4	69	–
Diabetes mellitus (IDDM)	12	52	–
Pernicious anaemia	18	Rare	–
Ovarian failure (only females)	60	2	–
HLA association	No HLA association	DRB1*0301 DQA1*0501 DQB1*0201	DRB1*0301 DQA1*0501 DQB1*0201

of the aforementioned three components. However, the syndrome includes several other clinical conditions such as chronic atrophic gastritis with or without pernicious anaemia, chronic active hepatitis, insulin-dependent diabetes mellitus (IDDM), autoimmune thyroid disease, alopecia, vitiligo or keratopathy, and in puberty, gonadal dysfunction [12].

Immunologically, the major findings are the presence of high-titre serum autoantibodies against the affected organs, antibodies against antigens of *Candida albicans*, and a low or absent T cell response toward candidal antigens [13]. The disease is not associated with any particular HLA haplotype and both males and females are equally affected, consistent with the autosomal recessive mode of inheritance.

Autoimmune polyglandular syndrome type 2 (APS 2)

APS 2, also known as Schmidt's syndrome, is more common and does not show the population restriction observed with APS 1. Clinical onset usually occurs in early adulthood, although it can start at any time during the lifespan. APS 2 is defined as a combination of Addison's disease with autoimmune thyroid disease [14] or IDDM [14], or both. Pernicious anaemia and hypogonadism may occur but less frequently than in APS 1 and not usually in childhood. This syndrome affects especially middle-aged Caucasoid women with a male/female ratio of 1:8. A multifactorial aetiology has been proposed, involving different genetic and environmental factors [16]. One clearly critical genomic region is the major histocompatibility complex (MHC). In contrast to APS 1, APS 2 is clearly associated with specific HLA risk haplotype [17,18].

Solitary Addison's disease

The solitary adult form of Addison's disease has the same age of onset and HLA association as APS 2. Although other immune diseases are not seen in these patients, the clinical picture and, especially, association with HLA suggest that this form is in fact a variant of APS 2. It is likely that the similar genetic background, in particular through the effect of HLA genes, can lead to any combination of the three main diseases seen in APS 2.

GENETICS

The genetic background of autoimmune Addison's disease depends on whether it occurs as a part of APS 1 or APS 2 or as a solitary form. It should be noted that some APS 1 cases may have Addison's disease as their only clinical manifestation and may therefore be difficult to classify if family records are not available. Furthermore, cases where the diagnosis of APS 1 is based on genetic studies or on family history, only some of the clinical conditions belonging to the syndrome may have appeared, depending largely on the age of the patient.

Because of the genetic differences in APS 1 and APS 2 or the solitary disease, the aetiology of the autoimmune process attacking adrenal cortex in these syndromes is probably different, but will eventually lead to a similar immunological destruction and clinical disease.

APS 1: an autosomal recessive genetic disease

APS 1 has a well-defined autosomal recessive form of inheritance, confirmed by several reports [10,19–21]. APS 1 in populations with a high incidence of the disease is likely to be the result of one or a few founder mutations. The prevalence of the disease among the Finns and Iranian Jews is estimated to be 1:25000 and 1:9000, respectively, whereas only a few cases in other parts of the world are found each year. The slight clinical variability of the disease between the populations, with relative infrequency of candidiasis among the Iranian Jews is presumably caused by different mutations in the defective gene or by other modifying genetic factors [13,22]. Nevertheless, environmental factors influencing the expression of APS 1 cannot be entirely excluded [22].

The localization of the APS 1 gene on chromosome 21p22.3 has been carried out using linkage analyses in Finnish families [23]. The analysis assigned the disease locus to a position between D21S49 and D21S171, with the peak value of lod score between markers PFKL and D21S171. This limited the APS 1 critical region to approximately 500 kb. Furthermore, the analyses of 9 Iranian Jewish and 21 other non-Finnish families revealed that APS 1 in different populations is probably due to different mutations in a single gene on 21q22.3 [24]. The haplotype analyses of Finnish family material suggest that >85–90% of cases are due to one major mutation that has been common in the ancestors of the Finnish population and that some minor mutations originating from different Finnish subpopulations are responsible for the remaining 10% of the APS 1 cases [24].

Recently, as part of the international efforts to generate the entire sequence of human chomosome 21, the partial sequence of the critical region for APS 1 was made available in GenBank by the Stanford Human Genome Center. The Center is currently carrying out the sequencing of 1.0 Mb around the region of APS 1 gene.

APS 2 and the solitary form of Addison's disease

Many cases of APS 2 and solitary Addison's disease are sporadic. However, similarly to other organ-specific autoimmune diseases the syndrome often shows familial aggregation [16]. It is likely that APS 2 does not have a strictly mendelian inheritance, but is triggered by some genetic predisposition combined with extrinsic factors.

APS 2 shows a strong association with the MHC locus (Figure 9.1), and was first found to be associated with HLA-B8 in the class I region [25,26]. Subsequent studies demonstrated that the primary association was with HLA-DR3 in the MHC class II locus and that HLA-B8 is involved secondarily

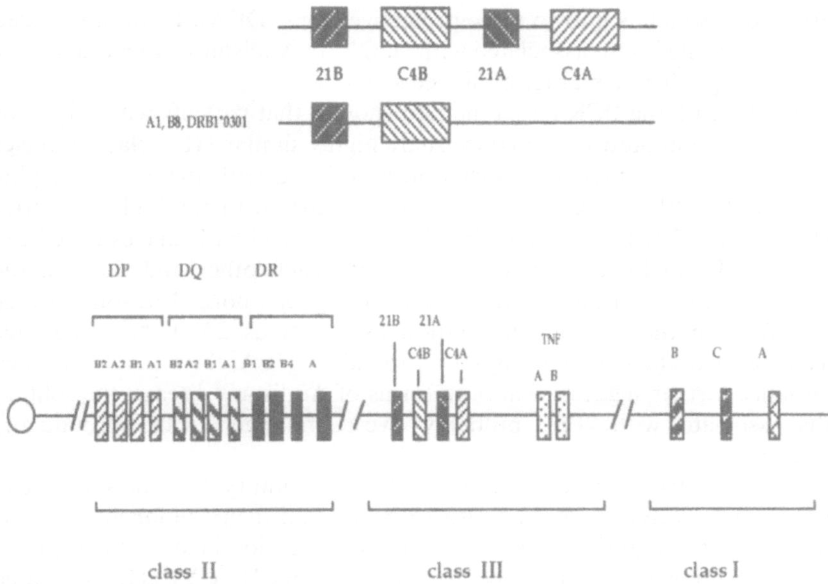

Figure 9.1 Map of the human MHC (adapted from Campbell and Trowsdale 1993)

through linkage disequilibrum between these two regions [27,28]. In a study with 34 Addison's disease patients, the frequency of DR3 was significantly increased with a relative risk factor of 3.4 [27]. When occurring as part of APS 2, the relative risk factor rose to 10. In another study of 45 patients DR3 but also DR4 carried a risk of 6 and 4.6, respectively [28]. Both HLA antigens are also associated with IDDM [29]. Despite this the relative risks in relation to Addison's disease of both molecules remained significant even when patients with co-existing IDDM were excluded from this series. Weetman and co-workers [17] confirmed the positive association with DR3 in 33 British patients (relative risk 3.6), but failed to find any increased frequency of DR4. A strong and significant association was also found for HLA-DQ2 but as DR3 and DQ2 are in linkage disequilibrium, the finding was thought to be a reflection of this fact. It is important to note that the presence of polyendocrinopathy in these Addison's disease patients did not increase the relative risk for HLA-DR3 and DQ2 molecules. Addison's disease patients in the German population also showed a DR3 association [30]. In this study the role of HLA-DQ was analysed by dividing DR4-positive Addison's disease patients into two groups: those with and without IDDM. Addison's disease with IDDM invariably showed an association with HLA-DQ8 (DQB1*0302 according to the new nomenclature), a high risk allele in isolated IDDM. In contrast, in the DR4-positive Addison's disease patients without IDDM the preferential HLA-DQ allele was DQ7

(DQB1*0301), which is known to be protective from IDDM. It was concluded that DQ8 molecule is also associated with IDDM in Addison's patients and may therefore be a predictive marker of diabetes [30].

Our results with the PCR-based method showed that patients with APS 2 or the solitary form of Addison's disease share highly similar HLA class II alleles [18]. A strong and significant association was found with three polymorphic alleles: DRB1*0301, DQA1*0501 and DQB1*0201, with the highest relative risk (RR) up to 27 with DQA1*0501 allele. All three class II alleles have been described to be in linkage disequilibrum with each other and, indeed, the frequency of the three alleles together remained higher among Addison's disease patients than in the random population (83% versus 20%). No difference between the two clinical subgroups was found in HLA class II alleles. Such concordance further suggests that both forms of Addison's disease, the solitary and that associated with APS 2, probably have a similar genetic background and aetiology.

In view of the strong association with APS 2 and solitary Addison's disease to specific HLA haplotypes, one can also speculate that the polymorphism of the identified major autoantigen, P450c21 (see the discussion below), could play a role in the pathogenesis. The gene coding for P450c21, CYP21B, is located within the HLA region, between class II and class III and known to be polymorphic. We therefore studied both the gene organization of the CYP21 gene as well as the polymorphism in the coding region [31]. We showed that patients with solitary Addison's disease or APS 2 had the HLA-B8, DRB1*0301, DQA1*0501 DQB1*0201 haplotype with specific alleles in the HSP70 and TNFB genes located approximately 200 kb and 450 kb, respectively, telomeric to MHC class III region. Furthermore, 11 of 12 patients had a deletion of the C4A and CYP21A (a pseudogene for P450c21) genes and thus carried only the remaining C4B and CYP21B gene pair. In the coding sequence of a CYP21B specific polymorphism was also seen to be associated with APS 2 and solitary Addison's disease. All patients studied had a particular CYP21B allele; an additional leucine was found in position 10, Lys→Arg transition at position 102 and an Asn→Ser transition at position 494 [31]. This polymorphism was present either homozygously or heterozygously in all patients studied. Based on these studies, one can conclude that in APS 2 and solitary Addison's disease a specific HLA haplotype, linked with an equally specific polymorphism in the CYP21B gene, is the key risk factor for developing Addison's disease.

IMMUNOLOGICAL FINDINGS

Immunofluorescence studies on adrenocortical autoantibodies

A large amount of information concerning the presence and nature of adrenal autoantibodies has been collected for four decades. Anderson *et al.* [32] were the first to report the presence of adrenocortical antibodies in patients with Addison's disease using complement fixation. This work was later confirmed by the immunofluorescence method [33] and showed that the reactivity of patient sera with adrenal cortex could be absorbed with an adrenal microsomal fraction but not with extracts from other tissue sources [13]. Using indirect immunofluorescence, adrenocortical autoantibodies (ACA) were found in 50–90% of patients with Addison's disease [13,34,35]. ACA have also been detected by immunodiffusion [36,37], ELISA [38] and radioimmunoassay [39]. The autoantibodies are mostly of the IgG class [36,40] and usually react with all layers of the adrenal cortex in immunofluorescence [41].

Differential centrifugation of subcellular fractions of adrenal cortex has been used to demonstrate that both microsomal and mitochondrial fractions contain adrenal autoantigens [40,42,43]. Other investigators have reported antibodies reacting with the adrenal cell surface [44a] and antibodies affecting the *in vitro* stimulation of cortisol secretion by ACTH have also been described [45,46]. Adrenal autoantigens have been further characterized by immunoprecipitation of ^{125}I labelled adrenal microsomes demonstrating that 57% of Addison's disease serum samples reacted with a 55 kDa adrenal-specific protein [47].

Immunofluorescence studies have revealed several antigens in the steroid producing cells, consistently present in the adrenal but with variable distribution in the ovary, testis and placenta. The sera of patients with Addison's disease and APS 1 react with the theca interna and corpus luteum of ovary, interstitial cells of testis, and placental trophoblasts [41,48–50]. To distinguish such antibodies from the ACA, they have generally been named steroid cell antibodies (StCA).

Destruction of adrenocortical cells and cell-mediated immunity

Adrenalitis appears to be largely diffuse, affecting all three layers of the cortex. It consists mainly of lymphocytes, but macrophages and plasma cells are also detected [15]. Small focal lymphocytic infiltrates are sometimes observed in elderly, apparently normal individuals. More than 60% of Japanese over the age of 60 were found to have focal adrenal infiltration at autopsy [51]. Immunohistochemical examinations revealed that the mononuclear cells were mainly $CD3^+$ $CD4^+$ T cells, whereas $CD3^+$ $CD8^+$ T cells were less in number. As judged by IL-2R expression, a considerable proportion of $CD4^+$ T cells were activated [51].

T cell responses toward adrenal tissue have been examined by the leukocyte migration inhibition test *in vitro*. Using adrenal extract as an antigen, positive findings have been reported in 40% of patients with autoimmune Addison's disease, while no response was found in patients with tuberculous Addison's disease [52]. However, the same antigen was unable to stimulate T cell proliferation in blast transformation experiments. The finding of leukocyte migration inhibition was confirmed later with positive reactivity in more than 80% of patients [52]. Leukocyte migration tests showed no correlation with the presence of adrenocortical antibodies or to the duration of the disease. A delayed type skin reaction was also demonstrated *in vivo* by intradermal injections of adrenal antigen [52]. An increased number of circulating activated and HLA class II$^+$ T lymphocytes has been reported among patients with a recent onset of the disease, whereas patients with Addison's disease of long duration have not been found to differ from normal individuals [53].

As a source of crude antigen, fractionated adrenal homogenate was used by Freeman and Weetman in a T cell proliferation assay [54]. Peripheral blood mononuclear cells from six out of ten patients tested showed proliferation in response to different fractions used and, in particular, to one with a molecular weight of 18–24 kDa. It was unclear whether this fraction represented a whole protein antigen with low molecular weight or whether it was a breakdown product.

Aberrant MHC class II molecule expression and antigen presentation has been proposed as an initiating mechanism in pathogenesis of autoimmune endocrine diseases [55]. According to this, up-regulation of MHC molecules on endocrine cells will induce the activation of CD4$^+$ T cells and consequently give rise to humoral and cytotoxic immune reactions against the tissue. The first findings were based on experiments in thyroid autoimmunity [56] and were later also described in pancreatic β cells in IDDM [57,58]. However, expression of class II molecules in non-lymphoid tissues can be physiological [59] or the result of an inflammatory process [60]. The expression of MHC class II molecules on adrenals was studied in eight patients who had died of recent-onset Addison's disease [61]. The majority of residual adrenocortical cells from these glands were positive for MHC class II molecules by immunohistochemistry, varying between 50 and 100% in different cases. In normal autopsy adrenals, by contrast, class II immunoreactivity was lacking or was variably observed in 5–50% of cortical cells, mostly restricted to the zona reticularis [44,61,62]. Interestingly, adrenals from patients with tuberculous Addison's disease also showed immunoreactivity similarly to those from patients with autoimmune adrenal disease. So far no evidence exists of virus-induced autoimmunity in Addison's disease.

TARGET ANTIGENS IN ADDISON'S DISEASE AND RELATED ENDOCRINOPATHIES

Steroidogenic P450 cytochromes, P450c17, P450c21 and P450scc and APS 1

The organ-specific reactivity of ACA and StCA suggested that the autoantigens recognized would be involved in steroid biosynthesis. In fact, early studies revealed that the autoantigens recognized by APS 1 sera resided in a protein fraction that bound radioactive cholesterol and converted it to cortisol [43]. In the early 1990s it was shown that the major autoantigens in Addison's disease were, in fact, members of the enzymatic pathway responsible for steroid hormone biosynthesis in the adrenal cortex and in other steroid producing cells. Krohn *et al* [63] screened a fetal adrenal expression library with sera from patients with APS 1 and demonstrated that one of the steroidogenic P450 cytochromes, steroid 17α-hydroxylase (P450c17), was a target autoantigen. Subsequently Winqvist *et al.* [64,65], Song *et al.* [66], Uibo *et al.* [67], Colls *et al.* [68] and Chen *et al.* [69] have reported that two other steroidogenic enzymes, steroid 21-hydroxylase (P450c21) and side-chain cleavage enzyme (P450scc), are also recognized by sera from APS1 patients with Addison's disease. All three enzymes are actively involved in the steroidogenic pathway in adrenal cortex.

Our analyses of P450c17, P450c21 and P450scc as autoantigens showed that 81% of the patients with Addison's disease reacted with at least one of the three proteins in immunoblotting [67] and up to 85% of the patients were positive in immunoprecipitation [70]. All three cytochromes were frequently recognized in immunoprecipitation by sera from APS 1 patients with Addison's disease, with no significant difference (55%, 52% and 56% respectively) for P450c17, P450c21and P450scc reactivity [70]. A high frequency of autoantibodies to the three steroidogenic enzymes in APS 1 was also found by Chen *et al.* [69] using immunoprecipitation in their patient series: 55%, 64% and 45% of patients reacted with P450c17, P450c21 and P450scc, respectively.

Other autoantigens recognized by APS 1 sera

Some recent studies have indicated that several other enzymes act as target antigens in APS 1. The autoantibodies to 65-kDa isoform of glutamic acid decarboxylase (GAD65), the major autoantigen in IDDM (Chapter 7), were originally described by Velloso *et al.* [72] and Seissler *et al.* [73]. In both studies relatively small number of patients were analysed but with high titres of GAD65 antibodies. High levels of circulating antibodies to GAD65 were also found in a large series of Finnish patients (47 individuals) with APS 1 [74]. All eight APS 1 patients with IDDM had GAD65 antibodies and also 41% of patients without clinical IDDM were positive for these autoantibodies.

Li *et al.* [75] reported that six out of 17 (35%) patients with acquired hypoparathyroidism in APS 1 reacted with the extracellular domain of calcium sensing receptor, a specific parathyroid enzyme. No reactivity with intracellular domain of this enzyme was observed.

The reactivity of APS 1 sera with a novel 51 kDa protein has been described [65,72]: this was later identified by screening of an expression library derived from rat insulinoma cells with APS 1 serum, as aromatic L-amino acid decarboxylase, expressed in several tissues including pancreatic β cells [76]. All seven sera studied precipitated from metabolically labelled Langerhans islets the 51 kDa protein that comigrated with a protein precipitated by a specific anti-aromatic L-amino acid decarboxylase antibody. However, despite the 100% reactivity in APS 1 patients, none of the patients with recent-onset IDDM or stiff-man syndrome reacted with this pancreatic antigen.

APS 1 patients have often autoimmune hepatitis and, therefore, the target autoantigens of this disease were studied by Manns and Obermayer-Straub (personal communication). They analysed a panel of ten different P450 cytochromes (P450 1A1, 1A2, 2A6, 2B6, 2C8, 2C9, 2C19, 2D6, 3A4 and 2E1) for reactivity in immunoblotting. Four of 64 Finnish patients had anti-P450 1A2 and nine anti-P450 2A6 antibodies, but positive reactivity was also found with P450 1A1 and P450 2B6 cytochromes. Interestingly, none of these APS 1 patients had autoantibodies to P450 2D6, the major target in autoimmune hepatitis and, in contrast, none of the patients with autoimmune hepatitis but without APS 1 recognized cytochrome P450 2D6 and P450 2A6 as the autoantigens.

We screened a *C. albicans* cDNA expression library with patient sera to characterize the antibody responses in APS 1 patients with chronic mucocutaneous candidiasis and found four reactive proteins – enolase, heat-shock protein 90, pyruvate kinase and alcohol dehydrogenase [77]. The reactivity to these antigens was studied further by immunoprecipitation which showed the highest response to enolase (80% of patients reactive), compared to heat-shock protein 90 (67%), pyruvate kinase (62.5%) and alcohol dehydrogenase (64%). Overall, 95.5% of the patients had detectable antibodies to at least one of these proteins, indicating that these four candidal proteins are the major antigens and, therefore, can be used as accurate markers of candidiasis in APS 1 patients [77].

Such a variety of different autoantibodies in APS 1 suggests that multiple autoimmune processes to different organs are occurring in these patients and that many of the autoantigens in this disorder remain to be identified. The reason and role of the autoantibodies in APS 1 pathogenesis remains unknown but will be resolved, hopefully, after the identification of the defective gene and its function.

P450c21 in APS 2 and solitary Addison's disease

In our own patient series, seven out of nine (78%) Addison's disease patients with APS 2 reacted only with P450c21, and one patient was simultaneously positive for P450c17 autoantibodies. P450c21 has also been identified as a major autoantigen in adult Addison's disease by three independent groups [78–80] reporting prevalences of 75%, 72% and 87%, respectively.

Using the immunoprecipitation assay of *in vitro* translated and ^{35}S-labelled P450c21, Colls *et al.* [68] found autoantibodies to P450c21 in 66% of patients with isolated Addison's disease and in 90% of those with APS 2. Immunoprecipitation results were reported to correlate well with the results obtained by immunoblotting of P450c21 protein expressed in yeast. The same group in their most recent report describes the presence of P450c21 autoantibodies in 96% of APS 2 and in 64% of patients with solitary Addison's disease [69,71]. Furthermore, they have also found P450c17 autoantibodies in 33% and 5%, and P450scc autoantibodies in 42% and 9% of patients with APS 2 and solitary Addison's disease, respectively [69,71]. A report by Falorni *et al.* [81] describes the use of a similar immunoprecipitation assay with an 86% prevalence of P450c21 autoantibodies among 28 patients with Addison's disease. Further studies by Falorni and collaborators with 48 patients obtained even higher sensitivity (92%) among Addison's disease patients (personal communication).

A new and sensitive method has been developed by Furmaniak and collaborators. Using the recombinant human P450c21 expressed in yeast, purified to 100% homogeneity and labelled with ^{125}I, they were able to detect P450c21 autoantibodies in 100% and 72% of patients with APS 2 and solitary Addison's disease, respectively (personal communication).

Other steroidogenic enzymes expressed in Addison's disease

As all three identified autoantigens in Addison's disease were enzymes primarily involved in steroidogenesis, one could assume that other enzymes participating in this pathway might also act as autoantigens. However, no reactivity of APS 1, APS 2 or solitary Addison's disease sera with *E. coli*-expressed 3β-HSD and P450c11 was detected by Song *et al.* [66]. Similarly, four enzymes tested by us, 3β-HSD, P450c11, adrenodoxin and adrenodoxin reductase, showed no reactivity with APS 1, APS 2 or solitary Addison's disease patient sera [70]. 3β-HSD autoantibodies have been detected, however, in 21% of patients with premature ovarian failure by Arif and collaborators [83] but the sera from their patients with Addison's did not recognize the enzyme. The lack of reactivity toward these steroidogenic enzymes proves also that the humoral autoimmune response is specific, and not provoked non-specifically by the destruction of the adrenal gland and the subsequent release of autoantigen proteins.

These findings do not definitely rule out the possibility that other steroidogenic enzymes or other adrenal and steroid cell antigens are recognized by Addison's disease sera. In immunoblotting using whole human adrenal homogenate as antigen, several bands with molecular sizes of 55, 48, 43, 39 and 19 kDa [67] were seen and this would suggest that other antigens are also involved.

Predictive markers of Addison's disease

A good correlation with clinical findings has already been observed when ACA and StCA have been determined with immunofluorescence or other non-specific methods. Thus, ACA have not been detected in the tuberculous form of Addison's disease [41]. Furthermore, the presence of ACA is perceived as a highly specific marker for autoimmune Addison's disease and with a low prevalence (0.1–0.6%) in the normal population [84–88].

In our studies, 85% of patients with APS 1 reacted with one of the three steroidogenic proteins [70]. This is consistent with previous findings, where 85% of Addison's disease sera in this syndrome exhibited autoantibody reactivity towards steroid producing cells by immunofluorescence [86,89]. As described earlier, even higher specificity and sensitivity has been obtained with P450c21 autoantibodies in APS 2 and solitary Addison's disease. This means that the autoantibodies to steroidogenic P450 cytochromes are important disease markers in Addison's disease and, as a sign of ongoing immune destruction, often precede the clinical onset of the disease and may be potentially useful predictive markers.

The ACA were considered as a good predictive marker for Addison's disease and have been found in patients with IDDM or other autoimmune diseases, but without clinical Addison's disease [34,36,84,85,87,88,90]. Betterle and collaborators have performed extensive analysis of ACA among 8840 adult and 808 children patients with organ-specific autoimmunity but without clinical Addison's disease [91,92]. ACA were found in 0.8% of adults and in 1.7% of children. During a follow-up study, 21% of ACA-positive patients developed Addison's disease and 29% developed subclinical hypoadrenalism, while 50% of patients maintained normal adrenal function [91]. In contrast, nine of 10 ACA-positive children developed clinical Addison's disease [92]. The majority of ACA-positive individuals were also positive for P450c21 autoantibodies. Thus the detection of ACA/P450c21 antibodies has a low value as a predictive marker in adults but high value in children [91,92]. As many of these children had also hypoparathyroidism, they may be considered as patients with APS 1. In our own series of APS 1 patients who had antibodies but no clinical signs of adrenocortical failure, several developed the disease within the three years' observation period.

Adrenocortical autoantibodies have been demonstrated in patients with IDDM without clinical signs of Addison's disease [34,84,87]. We studied the sera from 304 patients with IDDM for P450c21 autoantibodies by the immunoprecipitation assay and found them in 2.3% [82]. Six of these patients carried the HLA-DQB1*0201 allele which is associated with increased susceptibility to adrenal autoimmunity. The P450c21 antibody-positive IDDM patients were also studied for ongoing Addison's disease, but no signs of clinical disease were observed, even during the 4 year observation period. These findings do not rule out, however, that the antibody-positive cases will later develop their disease, as it has been demonstrated that some patients may remain in the subclinical phase of Addison's disease for years [88] or develop adrenocortical insufficiency more than five years after the first appearance of autoantibodies [86]. Therefore, it will be important to follow up this and similar patient series.

The enzymes P450c17 and P450scc are present in most steroidogenic cells and APS 1 patients usually have or develop signs of gonadal failure, while patients with solitary Addison's disease or APS 2 usually only have symptoms from adrenal gland insufficiency. However, an interesting difference is seen between the men and women with APS 1; women frequently have signs of ovarian insufficiency while in men gonadal failure is not often seen. It is unknown whether this finding relates to the immunologically protected status of the testes.

Autoantigenic epitopes on P450c17 and P450c21

Defining antigenic B cell epitopes of autoantigens is of interest both from the practical as well as the theoretical point of view. More specific antibody tests, such as peptide ELISAs, can be developed when the specific B cell epitopes are known. Theoretically, the general finding that autoantibodies frequently recognize enzymes is of interest and the reason for this is unknown. However, with several other autoantigenic enzymes, the region recognized by the corresponding autoantibody has been shown to be identical, or close to, the catabolic site or other functionally active domains. One explanation for the fact that autoantibodies react with active sites of the antigens, might just be their location of the outer surface of the antigenic protein molecule.

In cases, where autoantibodies can be shown *in vitro* to inhibit the enzymatic activity of the autoantigen, it is temping to speculate that this activity could also have pathogenic significance, as is the case with antibodies recognizing receptor molecules on cell membranes. When the antigen is localized entirely inside a cell, as seems to be the case with the steroidogenic enzymes, it is however difficult to see how an antibody, localized outside, could have an effect *in vivo*.

Analysis of the autoantigenic epitopes of P450c17 and P450c21 shows that the major epitopes are also located closely to the active sites of the enzyme. The P450c17 cDNA fragments of different length were expressed in *E. coli* bacteria and patient sera were subsequently tested by immunoblotting [93]. Four epitope regions were found at amino acids 122–148, 280–304, 396–432 and 466–508, which all located in the regions with computer-predicted antigenicity. The first two epitope regions localized close to the region contributing to the substrate binding site, and the other two to the haem binding site [94]. As we found sera from APS 1 patients contained high titres of autoantibodies against P450c17, these autoantibodies can likely inhibit the enzyme activity *in vitro* [93].

Epitope mapping of P450c21 [95] with 11 Addison's sera revealed that deletions in the N-terminal part of the P450c21 polypeptide (amino acids 1–280) did not affect autoantibody binding. The central and C-terminal part (281–494) of P450c21 were important for autoantibody binding, and the authors suggested that two protein fragments, amino acids 281–379 and 380–494, interact to form at least one major conformational epitope. A series of more extensive modifications of P450c21 [96] showed that most of the amino acid sequence in region 241–494 is needed for autoantibody binding. In another study [79] the major antigenic region was found between amino acids 164 and 356, and by a further narrowing of this epitope, between amino acids 298 and 356. Only two of 30 patients reacted with amino acid fragments 1–162 and 344–494. These experiments also suggested the presence of conformational epitopes on P450c21. In conclusion, the main epitope regions recognized by sera from patients with Addison's disease seem to locate in a large segment in the central and C-terminal part of the protein.

The cross-reactivity between evolutionarily-related steroidogenic enzymes might be considered as a mechanism for autoimmunity in APS 1. Although the overall amino acid homology between P450c17 and P450c21, two adrenal steroidogenic enzymes of highest similarity, is only 29%, there is a considerable similarity in the regions predicted to form α-helices or β-sheets and also in the hydropathy profiles. In particular, similarity of protein conformation is found in the region of the presumed substrate binding site near amino acid 350 and downstream from the cysteine residue of haem binding site near amino acid 450 in the C-terminal half of the proteins. Furthermore, the catalytic regions on C-terminal part of P450c17 possess high amino acid sequence homology with P450c21, such as between amino acids 345 and 370 (76%), and between amino acids 435 and 465 (77%). To find out the eventual cross-reactivity between P450c17 and P450c21, the C-terminus corresponding protein regions (overall homology 64%) were used to preabsorb patient sera that were subsequently tested in immunoprecipitation assays [70]. The absorption experiments demonstrated that the preincubation with P450c17 or P450c21 inhibited specifically autoantibody binding to corresponding *in vitro* translated antigen but did not significantly influence the reactivity to the second antigen. The lack of extensive cross-reactivity between P450c17 and P450c21 supports the idea of independent autoantibody responses against steroidogenic P450 cytochromes and suggests that each enzyme is the individial target of humoral immunity in APS 1. However, cross-reactivity may occur on the T cell level.

Animal models

With the identification of the target autoantigens in Addison's disease, generation of an animal model would be advantageous in order to study in more detail the pathogenetic mechanism leading to the disease. In addition, this may also enable eventual testing of therapeutic and preventive strategies.

Spontaneous Addison's disease has been described in cats and dogs [96]. Experimental adrenal infiltration has been produced in guinea pigs by the intramuscular injection of adrenal homogenate with Freund's complete adjuvant, first described by Colover and Glynn [97]. Both the cortex and medulla were affected by infiltration and destruction. These and other similar experiments with guinea pigs were repeated with rabbits [98–100]. In addition to infiltration, the autoantibodies in immunized animals were found to react with homologous and heterologous adrenal organs [98–100]. Adrenalitis and adrenocortical autoantibodies have been obtained in Balb/c mice following cyclosporin A administration to newborn animals, coupled with thymectomy [101]. Multiple other organ-specific lesions such as gastritis, oophoritis, thyroiditis, sialoadenitis, insulitis and orchitis were also observed in these mice.

The lipopolysaccharide O3 from *Klebsiella* has been used as a powerful adjuvant to obtain lymphocytic infiltration of adrenals [102]. Immunization of SMA mice eight times with adrenal homogenate mixed with O3 lipopolysaccharide resulted in an adrenal infiltration of polymorphonuclear leukocytes, and after the ninth injection, infiltration of mononuclear cells such as lymphocytes and macrophages was observed. In addition, the adrenal tissue was replaced by fibrous connective tissue. No histological changes were found in the medullary regions suggesting that the adrenal cortex is more susceptible to immunological reaction. Both humoral and cell-mediated immunity were involved as the immunized mice produced adrenocortical autoantibodies and the adrenalitis could be produced in normal mice by transfer of spleen cells.

In preliminary experiments, we immunized Balb/c mice with DNA vectors expressing the P450c21 antigen and showed development of P450c21-specific antibodies linked with lymphocytic infiltration of the adrenal gland. This model could in the future be used to identify the T cell epitopes recognized by immune cells in the immunized animals, and furthermore to test whether antagonistic peptides could prevent the disease or affect the outcome of the disease process. An eventual mouse model for APS 1 could be a knock-out mouse of the analogous defective gene in this syndrome.

Possible pathogenic mechanisms of Addison's disease

Although the clinical picture of adrenal cortical failure in APS 1 and APS 2 and solitary Addison's disease is similar, it is likely that the pathogenetic mechanisms leading to the syndromes vary. APS 1 is caused by a defect in one, as yet unknown gene and when this defect is revealed it will be of interest to learn how failure of one gene function can lead to such a variety of features. The major feature in APS 1 can be considered to be a strong humoral response toward a variety of potential autoantigens. Thus, an imbalance in the two helper T cell populations, T_H1 and T_H2, can be suspected to be a key factor in the pathogenesis of the two polyendocrinopathy syndromes. It is conceivable to believe that in APS 1 the immune response has a T_H2 dominance, with increased production of cytokines IL-10 and IL-4 leading to over-reactivity of the B cell compartment. In APS 2 and in solitary Addison's disease, the immunological features would fit better to a T_H1-dominated immune response. This assumption fits also with the observed HLA association. It could therefore be speculated that the immunological lesions in APS 1 are caused mainly by antibodies, while lesions in APS 2 could be the result of cell-mediated immune responses, presumably having cytotoxic T lymphocytes as effector cells.

However, as discussed earlier, an antibody recognizing an intracellular antigen can hardly result in cellular destruction directly, and other pathogenic reactions must be involved. Thus, both in APS 1 and APS 2, the direct pathogenic mechanism by which the adrenal cortex is destroyed is probably cell-mediated. Attempts to demonstrate clearly a cell-mediated immune response toward adrenal cortical cells or its compartments has, however, so far been less successful. The identification of steroidogenic enzymes as autoantigens should in future assist these experiments.

An open question is whether, on the cellular level, the main effector cell belongs to the $CD4^+$ helper or to $CD8^+$ cytotoxic lineage, or whether both are crucial to disease progression. Activation of autoreactive T cells seems to be necessary in Addison's disease. Autoreactive $CD4^+$ cells recognizing autoantigenic peptides on HLA will subsequently release various cytokines and recruit and activate $CD8^+$ cells and macrophages. Most likely the $CD8^+$ cells will then cause the tissue destruction by expressing perforin and granzymes, the molecules associated with cytotoxicity [103]. However, it is also possible that $CD4^+$ cells or macrophages have cytotoxic properties [104] involved in the pathogenesis of Addison's disease.

Cytotoxic T cell assays have so far not been performed or reported in

Addison's disease. In future it will be appropriate to focus research efforts on a better understanding of the cell-mediated immunity of the disease. The ligand motifs are now available for many HLA molecules, and equipped with the amino acid sequence of autoantigens and a computer programme, it is possible to generate putative HLA binding peptides and test their antigenicity in T cell assays. Furthermore, based on the information on T cell epitopes, it is possible to create modified peptides from the target amino acid sequence e.g. by changing the amino acids exposed to the T cell receptor or by using chemically altered peptides to tolerize the patient by antagonistic peptide immunization.

In conclusion, during the last five years, research on Addison's disease has entered the era of molecular immunology. The target autoantigens in Addison's disease, both when occuring alone or in combination with the two polyendocrinopathy syndromes, have mostly been identified. Furthermore, the genetic background of the disease, such as the risk HLA haplotype or the gene defect causing APS 1, has been revealed or will be revealed soon. It is now possible to identify both T and B cell epitopes on the autoantigens, and this information will soon be used to generate not only better diagnostic methods but also ways to prevent or treat this model disease for autoimmunity.

During the process of this paper, we and others have identified the gene for APS 1, which was named AIRE for autoimmune regulator [105,106]. A common Finnish mutation, R257X, was shown to be responsible for 82% of Finnish APS 1 alleles. In addition, five other mutations were identified.

References

1. Addison T. On the constitutional and local effects of disease of the suprarenal capsules. In a collection of the publishedwritings of the late Thomas Addison MD, Physician to Guy's Hospital. New Sydenham Society (1868) London (Reprinted in Medical Classics 2, 244–93, 1939), 1855.
2. Wilks S. On diseases of the suprarenal capsule or morbus addisonii. Guy's Hosp Rep. 1862; 8:1.
3. Burke CW. Primary adrenocortical failure. In: A. Grossman, ed. Clinical Endocrinology. Blackwell Scientific Publications: Oxford; 1992:393–404.
4. Mosser J, Douar AM, Sarde K et al. Putative X-linked adrenoleukodystrophy gene shares unexpected homology with ABC transporters. Nature. 1993;361:726–73
5. Baker JR. Endocrine diseases. In: Stites DP, Terr AJ, eds. Basic and Clinical Immunology. Appleton and Lange: Singapore; 1991:464–75.
6. Stuart-Mason A, Meade TW, Lee JAH, Morris JN. Epidemiological and clinical picture of Addison's disease. Br Med J. 1968;2:744–7.
7. Nerup J. Addison's disease. Clinical studies. A report of 108 cases. Acta Endocrinol. 1974;76: 127–41.
8. Baxter JD. Adrenocortical hypofunction. In: Wyngaarden JB, Smith LH, eds. Cecil Textbook of Medicine. Philadelphia: Saunders; 1985:1310–15.
9. Kong MF, Jeffcoate W. Eighty-six cases of Addison's disease. Clin Endocrinol. 1994;41:757–61.
10. Perheentupa J. Autoimmune polyendocrinopathy-candidosis-ectodermal dystrophy (APECED). In: A. Eriksson, H. Forsius, H. Nevanlinna, P. Workman, R. Norio, eds. Population Structure and Genetic Disorders. London: Academic Press; 1980:577–83.
11. Ahonen P, Myllärniemi S, Sipilä I, Perheentupa J. Clinical variation of autoimmune polyendocrinopathy-candidiasis-ectodermal dystrophy (APECED) in a series of 68 patients. N Engl J Med. 1990;322:1829–36.

12. Blizzard RM, Kyle M. Studies of the adrenal antigens and antibodies in Addison's disease. J Clin Invest. 1963;42:1653–60.
13. Zlotogora J, Shapiro MS. Polyglandular autoimmune syndrome type I among Iranian Jews. J Med Genet. 1992;29:824–6.
14. Schmidt MB. Eine biglanduläre erkrankung (Nebennieren und schilddruse) bei morbus Addisonii. Verh Dtsch Ges Pathol. 1926;21:212–21.
15. Carpenter CCJ, Solomon N, Silverberg SG et al. Schmidt's syndrome (thyroid and adrenal insufficiency): a review of the literature and a report of fifteen new cases including ten instances of co-existent diabetes-mellitus. Medicine. 1964;43:153–80.
16. Butler K. Linkage analysis in a large kindred with autosomal dominant transmission of polyglandular autoimmune disease type II (Schmidt syndrome) Am J Med Genet. 1984;19: 61–5.
17. Weetman AP, Zhang L, Tandon N, Edwards OM. HLA associations with autoimmune Addison's disease. Tissue Antigens. 1991;38:31–3.
18. Partanen, J., P. Peterson, P. Westman, S. Aranko, K. Krohn. MHC class II and III in Addison's disease. MHC alleles do not predict autoantibody specificity and no independent role for 21-hydroxylase gene polymorphism in disease susceptibility. Hum Immunol. 1994; 41:135–40.
19. Hung W, Migeon C, Parrot R. A possible autoimmune basis for Addison's disease in three siblings, one with idiopathic hypoparathyroidism, pernicious anemia and superficial moniliasis. N Engl J Med. 1963;269:658–63.
20. Spinner M, Blizzard R, Childs B. Clinical and genetic heterogeneity in idiopathic Addison's disease and hypoparathyroidism. J Clin Endocrinol Metab. 1968;28:795–804.
21. Ahonen P. Autoimmune polyendocrinopathy-candidosis-ectodermal dystrophy (APECED): autosomal recessive inheritance. Clin Genet. 1985;27:535–42.
22. Ahonen P. Autoimmune polyendocrinopathy-candidiasis-ectodermal dystrophy APECED. The thesis. University of Helsinki, Helsinki; 1993.
23. Aaltonen J, Björses P, Sandkuijl L, Perheentupa J, Peltonen L. An autosomal locus causing autoimmune disease: autoimmune polyglandular disease type I assigned to chromosome 21. Nat Genet. 1994;8:83–7.
24. Björses P, Aaltonen J, Vikman A et al. Genetic homogeneity of autoimmune polyglandular disease type I. Am J Hum Genet. 1996;59:879–86.
25. Thomsen M, Platz P, Andersen OO et al. MLC typing in juvenile diabetes mellitus and idiopathic Addison's disease. Transplant Rev. 1975;22:125–47.
26. Eisenbarth GS, Wilson P, Ward F, Buckley C, Lebovitz HE. The polyglandular failure syndrome: disease inheritance, HLA-type and immune function. Ann Intern Med. 1979;91: 528–33.
27. Latienne D, Vandeput Y, Bruyere MD, Bottazzo F, Sokal G, Crabbe J. Addison's disease: immunological aspects. Tissue Antigens. 1987;30:23–4.
28. Maclaren NK and Riley WJ. Inherited susceptibility to autoimmune Addison's disease is linked to human leukocyte antigens DR3 and/or DR4, except when associated with autoimmune polyglandular disease. J Clin Endocrinol Metab. 1986;62:455–9.
29 Todd JA. Genetic control of autoimmunity in type 1 diabetes. Immunol Today. 1990;11:122–9.
30. Boehm BO, Manfras B, Seidl S et al. The HLA-DQb non Asp-57 allele: a predictor of future insulin-dependent diabetes mellitus in patients with autoimmune Addison's disease. Tissue Antigens. 1991;37:130–2.
31. Peterson P, Partanen J, Aavik E, Salmi H, Pelkonen R, Krohn KJ. Steroid 21-hydroxylase gene polymorphism in Addison's disease patients. Tissue Antigens. 1995;46:63–7.
32. Anderson JR, Goudie RB, Gray KG, Timbury GC. Auto-antibodies in Addison's disease. Lancet. 1957;ii:123–4.
33. Blizzard RM, Kyle MA, Chandler RW, Hung W. Adrenal antibodies in Addison's disease. Lancet. 1962;ii:901–2.
34. Riley WJ, Maclaren NK, Neufeld M. Adrenal autoantibodies and Addison's disease in insulin-dependent diabetes mellitus. J Pediat. 1980;97:191–5.
35. Sotsiou F, Bottazzo GF, Doniach D. Immunofluorescence studies on autoantibodies to steroid producing cells, and to germline cells In endocrine disease and fertility. Clin Exp Immunol. 1980;39:97–111.
36. Krohn K, Perheentupa J, Heinonen E. Precipitating anti-adrenal antibodies in Addison's disease. Clin Immunol Immunopathol. 1974;3:59–68.

37. Heinonen E, Krohn K, Perheentupa J, Aro A, Pelkonen R. Association of precipitating anti-adrenal antibodies to monialis–polyendocrinopathy syndrome. Ann Clin Res. 1976;8:262–5.
38. Stechemesser E, Scherbaum WA, Grossman T, Berg PA. An ELISA method for the detection of autoantibodies to adrenal cortex. J Immunol Meth. 1985;80:67–76.
39. Kozowicz J, Gryczynska M, Bottazzo GF. A radioimmunoassay for the detection of adrenal autoantibodies. Clin Exp Immunol. 1986;63:671–9.
40. Goudie RB, McDonald E, Anderson JR, Gray K. Immunological features of idiopathic Addison's disease: characterization of adrenocortical antigens. Clin Exp Immunol. 1968;3: 119–31.
41. Irvine WJ, Barnes EW. Addison's disease, ovarian failure and hypoparathyroidism. Clin Endocrinol Metab. 1975;4:379–84.
42. Heinonen E. Variety of determinants in an adrenal antigen common to man and some animals. Med Biol. 1976;54:341–6.
43. Heinonen E, Krohn K. Studies on an adrenal antigen common to man and different animals. Med Biol. 1977;55:48–53.
44a Khoury EL, Hammond L, Bottazzo GF, Doniach D. Surface reactive antibodies to human adrenal cells in Addison's disease. Clin Exp Immunol. 1981;45:48–55.
44. Khoury EL, Greenspan JS, Greenspan FS. Adrenocortical cells of the zona reticularis normally express HLA-DR antigenic determinants. Am J Pathol. 1987;127:580–91.
45. Kendall-Taylor P, Lambert A, Mitchell R, Robertson WR. Antibody that blocks stimulation of cortisol secretion by adrenocortcotrophic hormone in Addison's disease. Br Med J. 1988; 296:1489–91.
46. Wulffraat NM, Drexhage HA, Bottazzo GF, Wiersinga WM, Jeucken P, van der Gaag R. Immunoglobulins of patients with idiopathic Addison's disease block the in vitro action of adrenocorticotropin. J Clin Endocrinol Metab. 1989;69:231–8.
47. Furmaniak JD, Talbot D, Reinwein G, Benker F, Creagh M, Smith BR. Immunoprecipitation of human adrenal microsomal antigen. FEBS Lett. 1988;231:25–8.
48. Anderson JR, Goudie RB, Gray K, Stuart-Smith DA. Immunological features of idiopathic Addison's disease: An antibody to cells producing steroid hormones. Clin Exp Immunol. 1968;3:107–17.
49. Irvine WJ, Chan MW, Scarth L. The further characterization of autoantibodies reactive with extra-adrenal steroid-producing cells in patients with adrenal disorders. Clin Exp Immunol. 1969;4:489–503.
50. Maclaren NK and Blizzard RM. Adrenal autoimmunity and autoimmune polyglandular syndromes. In: Rose NR, McKay, IR, eds. The Autoimmune Diseases. New York: Academic Press; 1985:201–25.
51. Hayashi Y, Hiyoshi T, Takemura T, Kurashima C, Hirokawa K. Focal lymphocytic infiltration in the adrenal cortex of the elderly: immunohistological analysis of infiltrating lymphocytes. Clin Exp Immunol. 1989;77:101–5.
52. Moulias R, Goust MJ, Deville Chabrolle A, Buffet C, Muller-Berat CN. Le test de migration des leucocytes du sang peripherique (TML). Un nouveau test d'hypersensibilité retardée in vitro chez l'homme. Presse Médicale. 1970;73:2315.
52. Nerup J, Bendixen G. Anti-adrenal cellular hypersensitivity in Addison's disease. 2. Correlation with clinical and serological findings. Clin Exp Immunol. 1969;5:341–54.
53. Rabinowe SL, Jackson RA, Dluhy RG, Williams GH. Ia-positive T lymphocytes in recently diagnosed idiopathic Addison's disease. Am J Med. 1984;77:597–601.
54. Freeman M, Weetman AP. T and B cell reactivity to adrenal antigens in autoimmune Addison's disease. Clin Exp Immunol. 1992;88;275–9.
55. Bottazzo GF, Pujol-Borrell R, Hanafusa T. Role of aberrant HLA-DR expression and antigen presentation in induction of endocrine autoimmunity. Lancet. 1983;ii:1115–19.
56. Hanafusa T, Pujol-Borrell R, Chiovato L, Russell RC, Doniach D, Bottazzo GF. Aberrant expression of HLA-DR antigen on thyrocytes in Graves' disease: relevance for autoimmunity. Lancet. 1983;ii:1111–15.
57. Bottazzo GF, Dean BM, McNally JM, MacKay EH, Swift PGF, Gamble DR. In situ characterization of autoimmune phenomena and expression of HLA molecules in the pancreas in diabetic insulitis. N Engl J Med. 1985;313:353–60.
58. Foulis AK, Farquharson MA. Aberrant expression of HLA-DR antigens by insulin containing beta cells in recent onset type I (insulin-dependent) diabetes mellitus. Diabetes. 1987;35: 1215–24.

59. Spencer J, Pugh S, Isaacson PG. HLA-D region antigen expression on stomach epithelium in absence of autoantibodies. Lancet. 1986;ii:983.
60. Khoury EL. Aberrant expression of class II HLA antigens by the target cell: cause or consequence of the autoimmune aggression? Acta Endocrinol. 1987;281:35–41.
61. Jackson R, McNicol AM, Farquharson M, Foulis AK. Class II MHC expression in normal adrenal cortex and cortical cells in Addison's disease. J Pathol. 1988;155:113–20.
62. McNicol AM. Class II antigen expression in adrenal cortex. Lancet. 1986;ii:1282.
63. Krohn K, Uibo R, Aavik E, Peterson P, Savilahti K. Identification by molecular cloning of an autoantigen associated with Addison's disease as steroid 17 alpha-hydroxylase (see comments). Lancet. 1992;339:770–3.
64. Winqvist O, Gustafsson J, Rorsman F, Karlsson FA, Kämpe O. Two different cytochrome P450 enzymes are the adrenal antigens in autoimmune polyendocrine syndrome type I and Addison's disease. J Clin Invest. 1993;92:2377–85.
65. Winqvist O, Gebre-Medhin G, Gustafsson J et al. Identification of the main gonadal autoantigens in patients with adrenal insufficiency and associated ovarian failure. J Clin Endocr Metab. 1995;80:1717–23.
66. Song Y-H, Connor EL, Muir A et al. Autoantibody epitope mapping of the 21-hydroxylase antigen in autoimmune Addison's disease. J Clin Endocrinol Metab. 1994;78:1108–12.
67. Uibo R, Perheentupa J, Ovod V, Krohn K. Characterization of adrenal autoantigens recognized by sera from patients with autoimmune polyglandular syndrome (APS) type I. Autoimmunity. 1994;7:399–411.
68. Colls J, Betterle C, Volpato M, Prentice L, Rees Smith B, Furmaniak J. Autoimmune adrenal disease – a new immunoprecipitation assay for autoantibodies to steroid 21-hydroxylase. Clin Chem. 1995;41:367–74.
69. Chen S, Sawicka J, Betterle C et al. Autoantibodies to steroidogenic enzymes in autoimmune polyglandular syndrome, Addison's disease, and premature ovarian failure. J Clin Endocrinol Metab. 1996;81:1871–6.
70. Peterson P, Uibo R, Peränen J, Krohn K. Immunoprecipitation of steroidogenic enzyme autoantigens with autoimmunen polyglandular syndrome type I (APS I) sera: further evidence for independent humoral immunity to P450c17 and P450c21. Clin Exp Immunol. 1997;107:335–40.
71. Chen S, Sawicka J, Betterle C et al. Autoantibodien to steroidogenic enzymes in patients with autoimmune adrenal disease and premature ovarian failure. J Endocrinol. 1996;148:62.
72. Velloso LA, Winqvist O, Gustafsson J, Kämpe O, Karlsson FA. Autoantibodies against a novel 51 kDa islet antigen and glutamate decarboxylase isoforms in autoimmune polyendocrine syndrome type I. Diabetologia 1994;37:61–9.
73. Seissler J, Bieg S, Yassin N et al. Association between antibodies to the mr 67,000 isoform of glutamate decarboxylase (GAD) and type 1 (insulin-dependent) diabetes mellitus with coexisting autoimmune polyendocrine syndrome type II. Autoimmunity. 1994;19:231–8.
74. Tuomi T, Bjorses P, Falorni A et al. Antibodies to glutamic acid decarboxylase and insulin-dependent diabetes in patients with autoimmune polyendocrine syndrome type I. J Clin Endocrinol Metab. 1996;81:1488–94.
75. Li Y, Song Y, Rais N, Connor E, Schatz D, Muir A, Maclaren N. Autoantibodies to the extracellular domain of the calcium sensing receptor in patients with acquired hypoparathyroidism. J Clin Invest. 1996;97:910–14.
76. Rorsman F, Husebye ES, Winqvist O, Bjork E, Karlsson FA, Kämpe O. Aromatic L-amino acid decarboxylase, a pyridoxal phosphate-dependent enzyme, is a beta-cell autoantigen. Proc Natl Acad Sci USA. 1995;92:8626–9.
77. Peterson P, Perheentupa J, Krohn KJ. Detection of candidal antigens in autoimmune polyglandular syndrome type I. Clin Diagn Lab Immunol. 1996;3:290–4.
78. Winqvist O, Karlsson FA, Kämpe O. 21-Hydroxylase, a major autoantigen in idiopathic Addison's disease. Lancet. 1992;339:1559–62.
79. Song YH, Connor E, Li Y, Zorovich B, Balducci P, Maclaren N. The role of tyrosinase in autoimmune vitiligo. Lancet. 1994;344:1049–52.
80. Bednarek J, Furmaniak J, Wedlock N et al. Steroid 21-hydroxylase is a major autoantigen involved in adult onset autoimmune Addison's disease. FEBS Lett. 1992;309:51–5.
81. Falorni A, Nikoshkov A, Laureti S et al. High diagnostic accuracy for idiopathic Addison's disease with a sensitive radiobinding assay for autoantibodies against recombinant human 21-hydroxylase. J Clin Endocr Metab. 1995;80:2752–5.

82. Peterson P, Salmi H, Hyöty H et al. Steroid 21-hydroxylase autoantibodies in insulin-dependent diabetes mellitus. Clin Immunol Immunopathol. 1997;82:37–42.
83. Arif S, Vallian S, Farzaneh F et al. Identification of 3 beta-hydroxysteroid dehydrogenase as a novel target of steroid cell autoantibodies: association of autoantibodies with endocrine autoimmune disease. J Clin Endocrinol Metab. 1996;81:4439–45.
84. Scherbaum WA, Berg PA. Development of adrenocortical failure in non-addisonian patients with antibodies to adrenal cortex. A clinical follow-up study. Clin Endocrinol. 1982;16:345–52.
85. Ketchum CH, Riley WJ, Maclaren NK. Adrenal dysfunction in asymptomatic patients with adrenocortical autoantibodies. J Clin Endocrinol Metab. 1984;58:1166–70.
86. Ahonen P, Miettinen A, Perheentupa J. Adrenal and steroidal cell antibodies in patients with autoimmune polyglandular disease type I and risk of adrenocortical and ovarian failure. J Clin Endocrinol Metab. 1987;64:494–500.
87. Betterle C, Scalici C, Presotto F et al. The natural history of adrenal function in autoimmune patients with adrenal autoantibodies. J Endocrinol. 1988;17:467–75.
88. De Bellis A, Bizzarro A, Rossi R et al. Remission of subclinical adrenocortical failure in subjects with adrenal autoantibodies. J Clin Endocr Metab. 1993;76:1002–7.
89. Elder M, Maclaren, Riley W. Gonadal autoantibodies in patients with hypogonadism and/or Addison's disease. J Clin Endocr Metab. 1981;52:1137–42.
90. Betterle C, Zanette F, Zanchetta R et al. Complement fixing adrenal autoantibodies as a marker for predicting onset of idiopathic Addison's disease. Lancet. 1983;i:1238–41.
91. Betterle C, VolpatoM, Rees Smith B et al. I Adrenal cortex and steroid 21-hydroxylase autoantibodies in adult patients with organ-specific autoimmune diseases: markers of low progression to clinical Addison's disease. J Clin Endocrinol Metab. 1997a;82:932–8.
92. Betterle C, VolpatoM, Rees Smith B et al. II Adrenal cortex and steroid 21-hydroxylase autoantibodies in children with organ-specific autoimmune diseases: markers of high progression to clinical Addison's disease. J Clin Endocrinol Metab. 1997b;82:939–42.
93. Peterson P., K. Krohn. Mapping of autoantigenic B-cell epitopes on steroid 17α-hydroxylase, in autoimmune Addison's disease, using recombinant proteins. Clin Experiment Immunol. 1994;98:104–9.
94. Laughton CA, Neidle S, Zvelebil MJ, Sternberg MJ. Biochem Biophys Res Commun. 1990; 171:1160–7.
95. Wedlock N, Asawa T, Baumann-Antczak A, Smith BR, Furmaniak J. Autoimmune Addison's disease. Analysis of autoantibody binding sites on human steroid 21-hydroxylase. FEBS Lett. 1993;332:123–6
96. Asawa T, Wedlock N, Baumann-Antczak A, Smith BR, Furmaniak J. Naturally occuring mutations in human steroid 21-hydroxylase influence adrenal autoantibody binding. J Clin Endocrinol Metab. 1994;79:372–6.
96. Kaufman J. Diseases of the adrenal cortex of cats and dogs. Mod Vet Pract. 1985;65:513–16.
97. Colover J, Glynn LE. Experimental iso-immune adrenalitis. Immunology. 1958;2:172–8.
98. Barnett EV, Dumonde DC, Glynn LE. Induction of autoimmunity to adrenal gland. Immunology. 1963;6:382–402.
99. Steiner JW, Langer B, Schatz DL, Volpe R. Experimental immunologic adrenal injury. J Exp Med. 1960;112:187–202.
100. Witebsky E, Milgrom F. Immunological studies on adrenal glands. Immunization with adrenals of the same species. Immunology. 1962;5:67–78.
101. Sakaguchi S, Sakaguchi N. Organ specific autoimmune disease induced in mice by elimination of T cell subsets. J Immunol. 1989;142:471–80.
102. Fujii Y, Kato N, Kito J, Asai J, Yokochi T. Experimental autoimmune adrenalitis: a murine model for Addison's disease. Autoimmunity. 1992;12:47–52.
103. Lowin B, Peitsch MC, Tschopp J. Perforin and granzymes: crucial effector molecules in cytolytic T lymphocyte and natural killer cell-mediated cytotoxicity. Curr Top Microbiol Immunol. 1995;198:1–24.
104. Squier MKT, Cohen JJ. Cell-mediated cytotoxic mechanisms. Curr Opin Immunol. 1994;6: 447–52.
105. Nagamine K, Peterson P, Scott HS et al. Positional cloning of the APECED gene. Nature Genet. 1997;17:393–8.
106. Finnish–German APECED Consortium. An autoimmune disease, APECED, caused by mutations in a novel gene featuring two PHD-type zinc-finger domains. Nature Genet. 1997;17:399–403.

10
Premature ovarian failure

J. N. ANASTI

Premature ovarian failure (POF) is a condition causing amenorrhoea, low oestrogens and elevated gonadotrophins in young women. In the USA, the mean age of menopause is 50.8 years and cessation of menses prior to age 40 is considered premature. Early ovarian failure can be a traumatic experience for a young woman, especially those interested in future fertility. To be told that your ovaries are similar to those of someone in their fifties can play havoc with any young female's body image. The inability to explain the aetiology of this condition increases the frustration and hopelessness to both patient and physician. In this chapter, we will explore many facets of POF but we will concentrate on the immunological aspects of this condition. The initial discussion will include a historical review of POF and its definition, as well as a brief overview of ovarian embyrology. This background is essential to understand the pathophysiology, diagnosis and treatment of POF. For completeness, a cursory review of the non-immunological causes will precede the section on the immunologic aetiologies of POF. The final section will include a discussion of the diagnosis, treatment options, and future direction of POF research.

HISTORY

As early as the 1930s clinicians noted abnormally elevated urinary gonadotrophins in premature menopause [1]. Atria, in 1950, published one of the first reports of patients with ovarian failure [2]. In his series of 20 patients with precocious menopause, he described the basic clinical characteristics of POF, including amenorrhoea before the age of 40, symptoms and signs of hypo estrogenism, the effectiveness of hormonal replacement therapy, and the associations with a viral illness. Hertz, in 1961, reported on four interesting

A.P. Weetman (ed.), Endocrine Autoimmunity and Associated Conditions. 183–221.

amenorrhoeic patients with elevated urinary gonadotrophins and follicles noted on ovarian biopsy [3]. Jones and de Moraes-Ruehsen observed three patients with similar findings and resistance to ovulation induction with normal doses of gonadotrophins. The clinicians were able to achieve ovulation in one patient with massive doses of gonadotrophins. They called this the resistant ovary syndrome and named it after their first patient, Savage syndrome [4]. The above work provided the impetus for the search for aetiologic factors and treatment for POF.

TERMINOLOGY AND PREVALENCE

The initial terms of precocious and premature menopause are inappropriate on a psychological and physiological basis. The stigmata associated with the diagnosis of menopause in a young female interested in fertility can be psychologically devastating [5]. The designation POF [6] was applied to dispense the negative connotation suggested by the label of menopause. Furthermore, POF may itself be a misnomer. When followed serially, as many as 65% of the patients exhibit evidence of ovarian function, with documented ovulation in 20–30% [7–12]. Consequently, some authors have suggested the term hypergonadotrophic hypogonadism or even premature ovarian dysfunction to describe these patients more accurately [13].

The estimation of prevalence of POF in the general population is fraught with difficulties and has the potential of being under-reported. Women in their thirties with secondary amenorrhoea who have had a prior successful pregnancy may not seek medical treatment. In an attempt to generate an estimated prevalence, Aimak and Smentek combined their POF experience with that of several investigators. Of the 43 million women in the USA, about 3% have primary or secondary amenorrhoea, of whom 10% have POF, thus giving a frequency of 0.3% [14]. Coulam *et al.* [15], examining the medical records of 1858 women living in Rochester, Minnesota in 1950, calculated the risk of developing POF to be 0.9%, with an incidence of 10 per 100 000 person-years for ages 15–29 years and 76 per 100 000 person-years for ages 30–39 years. In women with primary amenorrhoea, the prevalence of POF is 10–28% and women with secondary amenorrhoea have a frequency of 4–18% [16]. In light of the potential under-reporting, POF is not uncommon.

EMBRYOLOGY, ANATOMY, PHYSIOLOGY

Understanding the potential pathophysiologies of POF requires a brief review of selected aspects of ovarian development and regulation of follicular growth. Readers interested in more information should consult the excellent reviews by Adashi and others [17,18]. Ovarian follicle development occurs *in vitro* and continues throughout a woman's reproductive life. Starting at the fifth gestational week, primordial germ cells originating from the endoderm of the yolk sac, migrate by amoeboid movements to the genital ridge [19]. In the following 3 weeks, these premeiotic germ cells, known as oogonia, increase mitotically to about 600 000 [20]. To determine further oogonial endowment the following three processes must remain in delicate balance:

(1) mitosis that increases oogonial number,

(2) meiosis which converts oogonia to non-dividing primary oocytes,

(3) oogonial atresia.

The net effect is a germ cell peak of 6–7 million by gestational week 20 [21]. During the subsequent 20 weeks, germ cell atresia reaches its peak. Oogonia enter meiosis which provides a temporary escape from oogonial atresia. Furthermore, they become invested by pregranulosa cells to form the primordial follicles. Interestingly, growth and development of these follicles are gonadotrophin independent. By the eighth month of gestation, oogonial atresia ends and the newly formed primordial follicles are the next victim of the atretic process [22]. Thus, the new born female has lost over 80% of her original germ cell endowment in a mere 20 weeks [23]. This number decreases to 300 000 by puberty, of which only 400–500 will be ovulated over the next 35 to 40 years (Figure 10.1).

As early as 6 months gestation, the primordial follicle's spindle shaped pregranulosa cells become cuboidal and secrete mucopolysaccarides forming a translucent vest around the oocyte, known as the zona pellucida [22]. These follicles are now primary follicles. Preantral follicles, with their granulosa cell mass separated by a basal lamina from the differentiating pretheca interna layer, continue to proliferate. Although originally thought to be gonadotrophin independent, experiments in the hypophysectomized fetal rhesus monkeys (with absent levels of gonadotrophins) revealed massive oocyte depletion secondary to atresia, suggesting an important role of gonadotrophins in early follicular development [24]. As growth continues to secondary follicles, the granulosa cells acquire cell surface follicle stimulating hormone (FSH) receptors and oestrogen and androgen nuclear receptors [25]. In addition, the theca interna cells develop luteinizing hormone (LH) cell surface receptors [26]. The secondary follicles increase their granulosa cell complement by 600-fold and enlarge to 15 times their original primordial germ cell diameter. They develop a central antrum filled with sex steroids, granulosa-derived proteins, and electrolytes. The growth from primordial to late antral follicle occurs over 60–70 days. All of these stages of ovarian development are observed in the postnatal prepubescent female.

The final road to oocyte maturation and ovulation is present in the postpubertal woman (Figure 10.2). The rising level of FSH stimulates expansion of the granulosa cells of the antral follicle. This FSH stimulation of granulosa cell aromatase results in an increase of oestradiol from the conversion of the theca-derived androgens. By menstrual cycle day 5–7, several follicles will increase in size, but only one or two will become the dominant follicle(s) (graffian follicle).

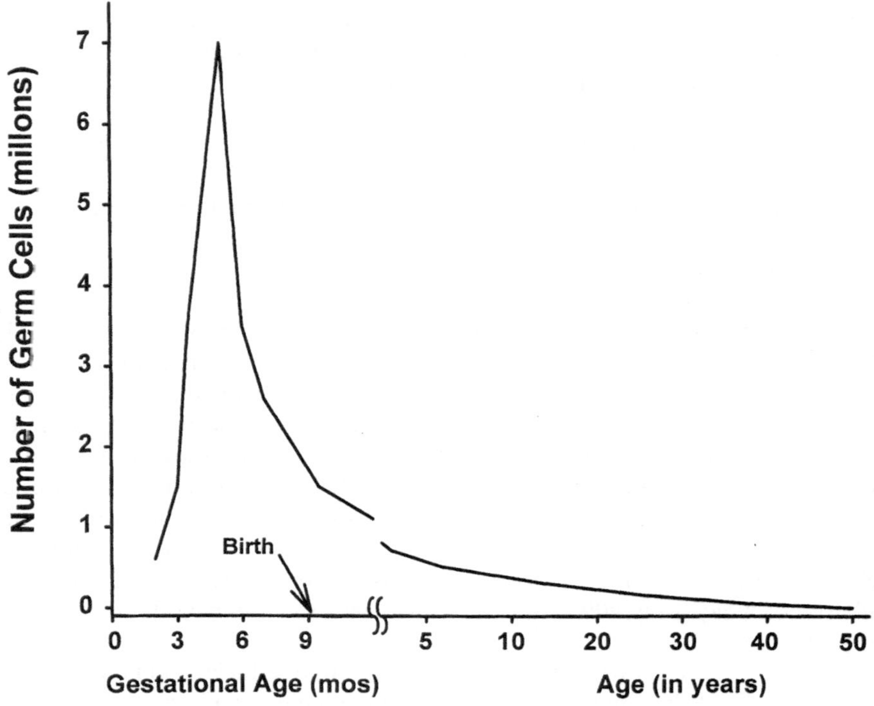

Figure 10.1 Germ cell loss in the ovary. Primordial germ cells reach a peak of 7 million at 20 weeks gestation. As a result of apoptosis greater than 90% of original germ cell complement is lost prior to puberty (age 13)

This selection process still remains an enigma. Many factors including, ovarian follicle endowment, appearance and number of gonadotrophin receptors, sex steroids, steroid enzyme activity, inhibin, activin, and other putative growth substances influence the selection process. Over the next 5–7 days, the dominant follicle, with its increased vascular network, expands to a diameter of 18–25 mm, while other smaller follicles in the original cohort become atretic. A massive and sudden release of LH caused by a sustained level of oestradiol initiates the trigger for ovulation [27]. The direct and indirect effects of LH release include

(1) oocyte resumption of meiosis,

(2) local synthesis of prostaglandins,

(3) conversion of the ruptured follicle apparatus to the corpus luteum (CL),

(4) induction of the enzymes required for progesterone production [28].

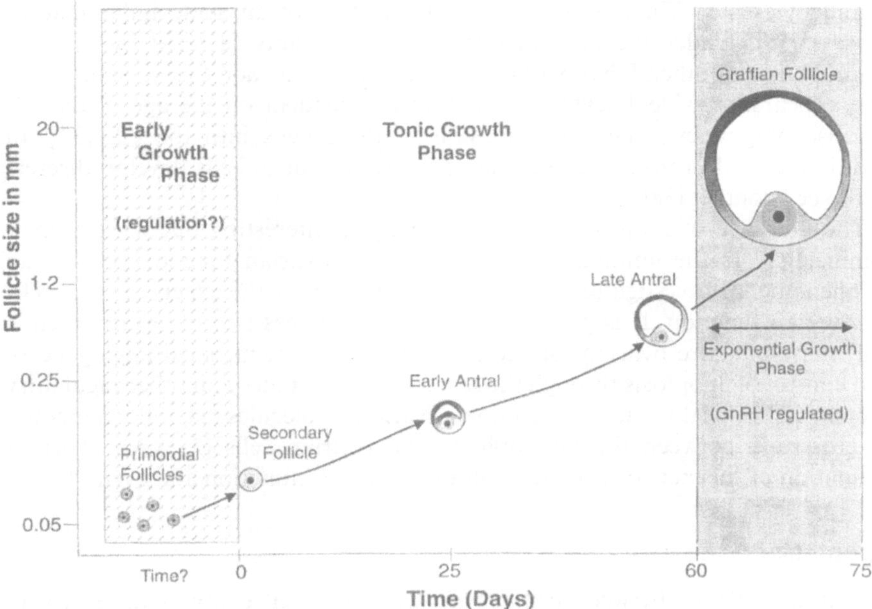

Figure 10.2 Follicular growth phases. The control of early follicle growth is not well defined. Tonic growth phase (lasting 60–70 days) is, at least in part, regulated by gonadotropins, and antral follicles are noted in prepubertal ovaries. Exponential growth phase (lasting 10–15 days) which occurs in the post-pubertal ovary is characterized by rapid growth regulated by gonadotropin releasing hormone (GnRH)

Without the human chorionic gonadotrophin (hCG) produced by a pregnancy, the CL regresses. The control of this luteolysis is uncertain, but appears to include prostaglandins, the immune system and reactive oxygen species. This monthly cycle repeats itself some 300–400 times until the menopause. Biopsies of post-menopausal ovaries are not always devoid of oocytes, suggesting that these ovaries may represent a state of granulosa cell failure and require a finite number of oocytes to effect efficient ovarian function.

Resident ovarian leukocytes

As boundaries between the endocrine and the immune system become less distinct [29,30], lymphocytes in the ovary are being investigated for their possible complementary role in ovarian regulation. Recent reviews by Adashi and Brannstrom focus on the function of these ovarian-based cells [31–34]. The ovary, unlike its male counterpart (testis), is not an immunologically privileged site. In the resting ovary, the macrophage is the predominate leukocyte present. However, as the follicle develops under gonadotrophin control, there is a five-fold increase in macrophages and an eight-fold increase in neutrophilic granulocytes [34]. These events are similar to that of an acute inflammatory process [35]. Under the influence of chemoattractants secreted by the CL, eosinophils and other T lymphocytes are the next to invade this structure [36]. The appearance of leukocytes is not simply dependent on the age of the CL because pregnancy delays the invasion of these cells into the CL [37]. In addition, co-cultures of ovarian macrophages and luteal cells develop discrete cell to cell contact [38].

The presence of immune cells in the ovary is interesting but what is their significance? Is the immune system modulating ovarian function or is it an epiphenomena? Investigators have just begun to explore the effects of these cells on ovarian function. It is postulated that macrophages and other activated T cells may influence ovarian function, oocyte development, local angiogenesis, and control of apoptosis through the secretion of cytokines and other regulatory proteins. This local paracrine secretion of various molecules may offer a method of cross-talk between the macrophage and ovarian cells [39]. An aberrant regulation of this network could result in ovarian dysfunction and even POF.

Apoptosis

A delicate balance between cell proliferation and cell death is necessary to achieve homeostasis in fetal and adult organ systems [40]. Apoptosis, or programmed cell death, is a physiologic process different from necrosis [41]. The ovary, from gestational week 20 to puberty, loses 90% of its original oocyte endowment. Apoptosis, at least in part, regulates the oocytes' fate [42]. In the mouse model, the oocyte's c-kit receptor and the ovarian stoma's stem cell factor (SCF) appear to be important in the control of apoptosis. The murine defect in c-kit and/or SCF protein that causes rapid oocyte loss and early menopause corroborates this hypothesis [43,44]. This programmed cell death also regulates the post-pubertal ovarian development from the antral follicle to CL regression. Specifically, the granulosa cells of the non-dominant antral follicles and luteal cells undergo apoptosis, with the classic findings of 180 bp oligonucleosomal DNA fragments resulting from Ca^{2+}/Mg^{2+} dependent endonucleases [45]. A myriad of factors controls apoptosis, including bcl-2 gene products [46], p53 protein [47] and growth factors [48]. Of particular interest is the regulation of apoptosis by cytokines [49] and APO/Fas/CD95 cell surface molecules [50]. These are the same regulators of T cell repertoire apoptosis, thus suggesting another link between alterations in the immune system and its potential effect on ovarian function.

AETIOLOGY OF POF

Investigators, in an attempt to understand the possible aetiologies of POF, have subdivided it into two broad categories: those with follicle depletion and those with follicle dysfunction. The following section will briefly review the above categories based on non-immune processes (Table 10.1).

Follicle depletion

The original embryonic endowment and the rate of follicle atresia determine the follicle complement. Perturbation of either of these processes could result in POF failure.

Table 10.1 Classification of premature ovarian failure

Ovarian follicle depletion
Deficient initial follicle number
Pure gonadal dysgenesis
Thymic aplasia/hypoplasia
Idiopathic
Accelerated follicle atresia
X chromosome related
Turner's syndrome
X mosaics
X deletions
Galactosaemia
Iatrogenic
Chemotherapy
Irradiation
Environmental toxins
Viral agents
Autoimmunity
Oocyte-specific cell cycle regulation defect
Idiopathic
Ovarian follicle dysfunction
Enzyme deficiencies
17α-Hydroxylase
Desmolase (17-20)
Cholesterol desmolase
Galactose-1-phosphate uridyltransferase
Autoimmunity
Lymphocytic oophoritis
Gonadotrophin receptor blocking immunoglobulins
Antibodies to gonadotrophins
Signal defects
Abnormal gonadotrophin
Abnormal gonadotrophin receptor
Abnormal G protein
Iatrogenic
Idiopathic (resistant ovary syndrome)

Deficiency in initial follicle number

The mechanism controlling the steps of germ cell migration, proliferation, and formation of primordial follicles remains obscure. However, a defect in any of these steps could result in POF. A genetic defect that alters the normal mechanism controlling the above processes could explain the streak gonads of patients with 46,XXX gonadal dysgenesis. Women with Turner's syndrome (45,XO), the most common human chromosomal defect, also have streak gonads. Singh and Carr examining the ovaries of eight 45,XO stillborn individuals, noted that the germ cells migrate to gonadal ridge but these primary oocytes were lost by accelerated atresia during late prenatal and early neonatal life [51,52]. The oocytes must be enveloped by follicular stroma cells to survive, a process that appears to require two intact active X chromosomes [53,54]. Supporting this hypothesis is the DNA hybridization studies of several families with POF that reveal a partial deletion of the long arm of X chromosome (q26-27 locus) [55]. Somatic chromosomes (or subtle sex chromosome abnormalities) are important because several POF kindreds exist with apparently normal karyotypes [56]. Between 5–46% of POF patients have an X chromosome abnormality [10,14,57]. These different rates of abnormal karyotypes may related to selection and referral population bias. Recently, a germ cell-deficient autosomal recessive mouse has been described with a mutation in chromosome 11 A2-3 [58]. This murine model may provide insight into human disease. However, only when the specific responsible genes are determined will familial POF cases be diagnosed.

Metabolic: galactosaemia

Galactosaemia is a rare inherited autosomal recessive disorder due to a deficiency in the enzyme galactose-1-phosphate uridyl transferase (GALT) [59]. These patients develop hepatocellular, ocular, renal, and neurological damage as a result of the accumulation of galactose and its metabolites. According to one study, POF was present in 81% of patients with galactosaemia [60]. Autopsy reports on a neonate suffering from galactosaemia revealed normal ovarian histology, suggesting that accelerated atresia depletes the oocytes prior to puberty [61]. However, a debate exists as to the exact mechanism [62]. A recent genetic marker has been identified in some patients with galactosaemia, GALT Q188. Those individuals who are heterozygous for the GALT Q188R mutation are not at increased risk of the developing ovarian dysfunction [63].

Chemotherapy, irradiation and environmental toxins

The efficacy of most chemotherapeutic agents is derived from their ability to destroy rapidly dividing cells. In the ovary, these agents have their greatest effect on the proliferating granulosa and theca cells of mature follicles [64]. The histologic findings of decreased primordial/graffian follicles in young women receiving chemotherapy and the clinical observations of amenorrhoea during therapy and the return of ovulation, even conceiving, after therapy support this concept [65,66]. Other chemotherapy agents, especially the alkylating agents, cause permanent damage to the ovary. These alkylating agents destroy cells by altering cellular DNA [67], and they can, therefore, affect resting oocytes as well as proliferating cells. It is difficult to predict if or when ovarian failure will occur, since each ovary appears to respond differently to chemotherapy [68,69]. However, age, dose, and type of drug appear to be the major predicative factors. Women younger than 40 required twice the dose of cyclophosphamide needed for older individuals to become amenorrhoeic [70]. The apparent resistance of the prepuberal ovary to the effects of alkylating agents has led investigators to attempt suppressing ovarian function during chemotherapy [71]. Randomized controlled trials using oral contraception or gonadotrophin-releasing hormone analogues to inhibit ovarian follicle development have not been performed. Primate and non-primate studies have not shown a benefit to ovarian suppression [72–74]. Unlike animal models [75,76], more exotic methods of human oocyte or ovarian tissue preservation prior to starting chemotherapy have met with little success [77].

It is important to remember that irradiation to the head as well as the pelvis can cause ovarian dysfunction: the former causes destruction of gonadotrophins and the latter results in the oocyte disruption [78]. Radiation-induced ovarian failure, like chemotherapy, is dependent on the age of the patient and the dose received. The most pronounced effect of radiation is in the early phases of ovarian follicle development, thus destroying oocytes and sparing mature follicles [79]. It is for this reason that radiation is a more potent ovarian toxin. A radiation dose of 600 rads or more to the ovary produces ovarian failure in virtually all individuals more than 40 years old. Lower doses have a more variable effect depending on the patient's age: a documented pregnancy has occurred in a 20 year old who received 3000 rads to the pelvis [13]. Fetuses conceived after chemotherapy and/or irradiation are not at increased risk of congenital abnormalities [65], although a previously irradiated individual may have a slightly higher rate of miscarriage. Suppressing ovarian follicular development prior to irradiation, as in chemotherapy, has not proven beneficial in preserving ovarian function. However, surgically transposing the ovary out of the field of radiation has met with some success [80,81].

The influence of the environmental toxins on ovarian function and age of menopause has been reviewed by Vermulen [82], who considers ovarian dysfunction to be a consequence of alterations in the hypothalamic gonadotrophin releasing hormone pulse generator. Thus, the majority of aberrant ovarian function occurs as a result of environmental toxins affecting the hypothalamus and not in an alteration of oocyte number. Although stress, food intake, alcohol and various other factors may influence ovarian function, the major environmental influence in determining the age of menopause is smoking [83,84].

Ovarian follicle dysfunction

The mere presence of oocytes does not ensure normal ovarian function. In fact, some POF patients have normal appearing oocytes that fail to function despite adequate stimulation by high levels of gonadotrophins. These patients, as described in a previous section, have resistant ovary or Savage syndrome [85], and the majority go undetected due to the lack of evidence to support the use of routine ovarian biopsy and our inability to determine oocyte existence non-invasively. While the aetiology of POF in individuals with normal appearing follicles on biopsy is unknown, a small subset have a rare, yet specific, cause for their ovarian dysfunction, discussed in this section. This subset may increase as we develop new molecular techniques to investigate subtle defects in cellular functioning.

Enzyme deficiences

As described earlier, the granulosa and theca cells are the major producers of the gonadal steroids, oestrogen and progesterone. At puberty, granulosa/theca cell growth and the stimulation of enzymes responsible for ovarian steroid production requires an increase in gonadotrophin secretion. Thus, the net effect is a tremendous augmentation in the amount of oestradiol and post-ovulatory progesterone. Several specific enzyme defect, including cholesterol desmolase, 17α-hydroxylase, 17-20 desmolase, and aromatase can lead to diminished levels of oestrogen [86–88]. Delayed puberty, primary amenorrhoea, and elevated gonadotrophins are clinical manifestations of impaired oestrogen synthesis. Although primordial follicles are present in these patients, they are unable to mature.

Cholesterol is the initial building block of all ovarian and adrenal steroid, and a defect in cholesterol desmolase enzyme is associated with neonatal death. However, the ovaries in these neonates have the normal oocyte complement. The 17α-hydroxylase-deficient patient has impaired adrenal and ovarian steroid synthesis. This results in patients developing hypertension, hypokalaemia, and ovarian failure. 17-20 desmolase is catalysed by the same P450 cytochrome complex as 17α-hydroxylase. Despite this finding, 17-20 desmolase deficiency can occur without a concomitant 17α-hydroxylase defect [87]. Although these patients present with POF, they exhibit no clinical manifestations of adrenal failure. A case report demonstrated growth and development of ovarian follicles in an affected individual, despite impaired oestrogen synthesis. A pregnancy, using assisted reproductive techniques, was reported in a patient with a 17α-hydroxylase defect [87]. This finding challenges the dogma of the importance of oestrogen in oocyte development and conception. Recently, several families have been described with a deficiency in the aromatase enzyme [86]. The female siblings presented with delayed puberty, hypergonadotropic amenorrhoea, and multiple ovarian cysts. Molecular techniques revealed a point mutation in the aromatase gene.

Earlier we discussed the role of GALT deficiency in POF. Biopsy results in these patients revealed either the presence or absence of follicles [62]. Due to the rarity of GALT and other enzyme disorders, there is a paucity of correlating histologic information.

Signal defects

The glycoprotein gonadotrophins exert their effect on the granulosa cells and theca cells by binding to transmembrane receptors. These receptors, acting through G proteins, stimulate second messengers resulting in specific cellular functions. Alterations in gonadotrophins biopotency and/or abnormal receptor functioning would result in ovarian failure. The search for a patient with abnormal gonadotrophins continues, in the light of a report of a mutant form of LH in a hypogonadal man [89]. In contrast, abnormal FSH or LH receptors that fail to bind their respective ligands have already been documented [90–92]. In these reports, the sequences of the aberrant gonadotrophin receptors were obtained from the genomic DNA of siblings with hypergonadotropic hypogonadism. Using recombinant DNA procedures, these mutant receptors were unable to bind gonadotrophins. Lastly, ovarian resistance is noted in patients with pseudohypoparathyroidism due to a defect in the cyclic AMP second messenger system. Such patients present with normal menarche but subsequently develop hypoestrogenism and elevated gonadotrophins [93].

IMMUNOLOGY OF POF

Although the pathophysiology of POF is likely to be diverse, as presented in the previous sections, several lines of evidence indicate a role for a perturbed immune system (Table 10.2). Data supporting this hypothesis include:

(1) the clinical association of POF with other autoimmune disease;

(2) the presence of circulating antibodies to ovarian homogenates and/or specific ovarian antigens;

(3) the presence of immune stigmata in ovarian biopsies from some patients with POF;

(4) the assocation with infectious agents and ovarian failure;

(5) the immunological findings of altered cell mediated autoimmunity;

(6) the reports of recovery of ovarian function and pregnancy after immunosuppressive therapies;

(7) the finding of immunogenetic markers in some patients with POF;

(8) the murine neonatal thymectomy-induced oophoritis model.

Table 10.2 Evidence supporting an immunologic role in premature ovarian failure

Associations with other autoimmune diseases
Presences of circulating antibodies
Anti-ovarian antibodies
Gonadotrophin and gonadotrophin receptor antibodies
Steroid cell antibodies
Zona pellucida antibodies
Other organ-specific and non-specific antibodies
Histological evidence of oophoritis
Association with infectious aetiologies
Altered cell-mediated autoimmunity
Recovery of ovarian function with immunosuppressive therapies
Presence of immunogenetic markers
Murine neonatal thymectomy-induced ovarian failure model

In the following section, we will summarize the current literature on each of the above points in support of an immunological cause for POF. Furthermore, the strength and the weakness of each of these concepts will be discussed.

The association with other autoimmune disorders

Since Guinet and Pommatau reported a cause of a POF and myxoedema preceding Addison's disease [94], investigators have noted an association with autoimmune disorders and ovarian failure. Initial reports focused on the incidence of POF in patients with Addison's disease, suggesting that 10% of these patients have POF [95,96; see also Chapter 9]. POF, as described in these early reports, develops several years prior to the onset of Addison's disease, 14 years being the longest delay [97]. In addition, hypothyroidism develops concurrently or shortly after the hypoadrenalism [97,98]. Recent studies have demonstrated a shift toward other autoimmune endocrinopathies [11,99,100]. The frequency of co-existing autoimmune syndromes varies from 0 to 57%, with averages of 17–29.5% [101–103]. In the later reports, hypothyroidism appears to be the most commonly associated autoimmune disease. Concurrent polyendocrine autoimmunity syndromes type I and type II exist in as many as 3% of patients with POF [102,104] and are discussed further in Chapter 9.

Myasthenia gravis, like autoimmune endocrine disorders, is an organ-specific autoimmune disease associated with POF [105]. Interestingly, the return of ovarian function occurs in some myasthenia patients following a therapeutic thymectomy [106,107]. Other organ-specific autoimmune diseases co-existing with POF include Crohn's disease [108], vitiligo [109,110] and pernicious anaemia [111]. SLE and rheumatoid arthritis are non-organ specific autoimmune disorders associated with POF [109,112,113]. Of particular interest is the hypothesis of Monyaco that the non-pregnant elevated levels of human chorionic gonadotrophin (hCG) in SLE patients may correlate with severity of disease and ovarian dysfunction or failure in these patients [112,114].

The prevalence of concurrent autoimmune diseases is generated from combining retrospective observational studies, the majority of which include less than 30 patients. Therefore, the true figure is difficult to obtain. The wide variation may reflect different study design, diagnostic laboratory screening techniques, determination of subclinical thyroid disorders, different study populations of POF (normal karyotype versus abnormal karyotype) and biased referral patterns. Recently, we presented data on 119 prospectively screened POF patients [115]. The analysis excluded patients with abnormal karyotype and iatrogenic causes of ovarian failure. The patients were screened for thyroid, adrenal and parathyroid autoimmunity, type 1 diabetes mellitus and pernicious anaemia. Hypothyroidism was the most common disorder (27%), with Addison's disease (2.5%) and diabetes (2.5%) also diagnosed in our patients.

Antibodies to the ovary

The role of ovarian antibodies (OAb) in the pathogenesis of ovarian failure is complex. Their prevalence rate varies widely with OAb reported in 0–67% of patients [116]. Attempting to make a generalization is impossible due to the heterogeneity in investigational methodologies. Studies differ in many aspects including the differences in species of the antigen, the maturation state of antigen, the specific type of ovarian antigen, the detection technique employed, and the population studied. Thus the reader is encouraged to analyse present and future studies with this in mind. Our discussion will start with a review of non-specific ovarian antigens used to screen for OAb and then proceed to the specific ovarian proteins.

Ovary as a source of antigen

Our understanding of OAb is in its infancy when compared to antibodies to other endocrine organ such as thyroid, adrenal, and pancreatic β cell. Excellent reviews on the history and methodology of OAb are presented elsewhere by Monacayo [117] and Kim [102]. The following is a brief overview of the past and present status of OAb in the literature. Vallton and Forbes in 1966, while searching for anti-nuclear antibodies, are credited with the first report of OAb in POF [118]. Using cytoplasm of rabbit ova, they described positive indirect immunofluorescence in 4 of 45 POF patients and 1 of 45 controls. Interested in the clinical association of Addison disease and POF, investigators focused their efforts on this subset of patients. Irvine and others, employing human ovaries, adrenal and placental tissue, developed the concept of steroid cell antibodies (SCAb) [96]. These antibodies cross-reacted with all of the above steroid-producing organs. Many other studies employing human tissue followed, searching for OAb in POF patients with or without Addison's disease [108,119–124].

The previous immunocytochemical and ligand binding techniques were cumbersome, time consuming, and yielded only qualitative results. Monyaco in

1989 developed the first ELISA test using human CL. However, his original study population did not include patients with POF [125]. Luborsky *et al.*, using a similar single bridge ELISA derived from ovarian cell membranes, detected circulating OAb in 69% of 45 women with POF [124]. In an attempt to further increase sensitivity, Kim used four types of ovarian proteins to develop a double bridge ELISA incorporating a sensitive biotin-streptavidin system. They found that 15 of 51 patients with POF were positive for OAb [126].

Other organ-specific tissue autoantibodies have been recorded in the sera of POF patients including those directed gastric mucosa, skin, pancreas, and testis. Non-organ-specific antibodies have also been described in patients with POF, including rheumatoid factor, antinuclear factor, and antibodies against mitochondria and smooth muscle.

Specific OAb: gonadotrophin receptor antibodies

The clinical and histological finding of gonadotrophin-unresponsive primordial follicles (Savage syndrome) sparked investigators to look for specific ovarian antigens as inducers of ovarian dysfunction. Using the model of hypothyroidism and myasthenia gravis, they searched for receptor antibodies against the gonadotrophin receptors. Early follicles do not develop abundant gonadotrophin receptors and are unique to the maturing ovarian follicle, thus making FSH/LH receptors an ideal candidate as an inciting antigen. Chiauzzi *et al.* discovered an IgG that blocked binding of FSH to its receptor in two myasthenia gravis patients with POF [127]. Monayaco, using an ELISA, was able to identify antibodies that reacted against both the unoccupied and the occupied hCG/LH receptor [125]. Tang *et al.* found antibodies in one of nine patients to the FSH receptor [128] and van Weissenbruch described the presence of IgGs that inhibited the trophic action of FSH, but did not inhibit FSH binding to rat testicular FSH receptors [129]. This latter study suggests that antibodies may inhibit gonadotrophin action by a different mechanism, conceivably by interfering with post-receptor function.

All of these groups utilized non-human gonadotrophin receptors and this may be an experimental design flaw. Recent data from Hsueh's group suggest that human gonadotrophin receptors are species-specific, binding human ligands with higher affinity than non-human gonadotrophins [92,130]. Assuming a species specificity and thus an antibody specificity, we employed a recombinant human gonadotrophin receptor bioassay (LH/FSH) to identify gonadotrophin receptor IgG class antibodies [131]. We were unable to find an inhibitor of gonadotrophin and its receptor in 27 patients with POF, including one with myasthenia gravis. Others have used the human recombinant FSH receptor bioassay with mixed results [132].

Several investigators have identified the existence of non-immunoglobulin inhibitors of FSH binding [133,134]. These low molecular weight interfering molecules are FSH receptor binding competitors. Isolated from the sera of patients with POF, these inhibitors effectively block the action of FSH on the receptor, but their exact nature and pathophysiological role remain to be established.

Specific antibodies: SCAb

Irvine in the late 1960s first postulated the concept of antibodies directed against steroid producing cells [135]. Using tissue preparations from placenta, adrenal, and ovary, he found that sera from Addison's patients with POF reacted to all three of these antigens. Common to the adrenal and the ovary are the 17α-hydroxylase and p450 side chain cleavage enzymes that provide an antigenic link in these organs [136]. Recently, investigators employed recombinant techniques in autoimmune polyglandular syndromes to search for antibodies against 21-hydroxylase, 17α-hydroxylase and p450 side chain cleavage [137]. Patients with POF alone did not have SCAb but SCAb were positive in POF patients with evidence of adrenal failure.

Specific antibodies: zona pellucida

The zona pellucida (zp) is a glycoprotein secreted by the granulosa cells in early follicle development. This unique ovarian protein is an excellent candidate as an inciting antigen in the immune destruction of the ovary [138]. Important in sperm attachment and subsequent fertilization [139], the zp has been a central player in the search for an immunocontraceptive method [140] and as a cause for infertility [141]. Current research has focused on animal models and excellent reviews of its role in human diseases have been published by Caudle [142] and Dunbar [143]. In summary, there appears to be an inter-species cross-reactivity of zp antigens; zp antibodies in some species can inhibit sperm attachment, and these results vary depending on zp species. Nelson *et al.* [127], using a commercial immunofluorescence assay employing cynologomous monkey zp, noted a positive reaction in 50% of patients with POF and in 30% of the controls. With the advent of the cloning and expression of human zp, the construction of human recombinant assays may be useful in defining zp antibodies and their pathophysiology [144].

OAb: what do they mean?

The differences in the studied population and methods used to determine antibody status makes summarizing the OAb data difficult. Contradictory results are obtained even when similar methods are applied to different patient groups. WhWheatcroft *et al.* recently were unable to validate the study of Monacayo of increased binding to bovine LH/hCG receptor in patients with POF [145]. Although POF patients had an increased in antibodies to ovarian antigen, their sera also demonstrated significant increase in binding to non-ovarian antigen (fallopian tube). Thus, it is uncertain whether circulating OAbs are pathogenic and therefore have a clinical role or are simply an epiphenomenon secondary to antigen release following cellular damage [146]. The correlation of OAb status and chronologic onset or severity of disease is poor. Even in the well-studied autoimmune polyglandular syndrome patients, with documented SCAb, the exact mechanism of ovarian and adrenal destruction is unclear [146]. The use of a functional bioassay to search for a pathogenic mechanism for OAb has also not been fruitful [131]. The lack of OAb in many patients with POF could result from OAb being present in the initial stages of the disease but no longer being produced after destruction of ovarian tissue [147]. As techniques improve, OAb may eventually be helpful in our clinical management of POF. Currently, it appears that patients with POF have an increased incidence of OAb, but their clinical and diagnostic implications are undefined. The possible exception may be the prediction of POF in patients with pre-existing Addison's disease who are SCAb positive [148].

HISTOLOGICAL EVIDENCE OF OOPHORITIS

The diagnosis of oophoritis requires ovarian tissue with histologic evidence of a stromal lymphocytic infiltrate. As early as 1968, investigators noted an association of ovarian failure and oophoritis [96]. However, the incidence of lymphocytic infiltration of the ovary in POF is unknown, since most of the literature documentation is either case reports or small series [98,123,149–158].

Reviewing individual pathology reports can provide insight into a specific disease process, but to make a generalization from these case studies can be misleading. Consistent in many, but not all reports, is the localization of lymphocytes and plasma cells near the maturing follicle and CL, with the apparent sparing of primordial follicles [151,159,160]. This implies a unique antigen in the developing follicle and hence, gonadotrophin dependence. Investigators have attempted to characterize the infiltrate found in these ovaries. Pre-plasma B cells were seen around the developing follicles with mature plasma cells noted by the CL [157,161,162]. Although based on limited studies, Sedmark noted a proportionately higher number of $CD4^+$ than $CD8^+$ cells [156]. On rare occasions, patients may present with chronic oophoritis composed of a granulomatous inflammatory infiltrate with or without the presence of tuberculosis or sarcoidosis [153,158,163]. Lymphocytic oophoritis may present clinically with lower abdominal pain and enlarged ovaries [164]. This ovarian enlargement may be the result of local lymphokine production impairing follicle steroidogenesis, as has been reported in animal models [165]. Similar to enzyme deficiency, this dysfunctional oestrogen synthesis causes ovarian cystic enlargement due to the disruption of oestrogen's ability to provide the appropriate negative feedback on gonadotrophin.

The literature implies an association of lymphocytic oophoritis with other autoimmune diseases such as hypothyroidism, pernicous anaemia, and SLE. However, in many cases OAb are not present. The most common association of oophoritis appears to be with the concomitant finding of Addison's disease. The reason for this is unclear but may be due to the higher proportion of SCAb in these patients or that Addison's patients undergo closer scrutinization, which represents a sampling bias. Of interest is the discovery of increased levels of progesterone and LH, along with the histologic findings of luteinized ovarian cysts, in menopausal women [166–168]. Several investigators postulated that the oophoritis may lead to premature intense luteinization with elevated levels of progesterone. Intrigued by this finding, we recently found luteinized ovarian cysts, but without lymphocytic infiltrate, in a series of patients with POF and ultrasonic evidence of follicular development [169]. This histological evidence suggests that inappropriate non-oophoritic luteinization of graafian follicles may be a major physiological mechanism in patients with POF.

The clinical value, expense and risk to the patients are reasons why a large series of ovarian biopsies in POF patients has not been performed. It was originally hoped that ultrasound-guided or small laparoscopic biopsy of the ovaries would be helpful, but these limited biopsies do not provide a true representation of ovarian pathology [14,170,171]. The past reports in the literature have been purely observational without a well-defined criterion for biopsy of a POF patient. Thus, the true incidence of oophoritis, as well as the actual histology of POF, is unknown [172]. Somerville has proposed that the presence of lymphocytic oophoritis is merely an incidental finding [173]. Additional data are needed to understand the role of the immune response in the normal ovary for, as previously stated, there exists a normal resident leukocyte complement in the ovary. The need to perform selected ovarian biopsy in patients with POF is still worthy of future study because oophoritis is a documented cause of POF and case reports suggest that treatment may restore ovarian function. In attempt to answer these questions, we have recently set up an ovarian biopsy and treatment protocol at the National Institutes of Health.

INFECTIONS

The original description of a POF included the association with a viral infection (mumps). In a retrospective review of past medical histories, Rebar noted that 3.5% of patients reported a prior record of viral infection including varicella, shigella, and malaria [170]. Reed, studying patients in Alaska during a mumps epidemic, found clinical evidence of oophoritis in four of 59 females, while 15 of 60 males described orchitis [174]. Grasso, in a similar study, described oophoritis in five of 171 women during a mumps outbreak [175]. The onset of the oophoritis in relation to clinical symptoms appears inconsistent and is poorly studied. However, during mumps, the virus emerges in vaginal secretions shortly after the appearance of symptoms. Cytomegalovirus causes oophoritis in patients with immunosuppressive illnesses including AIDS, lymphomal and transplantation [176–178].

Unfortunately verification of lymphocytic oophoritis based on clinical criteria fails to account for subclinical oophoritis. These studies lack long-term follow up and documentation of subsequent ovarian failure. Although infections (especially viral) are a cause of POF, the actual incidence is most likely small.

The incidence of ovarian failure following a viral illness requires longitudinal prospective studies.

Cell-mediated immune responses

Considering the early findings of lymphocytic oophoritis and the association of autoimmune disorders in POF patients, characterization of cellular immunity was an obvious line of investigation. In the early 1970s, immunologists using crude methods performed cytotoxic and cell-mediated reaction studies of patients with POF [98]. These early investigators demonstrated the presence of sensitized T cells and sera-mediated destruction of granulosa cells using, at times, unspecified ovarian antigens. As techniques became more sensitive, the study of T cell population became possible. Perkonen noted enhanced release of leukocyte migration factor, a lymphokine released by activated T cells, in four patients [179].

Rabinowe documented, in five of 10 patients with POF, a slight (5.6% versus <3%) increase in the number of Ia^+ T cells. Patients with other autoimmune diseases, such as type I diabetes mellitus, Addison's disease, rheumatoid arthritis, Graves' disease and SLE, frequently have elevated numbers of circulated Ia^+ T cells [159]. Furthermore, immunosuppressive therapy resulted in a reduction in the Ia^+ T cells. Miyake studied the peripheral lymphocyte population in a group of 20 POF patients. Atrophic changes without a mononuclear infiltrate were observed in the ovaries in all 10 patients who underwent laparoscopic biopsy. The CD4/CD8 ratio was elevated in POF patients (1.68% versus 1.4% in controls) [180]. In a similar non-biopsy study, Ho *et al.* examined a group of 45 patients and 45 age-matched controls. They noted an increase in circulating $CD4^+$ and $CD8^+$ T cells in POF patients with autoantibodies [181]. The CD4/CD8 ratio, however, was significantly lower in women with POF. Additional reports have added little to resolving the change in the lymphocytes of patients with POF. Delayed hypersensitivity, a measure of abnormal cell-mediated function, has been tested in a small series of POF patients [182]. Mignot noted absent or delayed hypersensitivity to Candida antigen in 11 out of 20 cases and two out of 10 controls [103,183].

MHC class II molecules regulate the immune response to foreign antigens, and this makes them logical candidates to play a role in the pathogenesis of autoimmunity [184]. Initiated by antigen presenting cells (APC), the immune response activates T helper cells. APC process the inciting antigen by cleaving this protein into small peptides. These specific proteins bind to the MHC class II molecules, forming a complex that causes activation of specific T cell. POF patients, according to several investigators, demonstrate an increase in HLA-DR^+ T cells [180,185]. Even more interesting is the finding of Hill *et al.*, who noted, in the inflammed ovaries of POF patients, an inappropriate expression of class II molecules. These and other investigators demonstrated that gonadotrophins and interferon-α act synergistically to increase the expression of MHC class II molecules on luteinized granulosa cells [185–187]. Theoretically, this would suggest gonadotrophin stimulation may increase the change of autoimmune POF.

The conflicting results presented in the literature are discouraging. Several factors may account for the diverse results obtained in the cell-mediated function of POF patients. Ho postulated and proved that the low oestrogen of these patients could be responsible for some of the immune changes [188]. However, oestrogen replacement failed to correct the increase in the HLA-DR$^+$ cells. The onset of POF and the time of entry into the study may have a great effect on the immune alterations. Immunological changes may exist only in the earlier stages of ovarian failure. The majority of these studies include patients in whom the initial diagnosis of POF is made more than 12 years before the immune function studies [186]. Lastly, and more importantly, the clinical and pathophysiologic importance of these findings remains to be seen. Thus characterization of immune cellular function should be used in a research setting only.

Recovery after immunosuppressive therapy

Resumption of ovarian function after the resolution of a concomitant autoimmune disease or treatment with immunosuppressive therapies provides additional evidence for an autoimmune aetiology [106,189–200]. Corticosteroids have been the predominant form of immunosuppressive agent. The profile of a responding patient appears quite diverse. OAb status, presence of oophoritis, and existence of associated autoimmune disorders do not appear to predict who will respond to therapy. However, several case reports describe the return of ovarian function after the treatment of Addison's disease, myasthenia gravis, polyglandular failure, and SLE. In addition to corticosteroid immunosuppressive treatment, plasmapheresis and thymectomy in myasthenia gravis patients [106] and intravenous immunoglobulin therapy in polyglandular failure syndrome [201] have resulted in the restoration of ovarian function. Alterations induced by immunotherapy of POF cases have not been well documented. Rabinowe, however, did not show a decrease in Ia$^+$ T cells during corticosteroid treatment [159].

The weakness of this evidence is obvious. Most reports are anecdotal without determination of the pathophysiology. Attempts made to look at the value of immunosuppressive therapy suffer from poor study design. The major fault of these reports is the failure to realize the high rate of spontaneous resumption of ovarian function. A prospective randomized study examining the efficacy of steroid therapy in lymphocytic oophoritis is now underway at the Clinical Center of the National Instsitutes of Health.

Immunogenetic markers

Investigators have shown that autoimmune diseases occur in genetically susceptible individuals and patients with one autoimmune disease commonly develop additional autoimmune disorders. At the genetic level, there is the well-known association of autoimmune endocrinopathies and HLA-DR3/DR4. This has led to three studies of HLA typing in POF patients. Walfish *et al.* [202] found a significant association of POF and HLA-DR3 in 22 white females (relative risk of 4.3, $p<0.35$). We were unable to corroborate this study in our own investigation of over 100 patients with POF [100]. Lack of HLA correlation was also obtained in a subsequent report [203]. Thus the prediction of risk for POF depending on HLA type is suspect. Newer immunogenetic markers and application of transgenics are currently being used in other autoimmune endocrine diseases and may in the future be applied to the study of POF [203–205].

Animal models

As early as 1961, investigators noted that thymectomy in the neonatal mouse had a profound effect on the mature immune system [206]. Similar immune findings are present in human thymic disorders. Sakakaura and Nishizuka were the first to describe the occurrence of ovarian dysgenesis in mice thymectomized on day 3 of life (THX3) [207]. In susceptible strains, over 90% of the animals develop autoimmune oophoritis by the fourth week of life (day 24). OAbs to the oocyte of developing follicles, zona pellucida, granulosa cells, theca cells, luteal cells and steroid-producing cells appear after the onset of oophoritis (day 30). These antibodies, along with active oophoritis, are not detectable by the 25th week of life. The resulting ovaries are reduced in weight and lack follicles and CL. This is consistent with the hypothesis that OAb and oophoritis are present only in the early acute phase of ovarian failure. In addition to the ovarian effects, THX3 induces inflammatory changes in the thyroid, pituitary, testis, salivary glands, prostate, and gastric mucosa. The affected organ and extent of the reaction are strain-specific.

Although many aspects of this model are undergoing intensive study, the following is a review of the pertinent findings. Donor cells from THX3 animals were able to transfer disease in young, but not adult mice and spleen cells from adult animals prevented oophoritis in susceptible strains [208]. Investigators noted, in THX3 mice, a deficiency of a T cell subpopulation [209] and an enrichment of a T cell line normally deleted from the adult thymus [210,211]. Using intrathymic injection of organ-specific antigens, Murakami suggested that the recognition of an autoantigen in the thymus is necessary for the induction of tolerance [212]. The development, however, of thymus and gonads is different among species. In the mouse, the thymus and gonads continue to develop for the first 14 days after birth, while in man, the thymus and ovary are fully developed *in utero*. It is for this reason that interpretation of the murine model and human disease remains speculative.

Despite these differences, Hodgen noted similar findings in primates who were thymectomized *in utero* at midgestation [213]. Furthermore, human thymic disorders, presenting clinically as thymic aplasia and myasthenia gravis, are associated with ovarian dysfunction. Miyake *et al.* [155] noted seven common features in the animal model and premature ovarian failure: infiltration of ovaries, end organ fibrosis, loss of oestrous cycle, elevated gonadotrophins, OAb, other organ-specific antibodies, and occurrence at a young age. As in man, the relative contribution of antibodies and the T cell response to experimental autoimmune oophoritis remains obscure. This has not deterred investigators in pursuing the THX3 mouse as a model of immune-related ovarian failure. Investigators have also induced ovarian dysfunction in animal models by immunizing them with ovarian antigens [140,214]. Although crude ovarian abstracts can serve as an antigen, current research employs the unique zp ovarian protein. Active immunization of rabbits, squirrel monkeys, and mice with zp proteins lead to ovarian dysfunction and, in the mouse, oophoritis [143,215–217]. Investigators continue to explore these models in the hope of developing a reversible immunocontraceptive method. The value of these models in the study of POF remains to be seen [218].

CLINICAL ASPECTS

Signs and symptoms

The cardinal finding in POF patients is the cessation of menses before the age of 40. In our experience with over 150 POF patients, there appears to be no characteristic antecedent menstrual history. Others have reported similar findings [170]. The majority of POF patients develop amenorrhoea acutely after having established a pattern of regular menses, and it is common for patients to report failure of menstruation after stopping oral contraceptives or completing a pregnancy. However, some patients may present with irregular bleeding prior to becoming amenorhoeic. Prodromal POF, although rare, may present with hot flushing before menstrual dysfunction. In addition to the amenorrhoea, vaginitis, dyspareunia and vasomotor symptoms can occur as a result of the hypoestrogenic state. Women with POF presenting as secondary amenorrhoea do not exhibit decrease fecundity [219]. However, infertility occurs in patients with POF who present with primary amenorrhoea (10–15%). A chromosomal defect is present in as many as 40% of POF patients with primary amenorrhoea [220]. Longitudinal studies of patients with POF demonstrate the sporadic return of ovarian function and even pregnancy. Thus, the clinical dictum of the permanent cessation of ovarian function is not corroborated by various studies, and prior diagnosis of POF does not exclude the occasional return of regular menstruation.

Making the diagnosis

The major aetiology of premature ovarian failure appears to be idiopathic. However, a specific disease process may exist in a small percentage of POF patients. Specific aetiologies may alter treatment plans and thus, it is prudent for the clinician to uncover them (Table 10.3).

Table 10.3 Differential diagnosis of premature ovarian failure

- Prodromal premature ovarian failure
- Abnormal karyotype
- Pure gonadal dysgenesis
- Iatrogenic ovarian failure
- Autoimmune ovarian failure
  - In assocation with other syndromes
  - Autoimmune polyglandular syndrome
  - Non-organ-specific autoimmunity
  - IgA deficiency
  - Isolated
- Miscellaneous rare causes
  - Perrault's syndrome
  - Enzyme deficiences
    - 17α-Hydroxylase
    - 17-20, Desmolase
    - Cholesterol desmolase
    - Galactosaemia
  - Pseudohypoparathyroidism
  - Thymic disorders
    - DiGeorge's syndrome
    - Ataxia telangiectasia
    - Tumour
  - Idiopathic
  - Pseudo-ovarian failure
    - Gonadotrophin-producing pituitary adenoma
    - Antibodies to gonadotrophins
    - Isolated gonadotrophin deficiency
    - Hypothyroidism

History

To exclude iatrogenic causes of ovarian failure, a detailed past history of prior ovarian surgery, chemotherapy and irradiation should be obtained. Specific infectious diseases need to be addressed, especially mumps and AIDS. Although serious systemic illness should be obvious, a history of past or current autoimmune disorders should be obtained. Inquiries as to the presence, in themselves or family, of Addison's disease, thyroid disease, diabetes, SLE, rheumatoid arthritis, vitiligo, Crohn's disease and Sjögren's disease need to be made. A thorough review of systems requires specific emphasis on the signs and symptoms of related disorders, with additional emphasis on autoimmune endocrine dysfunction. Attention should be paid to the subtle and insidious symptoms of Addison's disease. Therefore questions pertaining to weight loss, anorexia, vague abdominal pain, weakness, increased skin pigmentation, and salt craving are important. The ovarian failure and the subsequent hypo-estrogenism will lead to the complaints of vaginal dryness, dyspareunia and infertility.

Epidemiological studies have noted a possible familial relationship of POF among sisters and mothers, although recall bias may be a factor in these studies [221]. Coulam described an autosomal dominant form that traced through four generations [222].

Physical examination

Patients with POF can present with several rare familial disorders with unique physical manifestations. Deafness in patients with POF suggests the autosomal recessive disorder known as Perrault's syndrome [149]. Congenital dysplasia of the eyelids is an autosomal dominant inherited trait that can occur with ovarian failure [223,224]. The most common abnormal karyotype associated with POF is that of Turner's syndrome. The stigma of Turner's syndrome are well described and include many organ systems [225].

A search should be made for the physical characteristics of autoimmune disorders. Premature greying of the hair, as noted in pernicious anaemia, or the skin pigmentation disorder of vitiligo may be present. In existing Addison's disease one may note increased pigmentation of the hand skin folds and/or gums. In addition, the loss of adrenal androgen production results in sparse axillary and pubic hair. Other manifestations include the malar skin rash and alopecia areata of SLE. Careful thyroid examination may reveal enlargement.

Assessment of breast and pubic hair development according to the stages of Tanner are important in those individuals that present with primary amenorrhoea. Breast development is the first sign of sexual maturation (9.5 years) in 85% of girls, with the onset of menses at the mean age of 12.8 years. Amenorrhoea in girls older than 16, and in those who experience breast development but fail to menstruate during the succeeding 4 years, should undergo a careful assessment [136].

Pelvic examination may demonstrate atrophic vaginitis due to the lack of adequate oestrogen. It is important to remember, however, that POF patients may intermittently produce enough oestrogen to keep the vaginal mucosa normal. As a result of lymphocytic oophoritis or steroid enzyme defects, bimanual examination may reveal ovarian enlargement, with or without tenderness [123,151,226]. Neurological examination concentrating on pituitary mass effects, should be performed.

Laboratory evaluation

We require the following before diagnosing POF: at least 4 months of amenorrhoea and two circulating FSH values greater than 40 IU/L obtained at least one month apart in a woman younger than 40 years of age [100]. Some clinicians recommend the use of a progestin challenge test in all amenorrhoeic women. Patients are examined for withdrawal bleeding 4–7 days after the progesterone dose. If bleeding occurs, this is evidence of adequate oestrogen and ovarian function. Despite markedly elevated gonadotrophins, some patients with POF may have intermittent ovarian function and, hence, generate sufficient oestrogen to produce endometrial withdrawal bleeding. Thus, women with oligomenorrhoea and or prodomal phase POF patients may inadvertently be missed on the progesterone test alone [170]. We, therefore, do not recommend the progesterone withdrawal test. In those patients with amenorrhoea, oligomenorrhoea, or polymenorrhoea who plan to delay childbearing, serum FSH level should be measured. Elevated gonadotrophin levels imply possible ovarian dysfunction. Serum FSH, however, does not reflect the number of primordial follicles remaining in the ovary but only the lack of oestrogen/inhibin feedback from developing antral follicles. Thus non-invasive determination of follicle depletion or follicle dysfunction is not currently possible. Recently, several stimulation tests employing gonadotrophin releasing hormone antagonists or the antioestrogen, clomiphine citrate, have been used to measure ovarian reserve [227]. These stimulation tests are performed in an attempt to predict the success of ovarian stimulation protocols, but their diagnostic utility in patients with prodromal POF has not been studied.

A karyotype should be performed as a part of a basic laboratory evaluation for all patients with POF. It has been suggested that only those younger than 35 years undergo chromosomal analysis, but women with X chromosome abnormalities have delivered normal children and developed POF after the age of 35 [55]. Furthermore, patients are reassured by a normal karyotype and those with abnormal karyotypes will be relieved to find an explanation for their problems. In addition, certain karyotypes may have important implications for other family members.

POF can be a component of the autoimmune polyglandular syndromes and, therefore, many clinicians have recommended screening for other endocrine disorders [104,228,229]. Recently, we examined the results of our prospective screening programme in 119 patients with spontaneous POF with normal karyotype. No new cases of Addison's disease, pernicious anaemia, or hypoparathyroidism were uncovered. Screening studies did reveal 12 new cases of thyroid disease and two new cases of diabetes mellitus [115]. We no longer perform laboratory screening tests with exception of a TSH level.

To exclude non-organ-specific autoimmune disorders a complete blood count and urine analysis should be obtained. Sedimentation rate, antinuclear antibodies, and rheumatoid factor should be measured only as clinically indicated. Interestingly, we have identified an isolated IgG-deficient patient who presented with recurrent upper respiratory infection and POF. IgA deficiency, which is associated with autoimmune disorders, is the most common immunoglobulin deficiency [230]. Screening for this disease has not been clinically useful.

The evaluation of patients who present with the lack of secondary sexual characteristics is beyond the scope of this chapter, but several excellent reviews are available [136]. Screening for other unusual disorders, such as thymomas, in patients with POF is not warranted, unless there is co-existing myasthenia gravis. Gonadotrophin-producing pituitary tumours may be associated with menstrual irregularities and elevated gonadotrophins. Although these tumours are rare in women less than 40 years old, they should be suspected in the patient with amenorrhoea, elevated gonadotrophins and symptoms indicating a central nervous system mass lesion. Gadolinium-enhanced magnetic resonance imaging confirms the existence of a pituitary lesion. Measuring the response of intact FSH and α and β subunits of LH/FSH to a stimulatory dose of TRH will identify most (80%) patients with a gonadotrophin adenoma [231].

The clinical usefulness of other diagnostic procedures is suspect. These include measuring OAb, performing pelvic ultrasound, and laparoscopic ovarian biopsies. In fact, a commercially available test for OAb was positive in nearly one-third of normal women [127]. Several clinicians have used the presence of OAb to determine the type and success of treatment regimes [124,199,232]. However, these studies have not been carried out in a controlled manner. Likewise, the clinical utility of using ultrasound as a screening test is unfounded. The presence or absence of ultrasonically proven follicle structures does not change prognosis or clinical management [12]. Ovarian biopsy for the diagnosis of oophoritis, or the determination of afollicular versus follicular forms of POF has not been fruitful [14,170–172]. Due to problems in sampling error, pregnancies have occurred despite biopsies revealing ovarian tissue devoid of follicles.

Treatment and prognosis

When anticipating the diagnosis of POF, even before the confirmatory results are in hand, we schedule a follow up appointment to discuss the laboratory findings (Table 10.4). The busy clinician may forget the psychological and physical implications of such a diagnosis in a young, otherwise healthy, infertile woman [5]. Once the diagnosis is made, it is important to determine the wishes of the patient: is she considering pregnancy? A discussion of hormone relacement should follow in those individuals not presently interested in child bearing. Numerous epidemiological studies confirm the benefits and risks of hormone replacement therapy (HRT) [233,234]. A National Institutes of Health-sponsored prospective study is currently investigating the effects of HRT [235], but, the majority of these patients are older postmenopausal women and thus, the effect of HRT on young POF patients has not been studied. Physiologically, it appears safe to extrapolate to the young POF patient the most important benefits of HRT, namely protection against osteoporosis and prevention of cardiovascular disease. We and others have noted that these patients have lower bone densities (Figure 10.3), despite apparently adequate hormone replacement therapy [236,237]. This observation alone suggests the importance of early diagnosis, treatment and follow up in patients with POF.

Many types and methods of HRT are available [238]. Conjugated equine oestrogen (CEO), which has demonstrated safety and efficacy for more than 40 years, is our initial therapy. Although a daily oestrogen dose equivalent to 0.625 mg of CEO is sufficient to maintain bone density, most young women will require a higher dose (1.25 mg) to control vasomotor symptoms and oestrogen-

Table 10.4 Management of karyotypically normal spontaneous premature ovarian failure

Inform
Spontaneous remission can occur
Gonadotrophin therapy has a theoretic risk of exacerbating unrecognized autoimmune ovarian failure
Counsel
Time to allow spontaneous remission may be in order
Adoption or a change in life plans may resolve infertility for some couples
Ovum donation, after an appropriate delay, is an option for other couples
Replace
Cyclic oestrogen and progestogen therapy is indicated
Full replacement is needed to alleviate symptoms, not just for prophylaxis for osteoporosis
Follow-up
Vigilance to identify the few patients who will subsequently develop other component of the autoimmune polyglandular syndrome or non-organ-specific autoimmunity
Forewarning regarding the early symptoms of adrenal insufficiency

ize the vaginal epithelium. The cyclic addition of progesterone is required to counteract the stimulatory effects of CEO and prevent the occurrence of endometrial cancer. The most common cyclic progesterone method employs medroxyprogesterone acetate (MPA 5–10 mg daily) for 10–14 days per month. In 75% of women, cyclic progesterone leads to a monthly withdrawal bleed which may be important psychologically to the patient [238]. Some patients experience side effects from this high dose cyclic MPA, and may benefit from continuous CEO and low dose MPA (2.5 mg daily). This regimen is associated with less, but irregular, uterine bleeding and the long term effects of MPS on lipid profiles remain to be determined.

In counselling the POF patients, it is important to discuss the intermittent return of ovarian function and hence, the chance of irregular bleeding and pregnancy. For this reason, patients not desiring even the remote chance of pregnancy should be offered a low dose oral contraceptive (20–30 μg of ethinyl oestradiol). Pharmacologically, one must remember that the amount of ethinyl oestradiol contained in birth control pills is 7–10 times that needed to prevent osteoporosis and cardiac disease. This additional oestrogen, theoretically, could be associated with an increased risk of thrombolytic events and patients, especially those who smoke, should be so advised [239]. New regimens and formulations are being employed as alternatives to standard CEO/MPA HRT. If patients opt for a non-oral HRT, a transdermal delivery of 17β-oestradiol is available in a alcohol-based reservoir and in a controlled release matrix delivery patch [240,241]. The oral administration of a progestin is still required, but prototypes of transdermal progesterone delivery system will soon be released [242].

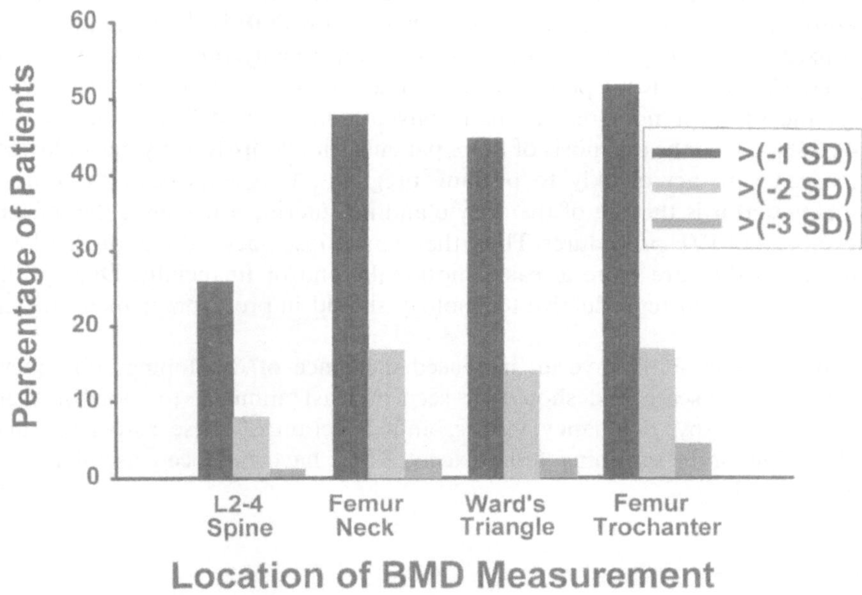

Figure 10.3 Percentage of POF patients with bone mineral densities (BMD) greater than 1, 2 and 3 standard deviations (SD) below age matched controls. Eighty-five percent of the 89 study patients were on hormone replacement therapy

The woman who desires a pregnancy is a more complicated problem and is affected not only emotionally but also fiscally. Numerous reports of pregnancy occurring in POF patients exist, but predicting the likelihood of spontaneous remission in a specific individual is impossible. When patients with POF are serially tested over a 4–6 month period, ovulation is noted in 20% of the cases [7,9,169]. Most pregnancies occur in individuals during HRT, but this may not be a cause and effect relationship, since statistically most patients are on HRT for reasons other than achieving pregnancy. The premise that gonadotrophin suppression may decrease the antigen load and help restore ovulation has been tested using gonadotrophin releasing hormones analogues or danocrine, a weak androgen [7,9]. Neither has been shown to be more effective than placebo.

Uncontrolled studies and anecdotal cases of the return of ovarian function after using a high dose steroid immunosuppression have been reported [243] but presently have no proven benefit and carry a significant risk. A prospective study of alternate-day prednisone therapy for lymphocytic oophoritis is now underway at the Clinical Center of the National Institutes of Health. Futile attempts at high dose gonadotrophin therapy, in the hope of stimulating the remaining follicles in POF patients, have been attempted. The success achieved with this method probably represents spontaneous remissions. The only proven therapy for obtaining a pregnancy in patients with POF is by implantation of fertilized donor oocytes into an exogenous hormonally prepared uterus. The success (22–33%) of this procedure continues to improve and the efficacy is at least the same, if not greater, than conventional *in vitro* fertilization (IVF) [244,245]. Given the diagnosis of POF, patients who desire fertility naturally feel an urgency to act quickly to become pregnant. It is important to counsel patients that it is the age of the oocyte and not uterine senescence that effects the success of IVF procedures. Thus, they can choose oocyte donation at a later date, when they are more at ease emotionally and/or financially. During this wait, advances in reproductive technology should improve pregnancy rates at reduced costs.

Patients with POF have an increased incidence of developing subsequent autoimmune disease and should be seen at least annually to monitor their hormone therapy, pregnancy wishes, and detection of these associated disorders. Elaborate screening tests, except TSH, have not been useful in our experience [115].

THE FUTURE

Heterogeneous populations (immunological versus non-immunological versus genetic), the status of the remaining follicles, immunologic regulation/dysregulation in the ovary, and the control of ovarian apoptosis are crucial unexplained factors in understanding POF. With the advent of new molecular and recombinant DNA technology, addressing these complex issues may be possible. The international impetus to sequence the entire human genome will increase our understanding of the genetic influence of ovarian development [246]. Recombinant production of oocyte-specific protein-based assays will help to identify those patients with remaining follicles. Adequately controlled immunological and non-immunological based therapies could be applied employing this subset of patients. Utilizing recombinant techniques, the isolation and production of ovarian antigens may permit immunotherapy designed to produce immunotolerance in autoimmune POF. These immunotherapies could employ the acquisition of tolerance following presentation of antigen through alternative routes, such as injection, intravenous infusion, and oral administration of specific ovarian antigens.

Advances in molecular immunology as a direct result of AIDS and diabetes research may further our understanding of POF. The existence of two different T helper cell activities had long been proposed to account for the divergence of humoral and cellular immunity in response to various stimuli. The cellular basis for this dichotomy is the segregation of $CD4^+$ T cells into two distinct phenotypes (T_H1/T_H2) based on their mutually exclusive cytokine production [247]. Therapies aimed at balancing the T cell subsets has been applied in other autoimmune animal models [248]. Is autoimmune POF a result of the dysregulation of T helper subsets, as in other autoimmune disorders [249]? Using the murine POF model some investigators have suggested a persistent T_H2 response in these neonatal thymectomized mice [250]. Thus, if a similar mechanism applies to human disease, the administration of appropriate cytokines could prevent POF.

The control of apoptosis appears to be a key piece to the POF puzzle [42]. The exploration of apoptosis and its interaction with the immune system will lead to crucial discoveries regarding the mechanisms involved in the control of follicle endowment and atresia [251]. Once the control of apoptosis is elucidated, manipulation of the regulatory factors of this programmed cell death could prevent the premature loss of oocytes and follicles.

New drugs for hormone replacement soon will be entering clinical trials, the first of which will be the antioestrogens. These drugs have positive effects on bone and the cardiovascular system and are without the associated risk of breast and endometrial stimulation [252,253]. For those patients desiring pregnancy, donor oocyte programmes will benefit from improved technology. Cryopreservation of oocytes as opposed to embryos could allow patients with the diagnosis of prodromal POF to have their oocytes saved for future fertilization. This technique has worked well in animals, but awaits future improvement before it can be applied to man [77].

References

1. Heller CG, Heller EJ. Gonadotrophic hormone: urine assays of normal cycling, menopausal, castrated and estrin treated human females. J Clin Invest. 1939;18:171–8.
2. Atria A. La menopausia precoz y tratamiento hormonal. Rev Med Chile, 1950;78:373–7.
3. Hertz R, Villee CA, eds. Control of Ovulation. New York: Pergamon Press; 1961:21.
4. Jones GS, De Moraes-Ruehsen M. A new syndrome of amenorrhea in association with hypergonadotropism and apparently normal ovarian follicular apparatus. Am J Obstet Gynecol. 1969;104:597–600.
5. Mahlstedt P. The psychological component of infertility. Fertil Steril. 1985;43:335–46.
6. De Moraes-Ruehsen M, Jones GS. Premature ovarian failure. Fertil Steril. 1967;18:440–61.
7. Anasti JN, Kimzey LM, Defensor RA, White B, Nelson LM. A controlled study of danazol for the treatment of karyotypically normal spontaneous premature ovarian failure. Fertil Steril. 1994;62:726–30.
8. Boyers SP, Luborsky JL, DeCherney AH. Usefulness of serial measurements of serum follicle stimulating hormone, luteinizing hormone and estradiol in patients with permature ovarian failure. Fertil Steril. 1988;50:408–12.
9. Nelson LM, Kimzey LM, Merriam GR. Gonadotrohin suppression for the treatment of karyotypically normal spontaneous premature ovarian failure: a controlled trial. Fertil Steril. 1992;57:50–5.
10. Rebar RW, Erickson GF, Yen SCC. Idiopathic premature ovarian failure: clinical and endocrine characteristics. Fertil Steril. 1982;37:35–41.
11. Conway GS, Kaltsas G, Patel A, Davies MC, Jacobs HS. Characterization of idiopathic premature ovarian failure. Fertil Steril. 1996;65:337–41.
12. Mehta AE, Matwijiw I, Lyons EA, Faiman C. Noninvasive diagnosis of resistant ovary syndrome by ultrasonography. Fertil Steril. 1992;57:56–61.
13. Taylor AE, Schneyer AL, Sluss PM et al. Ovarian failure, resistance and activation. In: Adashi EY, Leung CK, eds. The Ovary. New York: Raven Press; 1993:629–61.
14. Aiman J, Smentek C. Premature ovarian failure. Obstet Gynecol. 1985;66:9–14.
15. Coulam CB, Adamson SC, Annegers JF. Incidence of premature ovarian failure. Obstet Gynecol. 1986;67:604–6.

16. Alper MM, Garner PR, Seibel MM. Premature ovarian failure. Current concepts. J Reprod Med. 1986;31:699–708.
17. Adashi EY. The ovarian follicular apparatus. In: Adashi EY, Rock JA, Rosenwaks Z, eds. Reproductive Endocrinology, Surgery and Technology, 1st edn. New York: Lippincott-Raven; 1995:17–40.
18. Rabinovici J, Jaffe RB. Development and regulation of growth and differentiated function in human and subhuman primate fetal gonads. Endocrine Rev. 1990;11:532–57.
19. Witschi E. Migration of germ cells of human embryos from the yolk sac to primate gonadal folds. Contrib Embryol. 1948;32:67–8.
20. Ohno S, Klinger HP, Atkin NB. Human oogenesis. Cytogenetics. 1962;1:42–51.
21. Baker TG. A quantitative and cytological study of germ cells in the human ovaries. Proc Roy Soc Lond. 1963;158:417–33.
22. Chiquoine AD. The development of the zona pellucida in mammalian ovum. Am J Anat. 1960;106:149–69.
23. Peters H, Himelstein-Braw R, Faber M. The normal development of the ovary in childhood. Acta Endocrinol. 1976;82:617–30.
24. Gulyas BJ, Hodgen GD, Tullner WW, Ross GT. Effects of fetal and maternal hypophysectomy on endocrine organs and body weight in infant Rhesus monkeys (*Macaca mulatta*): with particular emphasis on oogenesis. Biol Reprod. 1977;16:216–27.
25. Huhtaniemi I, Yamamoto M, Ranta T, Jalkanen J, Jaffe RB. Follicle stimulating hormone receptors appear earlier in the primate testis than in the ovary. J Clin Endocrinol Metab. 1987;65:1210–4.
26. May JM, McCarty K, Reichert LE, Schomberg DW. Follicle stimulating-hormone-mediated induction of functional luteinizing/human chorionic gonadotrophin receptors during monolayer of porcine granulosa cells. Endocrinology. 1980;107:1041–9.
27. Hoff JD, Quigley ME, Yen SSC. Hormonal dynamics at midcycle: a reevaluation. J Clin Endocrinol Metab. 1983;57:792–7.
28. Speroff L, Glass RH, Kase NG. Regulation of the menstrual cycle. In: Clinical Gynecologic Endocrinology and Infertility, 5th edn. Baltimore: Williams & Wilkins; 1994:183–230.
29. Unanue ER, Allen PM. The basis for the immunoregulatory role of macrophages and other accessory cells. Science. 1987;236:551–7.
30. Harrison LC, Campbell IL. Cytokines: an expanding network of immuno-inflammatory hormones. Mol Endocrinol. 1988;2:1151–6.
31. Adashi EY. The potential relevance of cytokines to ovarian physiology. J Ster Biochem Mol Biol. 1992;43:439–44.
32. Norman RJ, Brannstrom M. White cells and the ovary – incidental invaders or essential effectors? J Endocrinol. 1994;140:333–6.
33. Adashi EY. The potential relevance of cytokines to ovarian physiology: the emerging role of resident ovarian cells of the white blood cells. Endocrine Rev. 1990;11:454–64.
34. Brannstrom M, Norman RJ. Involvement of leukocytes and cytokines in the ovulatory process and corpus luteum function. Hum Reprod. 1993;8:1762–75.
35. Espey LL. Ovulation as an inflammatory process. Biol Reprod. 1980;22:73–106.
36. Murdoch WJ, McCormick RJ. Production of low molecular weight chemoattractants for leukocytes by periovulatory ovine follicles. Biol Reprod. 1989;40:86–90.
37. Bagavandoss P, Wiggins RC, Kunkel SL, Remick DJ, Keyes PL. Tumor necrosis factor production accumulation of inflammatory cells in the corpus luteum of pseudopregnancy and pregnancy in rabbit. Biol Reprod. 1990;42:367–76.
38. Kirsch TM, Friedman AC, Vogel RL. Macrophages in corporea lutea of mice: characterization effects on steroid secretions. Biol Reprod. 1981;25:629–38.
39. Best CL, Pudney J, Welch WR, Burger N, Hill JA. Localization and characterization of white blood cell populations within the human ovary throughout the menstrual cycle and menopause. Hum Reprod. 1996;11:790–7.
40. Ueda N, Shah SV. Apoptosis. J Lab Clin Med. 1994;124:169–77.
41. Majno G, Joris I. Apoptosis, oncosis, and necrosis. An overview of cell death. Am J Pathol. 1995;146:3–15.
42. Hsueh AJ, Eisenhauer K, Chun SY, Hsu SY, Billig H. Gonadal cell apoptosis. Rec Prog Horm Res. 1996;51:433–55.
43. Spencer SJ, Cataldo NA, Jaffe RB. Apoptosis in the human female reproductive tract. Obstet Gynecol Surv. 1996;51:314–23.

44. Guo MW, Mori E, Xu JP, Mori T. Identification of Fas antigen associated with apoptotic cell death in murine ovary. Biochem Biophys Res Commun. 1994;203:1438–46.
45. Chun SY, Eisenhauer KM, Minami S, Billig H, Perlas E, Hsueh AJ. Hormonal regulation of apoptosis in early antral follicles: follicle-stimulating hormone as a major survival factor. Endocrinology. 1996;137:1447–56.
46. Tilly JL, Tilly KI, Kenton ML, Johnson AL. Expression of members of the bcl-2 gene family in the immature rat ovary: equine chorionic gonadotropin-mediated inhibition of granulosa cell apoptosis is associated with decreased bax and constitutive bcl-2 and bcl-xlong messenger ribonucleic acid levels. Endocrinology. 1995;136:232–41.
47. Tilly KI, Banerjee S, Banerjee PP, Tilly JL. Expression of the p53 and Wilms' tumor suppressor genes in the rat ovary: gonadotropin repression in vivo and immunohistochemical localization of nuclear p53 protein to apoptotic granulosa cells of atretic follicles. Endocrinology. 1995;136:1394–402.
48. Luciano AM, Pappalardo A, Ray C, Peluso JJ. Epidermal growth factor inhibits large granulosa cell apoptosis by stimulating progesterone synthesis and regulating the distribution of intracellular free calcium. Biol Reprod. 1994;51:646–54.
49. Simon C, Tsafrir A, Chun SY, Piquette GN, Dang W, Polan ML. Interleukin-1 receptor antagonist suppresses human chorionic gonadotropin-induced ovulation in the rat. Biol Reprod. 1994;51:662–7.
50. Hakuno N, Koji T, Yano T et al. Fas/APO-1/CD95 system as a mediator of granulosa cell apoptosis in ovarian follicle atresia. Endocrinology. 1996;137:1938–48.
51. Singh RP, Carr DH. The anatomy and histology of XO human embryos and fetuses. Anat Rec. 1966;155:369–84.
52. Carr DH, Haggar RA, Hart AG. Germ cells in the ovaries of XO female infants. Am J Clin Pathol. 1968;49:521–6.
53. Itu M, Neelam T, Ammini AC, Kucheria K. Primary amenorrhoea in a triple X female. Aust NZ J Obstet Gynaecol. 1990;30:368–8.
54. Powell CM, Taggart RT, Drumheller TC et al. Molecular and cytogenetic studies of an X; autosome translocation in a patient with premature ovarian failure and review of the literature. Am J Med Genet. 1994;52:19–26.
55. Krauss CM, Turksoy RN, Atkins L, McLaughlin C, Brown LG, Page DC. Familial premature ovarian failure due to an interstitital deletion of the long arm of the X chromosome. N Engl J Med. 1987;317:125–31.
56. Mattison DR, Evans MI, Schwimmer WB, White BJ, Jensen B, Schulman JD. Familial premature ovarian failure. Am J Hum Genet. 1984;36:1341–8.
57. Kinch RAH, Plunkett ER, Smout MS, Carr DH. Primary ovarian failure: a clinicopathological and cytogenetic study. Am J Obstet Gynecol. 1965;91:630–44.
58. Duncan MK, Lieman J, Chada KK. The germ cell deficient locus maps to mouse chromosome 11A2-3. Mam Genome. 1995;6:697–9.
59. Sardharwalla IB, Wraith JE. Galactosaemia. Nutrit Health. 1987;5:163–74.
60. Waggoner DD, Buist NRM, Donnell GN. Long-term prognosis in galactosaemia: results of a survey of 350 cases. J Inher Metab Dis. 1990;13:802–18.
61. Levy HL, Driscoll SG, Porensky RS, Wender DF. Ovarian failure in galactosaemia. N Engl J Med. 1984;310:50–3.
62. Fraser IS, Russell P, Greco S, Robertson DM. Resistant ovary syndrome and premature ovarian failure in young women with galactosaemia. Clin Reprod Fertil. 1986;4:133–8.
63. Kaufman FR, Reichardt JK, Ng WG et al. Correlation of cognitive, neurologic, and ovarian outcome with the Q188R mutation of the galactose-1-phosphate uridyltransferase gene. J Pediatr. 1994;125:225–7.
64. Gradishar WJ, Schilsky RL. Ovarian function following radiation and chemotherapy for cancer. Semin Oncol. 1989;16:425–36.
65. Averette HE, Boike GM, Jarrell MA. Effects of cancer chemotherapy on gonadal function and reproductive capacity. Can J Clin. 1990;40:199–209.
66. Apperly JF, Reddy N. Mechanism and management of treatment-related gonadal failure in recipients of high dose chemotherapy. Blood Rev. 1995;9:93–116.
67. Epstein RJ. Drug-induced DNA damage and tumor chemosensitivity. J Clin Oncol. 1990;8: 2062–84.
68. Barton C, Waxman J. Effects of chemotherapy on fertility. Blood Rev. 1990;4:187–95.
69. Shalet SM. Disorders of the endocrine system due to radiation and cytotoxic chemotherapy. Clin Endocrinol. 1983;19:637–59.

70. Koyama H, Wada T, Nishizawa Y et al. Cyclophosphamide-induced ovarian failure and its therapeutic significance in patients with breast cancer. Cancer. 1977;39:1403–9.
71. Chapman RM, Sutcliffe SB. Protection of ovarian function by oral contraceptive use in women receiving chemotherapy for Hodgkin's disease. Blood. 1981;58:849–51.
72. Ataya K, Rao LV, Lawrence E, Kimmel R. Luteinizing hormone-releasing hormone agonist inhibits cyclophosphamide-induced ovarian follicular depletion in Rhesus monkeys. Biol Reprod. 1995;52:365–72.
73. Glode LM, Robinson J, Gould SF. Protection from cyclophosphamide induced testicular damage with analogue of gonadotropin-releasing hormone. Lancet. 1981;1:1132–4.
74. Jarrell JF, McMahon A, Barr RD, Younglai EV. The agonist (d-leu-6,des-gly-10)-LHRH-ethylamide does not protect the fecundity of rats exposed to high dose unilateral ovarian irradiation. Reprod Toxicol. 1991;5:385–8.
75. Carroll J, Gosden RG. Transplantation of frozen-thawed mouse primordial follicles. Hum Reprod. 1993;8:1163–7.
76. Gosden RG. Restitution of fertility in sterilized mice by transferring primordial ovarian follicles. Hum Reprod. 1993;5:499–504.
77. Newton H, Aubard Y, Rutherford A, Sharma V, Gosden RG. Low temperature storage and grafting of human ovarian tissue. Hum Reprod. 1996;11:1487–91.
78. Ogilvy-Stuart AL, Shalet SM. Effect of radiation on the human reproductive system. Environ Health Perspect. 1993;101:109–16.
79. Baker TG. Radiosensitivity of mammalian oocytes with particular reference to the human female. Am J Obstet Gynecol. 1971;110:746–9.
80. Gabriel DA, Bernard SA, Lambert J, Croom RD III. Oophoropexy and the management of Hodgkin's disease. A reevaluation of the risks and benefits. Arch Surg. 1986;121:1083–5.
81. Thibaud E, Ramirez M, Brauner R et al. Preservation of ovarian function by ovarian transposition performed before pelvic irradiation during childhood. J Pediatr. 1992;121: 880–4.
82. Vermeulen A. Environment, human reproduction, menopause, and andropause. Environ Health Perspect. 1993;101:91–100.
83. Cooper GS, Baird DD, Hulka BS, Weinberg CR, Savitz DA, Hughes CL. Follicle-stimulating hormone concentrations in relation to active and passive smoking. Obstet Gynecol. 1995;85: 407–11.
84. Jick H, Porter J, Morrison AS. Relation between smoking and age of natural menopause. Lancet. 1977;1:1354–5.
85. Maxson WS, Wentz AC. The gonadotropin resistant ovary syndrome. Semin Reprod Endocrinol. 1983;1:147–60.
86. Morishima A, Grumbach MM, Simpson ER, Fisher C, Qin K. Aromatase deficiency in male and female siblings caused by a novel mutation and the physiological role of estrogens. J Clin Endocrinol Metab. 1995;80:3689–98.
87. Rabinovici J, Blankstein J, Goldman B et al. In vitro fertilization and primary embryonic cleavage are possible in 17α-hydroxylase deficiency despite extremely low intrafollicular 17β-estradiol. J Clin Endocrinol Metab. 1989;68:693–7.
88. Yanase T, Sanders D, Shibata A, Matusi N, Simpson ER, Waterman MR. Combined 17alpha hydroxylase/17,20 lyase deficiency due to a 7-basepair duplication in the N-terminal region of the cytochrome P450. J Clin Endocrinol Metab. 1990;70:1325–31.
89. Weiss J, Axelrod L, Whitcomb RW, Harris PE, Crowley WF, Jameson JL. Hypogonadism caused by a single amino acid substitution in the β subunit of luteinizing hormone. N Engl J Med. 1992;326:179–83.
90. Latronico AC, Anasti J, Arnhold IJ et al. Brief report: testicular and ovarian resistance to luteinizing hormone caused by inactivating mutations of the luteinizing hormone-receptor gene. N Engl J Med. 1996;334:507–12.
91. Aittomaki K, Lucena JLD, Pakarinen P et al. Mutation in the follicle-stimulating hormone receptor gene causes hereditary hypergonadotropic ovarian failure. Cell. 1995;82:959–68.
92. Tilly JL, Aihara T, Nishimoro K et al. Expression of recombinant human follicle-stimulating hormone receptor: species-specific ligand binding, signal transduction, and identification of multiple ovarian messenger ribonucleic acid transcripts. Endocrinology. 1992;131:799–806.
93. Wolfsdorf JI, Rosenfield RL, Fang VS, Kobayashi R, Razdan AK, Kim MH. Partial gonadotrophin-resistance in pseudohypoparathyroidism. Acta Endocrinol. 1978;88:321–8.
94. Guinet P, Pommatau E. Le pseudo-panhypopituitarisme par insuffisiences associees ovarienne, thyroidienne, et semenale. Ann Endocrinol. 1954;15:327–32.

95. Irvine WJ, Barnes EW. Addison's disease and autoimmune ovarian failure. J Reprod Fertil. 1974;21:1–31.
96. Irvine WJ, Chan MMW, Scarth L et al. Immunological aspects of premature ovarian failure associated with idiopathic Addison's disease. Lancet. 1968;2:883–90.
97. Turkington RW, Lebovitz HE. Extra-adrenal endocrine deficiencies in Addison's disease. Am J Med. 1967;43:499–507.
98. Edmonds M, Lamki L, Killinger DW, Volpe R. Autoimmune thyroiditis, adrenalitis, and oophoritis. Am J Med. 1973;54:782–7.
99. Coulam CB. The prevalence of autoimmune disorders among patients with primary ovarian failure. Am J Reprod Immunol. 1983;4:63–6.
100. Anasti JN, Adams S, Kimzey LM, Defensor RA, Zachary AA, Nelson LM. Karyotypically normal spontaneous premature ovarian failure: evaluation of association with the class II major histocompatibility complex. J Clin Endocrinol Metab. 1994;78:722–3.
101. LaBarbera AR, Miller MM, Ober C, Rebar RW. Autoimmune etiology in premature ovarian failure. Am J Reprod Immunol. 1988;16:115–22.
102. Kim JG, Moon SY, Chang YS, Lee JY. Autoimmune premature ovarian failure. J Obstet Gynecol. 1995;21:59–66.
103. Mignot MH, Schoemaker J, Kleingeld M, Rao BR, Drexhage HA. Premature ovarian failure. I: The association with autoimmunity. Eur J Obstet Gyn Reprod Biol. 1989;30:59–66.
104. Neufeld M, Maclaren N, Blizzard RM. Autoimmune polyglandular syndrome. Pediatr Ann. 1980;9:43–53.
105. Lundberg PO, Persson VH. Disappearance of amenorrhea after thymectomy. A case report. Acta Soc Med Upsalla. 1969;74:206–8.
106. Chung TK, Haines CJ, Yip SK. Case report: spontaneous pregnancy following thymectomy for myasthenia gravis associated with premature ovarian failure. Asia-Ocea J Obstet Gynaecol. 1993;19:253–5.
107. Bateman BG, Nunley WC, Kitchin JD III. Reversal of apparent premature ovarian failure in a patient with myasthenia gravis. Fertil Steril. 1983;39:108–10.
108. DeMoraes-Ruehsen M, Blizzard RM, Garcia-Bunuel R, Jones GS. Autoimmunity and ovarian failure. Am J Obstet Gynecol. 1972;112:693–703.
109. Collen RJ, Lippe BM, Kaplan SA. Primary ovarian failure, juvenile rheumatoid arthritis, and vitiligo. Am J Dis Child. 1979;133:598–600.
110. Herz KC, Gazze LA, Kirkpatrick CH, Katz SI. Autoimmune vitiligo: detection of antibodies to melanin-producing cells. N Engl J Med. 1977;297:634–8.
111. Blizzard RM, Gibbs JH. Candidiasis: studies pertaining to its association with endocrinopathies and pernicious anemia. Pediatrics. 1968;42:231–6.
112. Moncayo-Naveda H, Moncayo R, Benz R, Nat R, Wolf A, Lauritzen C. Organ-specific antibodies against ovary in patients with systemic lupus erythematosus. Am J Obstet Gynecol. 1989;160:1227–9.
113. Rose E, Pillsbury DM. Lupus erythematosus and ovarian function: observations on a possible relationship, with report of six cases. Ann Intern Med. 1944;21:1034.
114. Moncayo R, Moncayo HE. A new endocrinological and immunological syndrome in SLE: elevation of human chorionic gonadotropin and of antibodies directed against ovary and endometrium antigens. Lupus. 1995;4:39–45.
115. Anasti JN, Adams S, Zachary AA et al. Routine endocrine screening for patients with karyotypically normal spontaneous premature ovarian failure. Obstet Gynecol. 1997;89:777–9.
116. Moncayo R, Moncayo HE. Premature ovarian failure: evidence for the immunologic component. In: Ovarian Autoimmunity: Clinical and Experimental Data. Austin: Lanes Company; 1995:27–75.
117. Moncayo R, Moncayo HE. The association of autoantibodies directed against ovarian antigens in human disease: a clinical review. J Int Med. 1993;234:371–8.
118. Vallotton MB, Forbes AP. Antibodies to cytoplasm of ova. Lancet. 1966;2:264–5.
119. Coulam CB, Ryan RJ. Premature menopause. I. Etiology. Am J Obstet Gynecol. 1979;133:639–43.
120. Coulam CB, Ryan RJ. Prevalence of circulating antibodies directed toward ovaries among women with premature ovarian failure. Am J Reprod Immunol. 1985;9:23–4.
121. Mathur S, Melchers JT, Ades EW, Williamson HO, Fundenburg HH. Antiovarian and antilymphocyte antibodies in patients with chronic vaginal candidiasis. J Reprod Immunol. 1980;2:247–62.

122. Smith H, Lou Y, Lacy P, Tung KSK. Tolerance mechanism in experimental ovarian and gastric autoimmune disease. J Immunol. 1992;149:2212–8.
123. Case Records of the Massachusetts General Hospital C4. Case 46. N Engl J Med. 1986;315: 1336–43.
124. Luborsky JL, Visintin I, Boyers S, Asari T, Caldwell B, DeCherney A. Ovarian antibodies detected by immobilized antigen immunoassay in patients with premature ovarian failure. J Clin Endocrinol Metab. 1990;70:69–75.
125. Moncayo H, Moncayo R, Benz R, Wolf A, Lauritzen C. Ovarian failure and autoimmunity. J Clin Invest. 1989;84:1857–65.
126. Kim JG, Anderson BE, Rebar RW, LaBarbera AR. A biotin-streptavidin enzyme immunoassay for detection of antibodies to porcine granulosa cell antigens. J Immunoassay. 1991; 12:447–64.
127. Novosad-Oen JA, Tong ZB, Kimzey LM et al. Zona pellucida antibodies in patients with premature ovarian failure: a controlled analysis of a clinically available assay. [Abstract] SGI 1992. 39th Annual Meeting, San Antonio, TX, March 18–21, 1992.
128. Tang VW, Faiman C. Premature ovarian failure: a search for circulating factors against gonadotropin receptors. Am J Obstet Gynecol. 1983;146:816–21.
129. van Weissenbruch MM, Hoek A, van Vlietbleeker I, Schoemaker J, Drexhage H. Evidence for existence of immunoglobulins that block ovarian granulosa cell growth in vitro. A putative role in resistant ovary syndrome. J Clin Endocrinol Metab. 1991;73:360–7.
130. Jia X, Oikawa M, Bo M et al. Expression of human luteinizing hormone (LH) receptor: interaction with LH and chorionic gonadotropin from human but not equine, rat, and ovine species. Mol Endocrinol. 1991;5:759–68.
131. Anasti JN, Flack MR, Froehlich J, Nelson LM. The use of human recombinant gonadotropin receptors to search for immunoglobulin G-mediated premature ovarian failure. J Clin Endocrinol Metab. 1995;80:824–8.
132. Tano M, Minegishi T, Nakamura K, Karino S, Ibuki Y. Application of Chinese hamster ovary cells transfected with the recombinant human follicle-stimulating hormone (FSH) receptor for measurement of serum FSH. Fertil Steril. 1995;64:1120–4.
133. Sluss PM, Schneyer AL, Franke MA, Reichert LE Jr. Porcine follicular fluid contains both follicle-stimulating hormone agonist and antagonist activities. Endocrinology. 1987;120: 1477–81.
134. Schneyer AL, Sluss PM, Whitcomb RW, Hall JE, Crowley WF Jr. Development of a radioligand receptor assay for measuring follitropin in serum: application to premature ovarian failure. Clin Chem. 1991;37:508–14.
135. Irvine WJ, Barnes EW. Addison's disease, ovarian failure and hypoparathyroidism. Clin Endocrinol Metab. 1975;4:379–434.
136. Rosenfeld RL. Delayed puberty. In: Adashi EY, Rock JA, Rosenwaks Z, eds. Reproductive Endocrinology, Surgery and Technology, 1st edn. New York: Lippincott-Raven; 1995:1007–17.
137. Chen S, Sawicka J, Betterle C et al. Autoantibodies to steroidogenic enzymes in autoimmune polyglandular syndrome, Addison's disease, and premature ovarian failure. J Clin Endocrinol Metab. 1996;81:1871–6.
138. Ingram DL. Atresia. In: Zuckerman S, ed. The Ovary. New York: Academic Press; 1962:247–73.
139. Tachi J, Amino N, Iwatani Y et al. Increase in antideoxyribonucleic acid antibody titer in postpartum aggravation of autoimmune thyroid disease. J Clin Endocrinol Metab. 1988;67: 1049–53.
140. Murdoch WJ. Immunoregulation of mammalian fertility. Life Sci. 1994;55:1871–86.
141. Shivers CA, Dunbar BS. Autoantibodies to zona pellucida: a possible cause for infertility in women. Science. 1977;197:1082–4.
142. Caudle MR, Shivers CA. Current status of anti-zona pellucida antibodies. Am J Reprod Immunol. 1989;21:57–60.
143. Dunbar BS. Ovarian antigens and infertility. Am J Reprod Immunol. 1989;21:28–31.
144. Harris JD, Hibler DW, Fontenot GK, Hsu KT, Yurewicz EC, Sacco AG. Cloning and characterization of zona pellucida genes and cDNAs from a variety of mammalian species: the ZPA, ZPB and ZPC gene families. DNA Seq. 1994;4:361–93.
145. Wheatcroft NJ, Toogood AA, Li TC, Cooke ID, Weetman AP. Detection of antibodies to ovarian antigens in women with premature ovarian failure. Clin Exp Immunol. 1994;96:122–8.

146. Weetman AP. Autoimmunity to steroid-producing cells and familial polyendocrine autoimmunity. Baillières Clin Endocrinol Metab. 1995;9:157–74.
147. Belvisi L, Bombelli F, Sironi L, Doldi N. Organ-specific autoimmunity in patients with premature ovarian failure. J Endocrinol Invest. 1993;16:889–92.
148. Betterle C, Rossi A, Dalla Pria S et al. Premature ovarian failure: autoimmunity and natural history. Clin Endocrinol. 1993;39:35–43.
149. Nishi Y, Hamamoto K, Kajiyama M, Kawamura I. The Perrault syndrome: clinical report and review. Am J Med Genet. 1988;31:623–9.
150. Ayala A, Canales ES, Karchmer S, Alarcon D, Zarate A. Premature ovarian failure and hypothyroidism associated with sicca syndrome. Obstet Gynecol. 1979;53:98S–101S.
151. Biscotti CV, Hart WR, Lucas JG. Cystic ovarian enlargement resulting from autoimmune oophoritis. Obstet Gynecol. 1989;74:492–5.
152. Lewis J. Eosinophilic perifolliculitis: a variant of autoimmune oophoritis? Int J Gynecol Pathol. 1993;12:360–4.
153. Bannatyne P, Russell P, Shearman RP. Autoimmune oophoritis: a clinicopathologic assessment of 12 cases. Int J Gynecol Pathol. 1990;9:191–207.
154. Michael SD, De Angelo L, Kaikis-Astaras A. Plasma protein and hormone profiles associated with autoimmune oophoritis and ovarian tumorigenesis in neonatally thymectomized mice. Autoimmunity. 1990;6:1–12.
155. Miyake T, Taguchi O, Ikeda H, Sato Y, Takeuchi S, Nishizuka Y. Acute oocyte loss in experimental autoimmune oophoritis as a possible model of premature ovarian failure. Am J Obstet Gynecol. 1988;158:186–92.
156. Sedmak DD, Hart WR, Tubbs RR. Autoimmune oophoritis: a histopathologic study of involved ovaries with immunologic characterization of the mononuclear cell infiltrate. Int J Gynecol Pathol. 1987;6:73–81.
157. Wolfe CDA, Stirling RW. Premature menopause associated with autoimmune oophoritis. Case report. Br J Obstet Gynaecol. 1988;95:630–2.
158. Russell P, Bannatyne P, Shearman RP, Fraser IS, Corbett P. Premature hypergonadotropic ovarian failure: clinicopathological study of 19 cases. Int J Gynecol Path. 1982;1:185–201.
159. Rabinowe SL, Berger MJ, Welch WR, Dluhy RG. Lymphocyte dysfunction in autoimmune oophoritis. Am J Med. 1986;81:347–50.
160. Fox H. The pathology of premature ovarian failure. J Pathol. 1992;167:357–63.
161. Coulam CB. Autoimmune ovarian failure. Semin Reprod Endocrinol. 1983;1:161–7.
162. Gloor E, Hurlimann J. Autoimmune oophoritis. Am J Clin Pathol. 1984;81:105–9.
163. Papadopoulos KI, Hornblad Y, Liljebladh H, Hallengren B. High frequency of endocrine autoimmunity in patients with sarcoidosis. Eur J Endocrinol. 1996;134:331–6.
164. Lonsdale RN, Roberts PF, Trowell JE. Autoimmune oophoritis associated with polycystic ovaries. Histopathology. 1991;19:77–81.
165. Rivier C, Vale W. In the rat, interleukin-1α acts at the level of the brain and the gonads to interfere with gonadotropin and sex steroid secretion. Endocrinology. 1992;124:2105–9.
166. Stevens ML, Plotka ED. Functional lutein cyst in a postmenopausal woman. Obstet Gynecol. 1977;50:27s–9s.
167. Strickler RC, Kelly RW, Askin FB. Postmenopausal ovarian follicle cyst: an unusual cause of estrogen excess. Int J Gynecol Pathol. 1984;3:318–22.
168. Friedman CI, Gurgen-Varol F, Lucas J, Neff J. Persistent progesterone production associated with autoimmune oophoritis. J Reprod Med. 1987;32:293–6.
169. Nelson LM, Anasti JN, Kimzey LM et al. Development of luteinized graafian follicles in patients with karyotypically normal spontaneous premature ovarian failure. J Clin Endocrinol Metab. 1994;79:1470–5.
170. Rebar RW, Connolly HV. Clinical features of young women with hypergonadotropic amenorrhea. Fertil Steril. 1990;53:804–10.
171. Menon V, Edwards RL, Butt WR, Bluck M, Lynch SS. Review of 59 patients with hypergonadotropic amenorrhoea. Br J Obstet Gynaecol. 1984;91:63–6.
172. Barik S, Kushagradhi G. Ovarian biopsy for diagnosis of premature menopause. Br J Obstet Gynaecol. 1994;101:924–5.
173. Somerville JE, Iftikhar M, O'Sullivan JF, Hayes D. Autoimmune oophoritis. An incidental finding. Pathol Res Pract. 1993;189:475–80.
174. Reed D, Brown G, Merrick R, Sever J, Feltz E. A mumps epidemic on St. George, Alaska. J Am Med Assoc. 1967;199:655–9.
175. Grasso E. Parotiti epodemiche pluricomplicate. G Mal Infett Parassit. 1976;26:184–7.

176. Ribaux C, Gloor E. Ovarite necrosante a cytomeglovirus. Schweiz Med Woechschr. 1991; 119:160–3.
177. Familiari U, Larocca LM, Tamburrini E, Antiniori A, Ortona A, Capelli A. Premenopausal cytomegalovirus oophoritis in a patient with AIDS. AIDS. 1991;5:458–9.
178. Williams DJ, Connor P, Ironside JW. Pre-menopausal cytomegalovirus oophoritis. Histopathology. 1990;16:405–7.
179. Pekonen F, Siegberg R, Makinen T, Miettinen A, Yli-Korkala O. Immunological disturbances in patients with premature ovarian failure. Clin Endocrinol. 1986;25:1–6.
180. Miyake T, Sato Y, Takeuchi S. Implications of circulating autoantibodies and peripheral blood lymphocyte subsets for the genesis of premature ovarian failure. J Reprod Immunol. 1987;12:163–71.
181. Ho PC, Tang GWK, Fu KH, Fan MC, Lawton JWM. Immunologic studies in patients with premature ovarian failure. Obstet Gynecol. 1988;71:622–6.
182. Hoek A, van Kasteren Y, De Haan-Meulman M, Hooijkass H, Schoemaker J, Drexhage HA. Analysis of peripheral blood lymphocyte subsets, NK cells, and delayed type hypersensitivity skin test in patients with premature ovarian failure. Am J Reprod Immunol. 1995;33:495–502.
183. Mignot MH, Drexhage HA, Kleingold M, Van de Plassche-Boers EM, Rao BR, Schoemaker J. Premature ovarian failure. II. Considerations of cellular immunity defects. Eur J Obstet Gynecol Reprod Biol. 1989;30:67–72.
184. Todd JA, Acha-Orbea H, Bell JI et al. A molecular basis for MHC class II-associated autoimmunity. Science. 1988;240:1003–9.
185. Hill JA, Welch WR, Faris HMP, Anderson DJ. Induction of class II major histocompatibility complex antigen expression in human granulosa cells by interferon gamma: a potential mechanism contributing to autoimmune ovarian failure. Am J Obstet Gynecol. 1990;162: 534–40.
186. Tidey GF, Nelson LM, Phillips TM, Stillman RJ. Gonadotropins enhance HLA-DR antigen expression in human granulosa cells. Am J Obstet Gynecol. 1992;167:1768–73.
187. Nelson LM, Kimzey LM, Merriam GR, Fleisher TA. Increased peripheral T lymphocyte activation in patients with karyotypically normal spontaneous premature ovarian failure. Fertil Steril. 1991;55:1082–7.
188. Ho PC, Tang GW, Lawton JW. Lymphocyte subsets and serum immunoglobulins in patients with premature ovarian failure before and after oestrogen replacement. Hum Reprod. 1993;8: 714–6.
189. Shapiro AG, Rubin A. Spontaneous pregnancy in association with hypergonadotropic ovarian failure. Fertil Steril. 1977;28:500–1.
190. Shangold MM, Turksoy RN, Bashford RA, Hammond CB. Pregnancy following the 'insensitive ovary syndrome'. Fertil Steril. 1977;28:1179–81.
191. Wright CSW, Jacobs HS. Spontaneous pregnancy in a patient with hypergonadotrophic ovarian failure. Br J Obstet Gynaecol. 1985;153:154–5.
192. Amos WL Jr. Pregnancy in a patient with gonadotropin-resistant ovary syndrome. Am J Obstet Gynaecol. 1985;153:154–5.
193. Ohsawa M, Wu MC, Masahashi T, Asai M, Narita O. Cyclic therapy resulted in pregnancy in premature ovarian failure. Obstet Gynecol. 1985;66:64s–6s.
194. Ledger WL, Thomas EJ, Browning D, Lenton EA, Cooke ID. Suppression of gonadotrophin secretion does not reverse premature ovarian failure. Br J Obstet Gynaecol. 1989;96:196–9.
195. Finer N, Fogelman I, Bottazzo G. Pregnancy in a woman with premature ovarian failure. Postgrad Med J. 1985;61:1079–80.
196. Alper MM, Jolly EE, Garner PR. Pregnancies after premature ovarian failure. Obstet Gynecol. 1986;67:59s–62s.
197. Tang L, Sawers RS. Twin pregnancy in premature ovarian failure after estrogen treatment: a case report. Am J Obstet Gynecol. 1989;161:172–3.
198. Cowchock FS, McCabe JL, Montgomery BB. Pregnancy after corticosteroid administration in premature ovarian failure (polyglandular endocrinopathy syndrome). Am J Obstet Gynecol. 1988;158:118–9.
199. Corenblum B, Rowe T, Taylor PJ. High-dose, short-term glucocorticoids for the treatment of infertility resulting from premature ovarian failure. Fertil Steril. 1993;59:988–91.
200. Gossain VV, Carella MJ, Rovner DR. Pregnancy in a patient with premature ovarian failure. J Med. 1993;24:393–402.

201. Antonelli A, Gambbuzza C, Alberti B et al. Autoimmune polyendocrine syndrome. Treatment with intravenous immunoglobulins. Clin Ter. 1992;141:43–8.
202. Walfish PG, Gottesman IS, Shewchuk AB, Bain J, Hase BS, Farid NR. Association of premature ovarian failure with HLA antigens. Tissue Antigens. 1983;21:168–9.
203. Jaroudi KA, Arora M, Sheth KV, Sieck UV, Willemsen WN. Human leukocyte antigen typing and associated abnormalities in premature ovarian failure. Hum Reprod. 1994;9: 2006–9.
204. Yamane K, Yamamoto K, Yoshikawa Y, Sasazuki T. Effect of the expression of DR alpha E beta NOD molecule on the development of insulitis and diabetes in the non-obese diabetic (NOD) mouse. Clin Exp Immunol. 1996;103:141–8.
205. Rajalingham R, Mehra NK, Jain RC, Myneedu VP, Pande JN. Polymerase chain reaction-based sequence-specific oligonucleotide hybridization analysis of HLA class II antigens in pulmonary tuberculosis: relevance to chemotherapy and disease severity. J Infect Dis. 1996; 173:669–76.
206. Miller JFAP. Immunological function of the thymus. Lancet. 1961;2:748–9.
207. Nishizuka Y, Sakakura T. Thymus and reproduction: sex-linked dygenesia of the gonad after neonatal thymectomy in mice. Science. 1969;166:753–5.
208. Taguchi O, Nishizuka Y. Autoimmune oophoritis in thymectomized mice: T cell requirement in adoptive cell transfer. Clin Exp Immunol. 1980;42:324–31.
209. Sakaguchi S, Takahashi T, Nishizuka Y. Study on cellular events in post-thymectomy autoimmune oophoritis in mice II. J Exp Med. 1982;156:1577–86.
210. Smith H, Chem IM, Kubo R, Tung KSK. Neonatal thymectomy results in a repertoire enriched in T cells deleted in adult thymus. Science. 1989;245:749–52.
211. Bonomo A, Kehn PJ, Shevach EM. Post-thymectomy autoimmune: abnormal T-cell homeostasis. Immunol Today. 1995;16:61–7.
212. Murakami K, Maruyama H, Nishio A et al. Effects of intrathymic injection of organ-specific autoantigens, parietal cells, at the neonatal stage on autoreactive effector and suppressor T cell precursors. Eur J Immunol. 1993;23:809–14.
213. Healy DL, Bacher J, Hodgen GD. Thymic regulation of primate fetal ovarian-adrenal differentiation. Biol Reprod. 1985;32:1127–33.
214. Sacco AG. Immunocontraception: consideration of the zona pellucida as a target antigen. Obstet Gynecol Annu. 1981;10:1–26.
215. Skinner SM, Mills T, Kirchick HJ, Dunbar BS. Immunization with zona pellucida proteins results in abnormal ovarian follicular differentiation and inhibition of gonadotropin-induced steroid secretion. Endocrinology. 1984;115:2418–32.
216. Sacco AG, Subramanian MG, Yurewicz EC, DeMayo FJ, Dukelow WR. Heterimmunization of squirrel monkeys (*Saimeri sciureus*) with a purified zona antigen (PPZA): immune response and biological activity of antiserum. Fertil Steril. 1983;39:350–8.
217. VandeVoort CA, Schwoebel ED, Dunbar BS. Immunization of monkeys with recombinant complimentary deoxyribonucleic acid expressed zona pellucida proteins. Fertil Steril. 1995; 64:838–47.
218. Smith S, Hosid S. Premature ovarian failure associated with autoantibodies to the zona pellucida. Int J Fertil Menopausal Stud. 1994;39:316–9.
219. Nelson LM, Kimzey LM, White BJ, Merriam GR. Gonadotropin suppression for the treatment of karyotypically normal spontaneous premature ovarian failure: a controlled trial [see comments]. Fertil Steril. 1992;57:50–5.
220. Sarto GE. Cytogenetics of fifty patients with primary amenorrhea. Am J Obstet Gynecol. 1974;119:14–23.
221. Cramer DW, Xu H, Harlow BL. Family history as a predictor of early menopause. Fertil Steril. 1995;64:740–5.
222. Mattison DR, Evans MI, Schwimmer WB, White BJ, Jensen B, Schulman JD. Familial premature ovarian failure. Am J Hum Genet. 1984;36:1341–8.
223. Amati P, Gasparini P, Zlotogora J et al. A gene for premature ovarian failure associated with eyelid malformation maps to chromosome 3q22-q23. Am J Hum Genet. 1996;58:1089–92.
224. Panidis D, Rousso D, Vavilis D, Skiadopoulos S, Kalogeropoulos A. Familial blepharophimosis with ovarian dysfunction. Hum Reprod. 1994;9:2034–7.
225. Plouffe L, McDonough PG. Ovarian agensis and dysgensis. In: Adashi EY, Rock JA, Rosenwaks Z, eds. Reproductive Endocrinology, Surgery, and Technology, 1st edn. New York: Lippincott-Raven; 1995:1365–84.

226. Conte FA, Grumbach MM, Ito Y, Fisher CR, Simpson ER. A syndrome of female pseudohermaphrodism, hypergonadotropic hypogonadism, and multicystic ovaries associated with missense mutations in the gene encoding aromatase (P450arom). J Clin Endocrinol Metab. 1994;78:1287–92.
227. Scott RT Jr, Hofmann GE. Prognostic assessment of ovarian reserve. Fertil Steril. 1995;63:1–11.
228. Speroff L, Glass RH, Kase NG. Menopause and postmenopausal hormone therapy. In: Clinical Gynecologic Endocrinology and Infertility, 5th edn. Baltimore: Williams & Wilkins; 1994:583–650.
229. May ME, Carey RM. Rapid adrenocorticotropic hormone test in practice. Am J Med. 1985;79:679–84.
230. Nelson LM, Anasti JN, Flack MR. Premature ovarian failure. In: Adashi EY, Rock JA, Rosenwaks Z, eds. Reproductive Endocrinology, Surgery, and Technology, 1st edn. New York: Raven Press; 1995:1393–410.
231. Daneshdoost L, Gennarelli TA, Bashey HM et al. Recognition of gonadotroph adenomas in women. N Engl J Med. 1991;324:589–94.
232. Blumenfeld Z, Halachmi S, Peretz BA et al. Premature ovarian failure – the prognostic application of autoimmunity on conception after ovulation induction. Fertil Steril. 1993;59: 750–5.
233. Cooper A, Whitehead M. Menopause: refining benefits and risks of hormone replacement therapy. Curr Opin Obstet Gynecol. 1995;7:214–9.
234. Lobo RA. Benefits and risks of estrogen replacement therapy. Am J Obstet Gynecol. 1995; 173:982–9.
235. Effects of estrogen or estrogen/progestin regimens on heart disease risk factors in postmenopausal women. The Postmenopausal Estrogen/Progestin Interventions (PEPI) Trial. The Writing Group for the PEPI Trial. J Am Med Assoc. 1995;273:199–208.
236. Metka M, Holzer G, Heytmanek G, Huber J. Hypergonadotropic hypogonadic amenorrhea (World Health Organization III) and osteoporosis. Fertil Steril. 1992;57:37–41.
237. Anasti JN, Kalantrizdou SN, Kimzey LM, Defensor RA, Nelson LM. Bone loss in young women with karyotypically normal spontaneous premature ovarian failure. Obstet Gynecol. 1998;91:12–16.
238. Thorneycroft IH. Practical aspects of hormone replacement therapy. Prog Cardiovasc Dis. 1995;38:243–54.
239. Fruzzetti F, Ricci C, Fioretti P. Haemostasis profile in smoking and nonsmoking women taking low-dose oral contraceptives. Contraception. 1994;49:579–92.
240. Marty JP. New trends in transdermal technologies: development of the skin patch, Menorest. Int J Gynaecol Obstet. 1996;52:S17–20.
241. Sitruk-Ware R. Percutaneous and transdermal oestrogen replacement therapy. Ann Med. 1993;25:77–82.
242. Mitragotri S, Edwards DA, Blankschtein D, Langer R. A mechanistic study of ultrasonically-enhanced transdermal drug delivery. J Pharm Sci. 1995;84:697–706.
243. Coulam CB, Kempers RD, Randall RV. Premature ovarian failure: evidence for the autoimmune mechanism. Fertil Steril. 1981;36:238–40.
244. Lydic ML, Liu JH, Rebar RW, Thomas MA, Cedars MI. Success of donor oocyte in in vitro fertilization-embryo transfer in recipients with and without premature ovarian failure. Fertil Steril. 1996;65:98–102.
245. Dean NL, Edwards RG. Oocyte donation – implications for fertility treatment in the nineties. Curr Opin Obstet Gynecol. 1994;6:160–5.
246. Cui KH. Genome project and human reproduction. Hum Reprod. 1995;10:1275–9.
247. Mosmann T, Coffman R. Th1 and Th2 cells: different patterns of lymphokine secretion leads different functional properties. Ann Rev Immunol. 1989;7:145–73.
248. Rizzo LV, Caspi RR. Immunotolerance and prevention of ocular autoimmune disease. Curr Eye Res. 1995;14:857–64.
249. De Carli M, D'Elios MM, Zancuoghi G, Romagnani S, Del Prete G. Human Th1 and Th2 cells: functional properties, regulation of development and role in autoimmunity. Autoimmunity. 1994;18:301–8.
250. Maity R, Caspi RR, Nair S et al. Murine post-thymectomy autoimmune oophoritis is associated with a persistent neonatal-like TH2 response. Clin Immunol Immunopathol. 1997;83:230–6.

251. Baixeras E, Bosca L, Stauber C et al. From apoptosis to autoimmunity: insights from the signaling pathways leading to proliferation or to programmed cell death. Immunol Rev. 1994;142:53–91.
252. Yang NN, Bryant HU, Hardikar S et al. Estrogen and raloxifene stimulate transforming growth factor-beta 3 gene expression in rat bone: a potential mechanism for estrogen- or raloxifene-mediated bone maintenance. Endocrinology. 1996;137:2075–84.
253. Fuchs-Young R, Glasebrook AL, Short LL et al. Raloxifene is a tissue-selective agonist/antagonist that functions through the estrogen receptor. Ann NY Acad Sci. 1995;761:355–60.

[illegible]

[illegible]

[illegible]

11
Pituitary autoimmunity

H. A. SAWERS and J. S. BEVAN

INTRODUCTION

Lymphocytic hypophysitis is one of a number of different disorders affecting the pituitary gland to which has been ascribed a possible autoimmune pathogenesis. The condition was first recognized in an autopsy specimen by Goudie and Pinkerton in 1962 [1]. It soon became considered to be an autoimmune disorder, partly on account of its frequent association with other classical autoimmune disorders associated with organ specific antibodies [2], particularly thyroiditis. With over 80 cases now described it is clear that the inflammatory process is typically confined to the adenohypophysitis, more accurately termed lymphocytic adenohypophysitis, and the condition occurs mostly, but not exclusively, in the peripartum period.

When lymphocytic hypophysitis occurs outside the peripartum period or in men it may present a different clinical spectrum. The lymphocytic infiltrate appears not to respect the boundaries of the adenohypophysitis, so that there is more likely to be cavernous sinus involvement, possibly resulting in involvement of lower cranial nerves supplying the extraocular muscles, or infundibuloneurohypophyseal involvement causing diabetes insipidus. Some authors suggest that granulomatous hypophysitis is one end of the spectrum of the same process but others see it as a distinct clinicopathological entity [3]. A more recently described infundibulo-neurohypophysitis may account for some cases of idiopathic cranial diabetes insipidus and this too is possibly a distinct clinical entity, not affecting the adenohypophysitis [4]. Finally, some cases of empty sella, when it develops in adulthood, may have an autoimmune origin.

A.P Weetman (ed.), Endocrine Autoimmunity and Associated Conditions. 223–241

LYMPHOCYTIC HYPOPHYSITIS

In 1962 Goudie and Pinkerton described the autopsy findings in a 22-year-old woman who died following appendicectomy performed 14 months postpartum [1]. As well as lymphocytic thyroiditis and severely atrophic adrenals, the pituitary gland was atrophic with an extensive lymphocytic infiltrate. This case was followed by sporadic autopsy reports of lymphocytic hypophysitis [5], until Quencer's report of a live patient with biopsy proven lymphocytic hypophysitis in 1980 led to renewed interest in the condition [6].

Over the last 15 years there have been over 80 probable cases reported in the literature and it is evident that the condition is much more prevalent than previously recognized. Although a number of the early autopsy cases had been in post-menopausal women it became rapidly clear that this was primarily a condition arising peripartum, presenting particularly in the third trimester or within the first 6 months of delivery. It was not until 1987 that the first case was recognized in a man [7] and now approximately 14% of the cases described are in men. This figure probably reflects current reporting bias and is not a useful indicator of the relative prevalence in men, which is almost certainly smaller than this.

Doubtless many earlier cases of postpartum hypopituitarism, attributed to Sheehan's syndrome despite unconvincing evidence of a hypotensive episode at delivery, may well have been unrecognized cases of lymphocytic adenohypophysitis. Other cases may have been misdiagnosed as having a pituitary adenoma. It is now appreciated that there is wide spectrum of pituitary enlargement seen in this condition, those patients having no pituitary mass not normally being subjected to pituitary biopsy. Furthermore, amongst clinicians aware of the disorder, expectations regarding spontaneous resolution are now such that pituitary biopsy is not necessarily performed even if there is a substantial pituitary mass, so that increasingly the diagnosis may not be biopsy proven [2]. Even when biopsy is performed there may be difficulties in interpreting its significance since lymphocytic changes may be patchy and associated with other pathologies which are not revealed within the surgical specimen [8]. All these factors make it difficult to assess accurately the true incidence of this rare condition.

Bevan *et al.* [9] looking specifically at a group of 148 postpartum women who had antibodies to thyroid peroxidase, found 73 to have biochemical evidence of postpartum thyroiditis but only one developed mild secondary hypothyroidism which was then found to be associated with adrenocorticotrophic hormone (ACTH) deficiency and presumed to be due to autoimmune hypophysitis. It should be emphasized that pituitary function was not assessed in these patients other than with respect to TSH measurement, but certainly in one patient this proved to be an adequate marker of probable autoimmune hypophysitis. This would indicate that the incidence of postpartum hypophysitis is likely to be well below 1%.

CLINICAL PRESENTATION

Peripartum patients

The clinical presentation and clinical course appears to be rather different in peripartum individuals from others and indeed this may possibly be a distinct clinical entity, similar to postpartum thyroiditis. It therefore seems appropriate to describe these patients separately. Although representing approximately 70% of the total number of reported cases, they probably account for a rather larger majority of cases overall because of current reporting bias.

The spectrum of clinical presentation is wide, ranging from death in labour [10], probably due to hypoadrenalism, to almost symptomless glucocorticoid deficiency detected during a research study [9]. More than half the patients present with mass effects, particularly headache and visual field defects, but also reduced visual acuity and diplopia. This is the almost invariable mode of presentation during pregnancy itself which is not surprising since the pituitary gland is already substantially enlarged in normal pregnancy [11,12]. Symptoms such as nausea, anorexia, dizziness and, particularly in the postpartum patient, failed lactation and amenorrhoea indicate adenohypophyseal hypofunction and occur in approximately 65% of patients. Many fewer experience persistent galactorrhoea after lactation as a symptom of hyperprolactinaemia and a similar number experience symptoms attributable to hypothyroidism.

Diabetes insipidus occurs rarely, if ever, in this peripartum group of patients, although Nishioka *et al.* [13] reported a case in a 33-year-old 2 months postpartum in which histology revealed massive fibrosis as well as lymphocytic hypophysitis.

Men and non-peripartum women

A frequent presentation in a man is with reduced libido or impotence [7,14–19]. Headaches are less frequently reported although patients have presented with extraocular muscle palsy due to cavernous sinus involvement [15,16]. Symptoms of anterior pituitary deficiency may be overshadowed by clinical features of diabetes insipidus [19,20]. In non-peripartum women the most common anterior pituitary symptom is amenorrhoea, with occasional patients experiencing diabetes insipidus [21].

Very occasionally in these non-peripartum cases an episode of lymphocytic meningitis has been described. At least in Paja's case it seemed clearly to postdate the development of symptoms of pituitary dysfunction, making it unlikely that the aetiological factor in the lymphocytic hypophysitis was a putative viral agent, and more likely that the meningeal irritation was related to spread of an established inflammatory infiltrate [21].

Patients in either of the above groups may also have symptoms related to associated autoimmune disease, particularly autoimmune hypothyroidism and, in peripartum patients, postpartum thyroiditis. There are also a few reports of co-existing adrenalitis, pernicious anaemia and insulin-dependent diabetes mellitus, with small numbers of patients showing serum positivity for non-organ specific antibodies (to smooth muscle, nuclear antigens or mitochondria) [2,5].

INVESTIGATIONS

Blood tests

Routine biochemical testing may reveal hyponatraemia or hypoglycaemia due to hypoadrenalism, or hypercalcaemia reflecting either transient hyperthyroidism or hypoadrenalism. Routine haematology may demonstrate anaemia, which is likely to be due in part to hypocortisolism or hypothyroidism. There are occasional reports of an increase in the CD4/CD8 ratio amongst peripheral blood T lymphocytes [21].

Anterior pituitary hormone secretion is variably affected with isolated ACTH deficiency being the most common single abnormality. Random cortisol may be clearly subnormal; four of the five peripartum cases described by Patel *et al.* had random cortisol <50 nmol/L, but otherwise the abnormality is revealed by a subnormal cortisol response to tetracosactrin (Synacthen) and a low ACTH concentration, which is minimally or not responsive to corticotrophin releasing hormone (CRH). There is frequently secondary hypothyroidism, which may rarely occur as an isolated deficiency, but more characteristically occurs in association with ACTH deficiency. Prolactin secretion is rarely normal [5]. It may be subnormal or, in 50% of cases, elevated for a variety of reasons, including lactotroph hyperplasia of pregnancy and the puerperium, interruption of flow of hypothalamic dopamine by mass effects on the pituitary stalk, decreased dopaminergic activity secondary to hypothyroidism, or, more speculatively, an effect of the inflammatory process on the lactotrophs [14,22].

Recent work confirms that growth hormone (GH) secretion is likely to be subnormal in response to the stimulus of insulin-induced hypoglycaemia, but this is possibly difficult to interpret if there is pre-existing sex hormone deficiency [2]. A review by Hughes [23] of random GH levels in 18 patients with lymphocytic hypophysitis revealed that eight patients had undetectable levels but five had a random value in excess of 10 mU/L (5 μg/L) and they described a case with a similarly raised random GH level, a marginally elevated IGF1, but no clinical features of acromegaly. In this particular patient an oral glucose tolerance test was performed and showed non-suppressibility of GH. Gonadotrophin secretion is likely to be the best preserved of the anterior pituitary hormones, but if hyperprolactinaemia is present there may be secondary gonadotrophin suppression.

The extent of any anterior pituitary endocrine defect is highly variable ranging from normal function to panhypopopituitarism. Cosman's review of 30 probable cases is likely to be representative [5], showing a pattern of preferential impairment of ACTH and TSH secretion which seems to be characteristic of lymphocytic hypophysitis. There was normal pituitary function in 10%, panhypopopituitarism in 30%, hypoadrenalism with hypothyroidism in

27%, isolated hypoadrenalism in 10%, hypoadrenalism with hypogonadism in 7% and a variety of disorders not involving ACTH in the remaining 16% of cases. The extent of hormonal secretory loss seen with what is often a modest mass lesion is in marked contrast to the situation seen with pituitary tumours where loss of gonadotrophins and GH typically occurs first, this compressive loss occurring only when the size of the tumour is substantial.

Pituitary imaging

Although the spectrum is wide, most cases of lymphocytic hypophysitis show a sellar mass often with suprasellar extension. At its extreme the pituitary enlargement is significant, even with demineralization of the sella [2] and suprasellar extension may result in compression of the optic chiasm. Neuroimaging is often unable to differentiate lymphocytic hypophysitis from a pituitary adenoma preoperatively; in the pregnant patient further confusion may be caused by physiological pituitary hyperplasia of pregnancy. In lymphocytic hypophysitis it is recognized that computerized tomography (CT) scan appearances may be normal when pituitary magnetic resonance imaging (MRI) shows an abnormality [24].

Contrast enhanced MRI is now the pituitary imaging modality of choice and using this technique various workers have attempted to define imaging characteristics allowing a more confident diagnosis of lymphocytic hypophysitis. Many of the earlier reported cases have been subjected to much less sophisticated imaging so experience with this newer technique is limited. While not pathognomonic, an intensely uniformly enhancing pituitary mass associated with adjacent strips of enhancing dura mater is very suggestive of lymphocytic hypophysitis [25] (see Figure 11.1). In many cases there is suprasellar extension, but much more unusual is cavernous sinus extension and if there is any degree of diabetes insipidus there will be detectable thickening of the pituitary stalk as well as loss of the normal hyperintense signal from the neurohypophysis. When a pituitary adenoma is complicated by haemorrhage, necrosis or infarction there may be extensive inflammatory infiltration resulting in pituitary MRI features very similar to those of hypophysitis [25].

TREATMENT/COURSE

It seems likely that many mild self-limiting cases of lymphocytic hypophysitis are undiagnosed, although at the other extreme the condition is potentially life-threatening, particularly because of its propensity to interfere preferentially with control of adrenal function. Furthermore, where there is a substantial mass effect a real risk of visual loss exists which is most likely to be a presenting feature during pregnancy itself.

Although peripartum lymphocytic adenohypophysitis was typically thought to present within the first 4 months of delivery, with an extreme of 14 months [5], there are recent reports which reveal that the condition may run an indolent

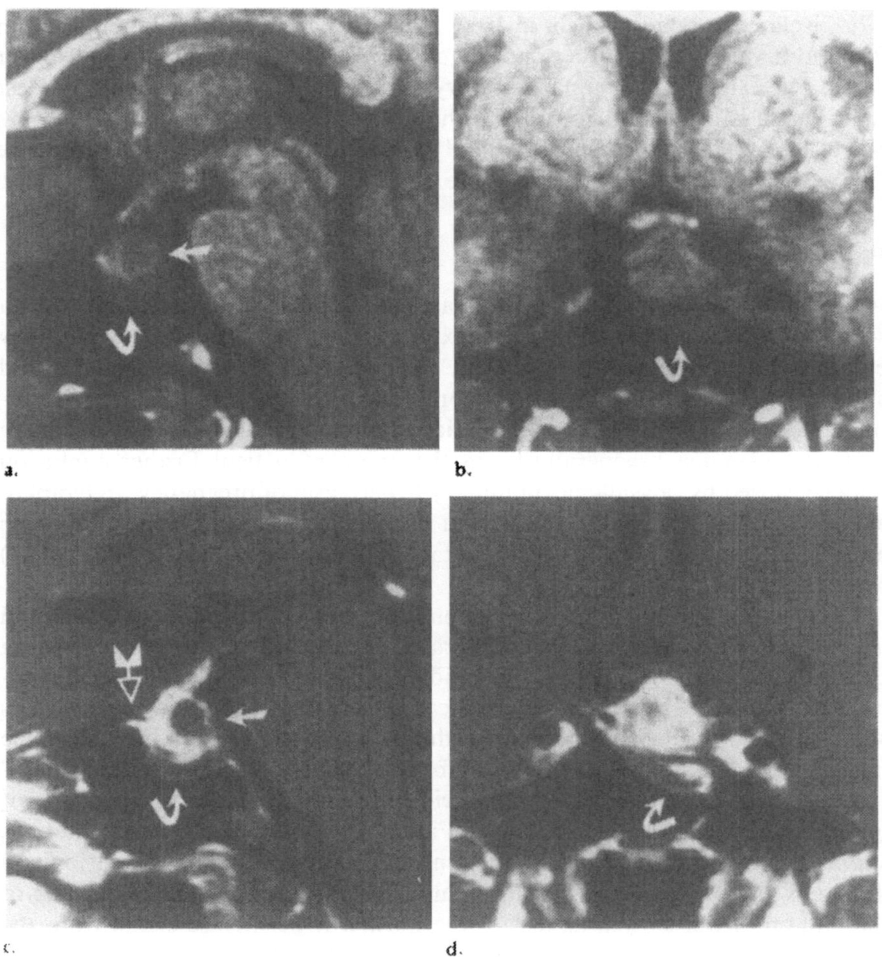

Figure 11.1 Lymphocytic hypophysitis in a 29-year-old woman with headaches, amenorrhoea and galactorrhoea. (a) Sagittal (400/18) and (b) coronal (400/18) pre-contrast T1-weighted magnetic resonance images demonstrate a pituitary masss abutting the optic chiasm with an immediately contiguous sphenoid sinus submucosal component (curved arrow). The mass is slightly hyperintense relative to grey matter. (c) Sagittal (500/16) and (d) coronal (500/16) post-contrast T1-weighted magnetic resonance images demonstrate intense but heterogeneous enhancement of the anterior pituitary gland extending along the infundibulum. There are enhancing strips of adjacent dura mater (open arrow in c). Focal area of non-enhancing tissue corresponds to the posterior pituitary lobe on both pre- and post-contrast sagittal images (straight arrow in a and c). Note enhancment of the extra-pituitary component of the lesion extending into the adjacent sphenoid sinus (curved arrow) without evidence of disruption of the sellar floor. [Figure reproduced with permission of the Radiological Society of North America]

course. For example, Jenkins reported a 23-year-old who developed severe frontal headache late in the third trimester of pregnancy [8]. Post-delivery CT scan showed a sellar mass with suprasellar extension. There was no endocrine deficit and transsphenoidal hypophysectomy was recommended, but the patient declined and was lost to follow up. Five years later she represented with symptoms of hypoadrenalism and hypothyroidism; repeat CT scan showed no change in the sellar mass which histologically proved to be due to lymphocytic hypophysitis. A similar patient is described by Naik [26], with a latent period of 8 years between first peripartum symptoms of a mass lesion and subsequent presentation with symptoms of adenohypophyseal deficiency. The final outcome and first presentation may be decades after pregnancy, with hypopituitarism and an empty sella, as discussed below. There are some reports of pregnant patients in whom improvement in a visual field defect was temporally associated with the use of bromocriptine to treat hyperprolactinaemia [27,28]. This was presumably achieved by reducing the physiological lactotroph hyperplasia of pregnancy. A further patient reported by Pestell received high dose steroids (to induce fetal lung maturity) as well as bromocriptine. Her visual field defect initially showed improvement before deteriorating, but in all these cases the dynamic changes in the pituitary due to pregnancy itself were superimposed on other factors [14]. In another patient [29] who first had symptoms 13 months postpartum, prednisolone in a dose of 60 mg/day for 3 months, progressively reduced over the subsequent 6 months, produced a gradual improvement in panhypopopituitarism as well as a reduction of two-thirds in the pituitary mass. Five months after discontinuing steroids the patient relapsed with an increase in the pituitary mass and panhypopopituitarism.

Many patients had shown spontaneous endocrine and radiological improvement without any immunosuppressive treatment [2,30,31], including one patient with total panhypopituitarism who recovered complete function after one year [32]. The patient described by Hughes presented 18 months postpartum with hypoadrenalism, hypothyroidism, hypogonadism, but hyperprolactinaemia and GH excess, and was submitted to transsphenoidal surgery which provided diagnostic pathological material. Within 6 months of surgery pituitary function was fully restored and has remained normal over 2 years of subsequent follow up [23]. Descriptions of spontaneous recovery are not confined to peripartum cases: Ozawa *et al.* reported a 50-year-old woman in whom panhypopituitarism and a sellar mass resolved spontaneously over an 18 month period [33]. Bevan's case of isolated ACTH deficiency developing and recovering spontaneously within 14 months of delivery, without hormone deficiency or sellar mass symptoms becoming evident [9] (see Figure 11.2) illustrates that not all patients will present for clinical diagnosis, her case only coming to light as she was participating in a monthly follow up programme as part of a study of postpartum thyroiditis. There may be many other such mild self-limiting cases.

This recent appreciation of the potential benign natural history of the condition, combined with the high quality neuroimaging which is now available for monitoring mass lesions, means that in most cases a conservative policy of

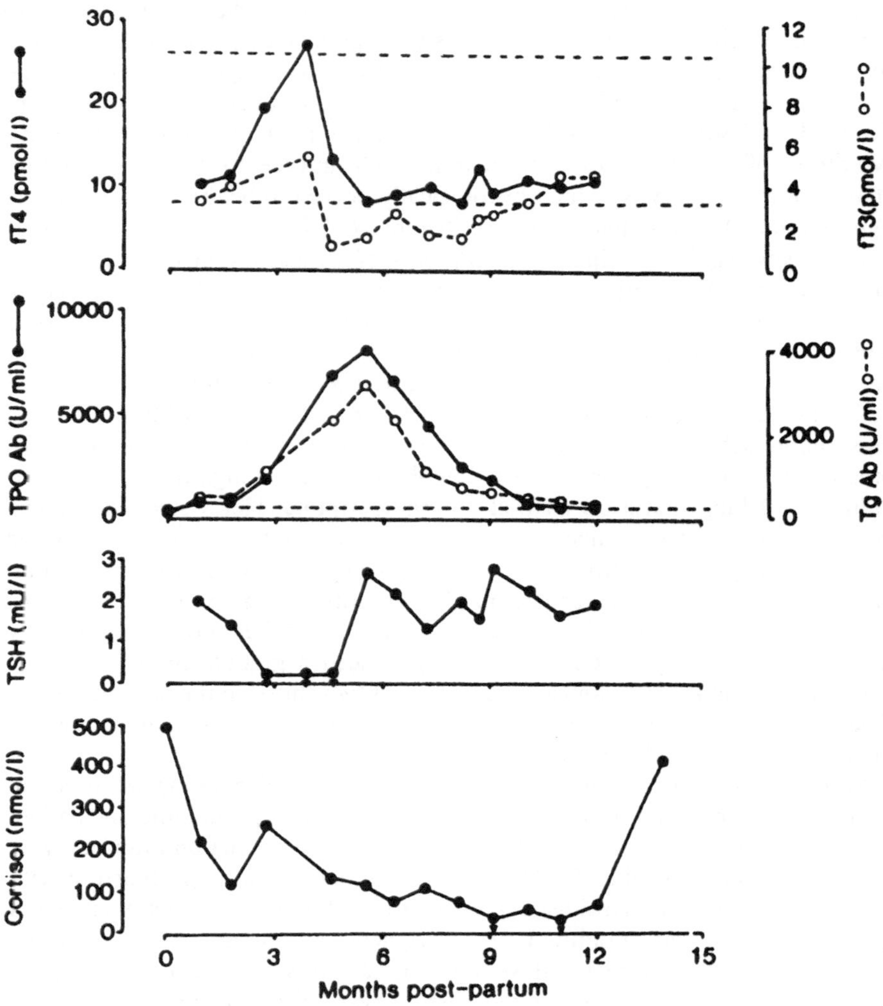

Figure 11.2 Free T_4 free T_3, thyroid peroxidase and thyroglobulin autoantibodies, TSH and mid-afternoon cortisol levels in a 34-year-old woman with postpartum thyroiditis and probable autoimmune hypophysitis [9]. Four months postpartum she developed mild hyperthyroidism and showed a rise in thyroid autoantibody titres. At nine months, the biochemistry suggested secondary hypothyroidism and serum cortisol was only 28 nmol/L. Retrospective analysis of stored samples showed developing hypocortisolism between 3 and 9 months postpartum. CT was normal and pituitary biopsy was not performed. The cortisol response to insulin-induced hypoglycaemia was subnormal at 9 months (peak cortisol 145 nmol/L), but had recovered at 18 months postpartum (590 nmol/L). Pituitary antibodies were undetectable throughout and she received no endocrine replacement therapy. [Figure reproduced with permission of the Endocrine Society.]

management can be pursued. There is definitely a role for transsphenoidal surgery where there is a need to decompress in the case of visual failure, particularly if a brief course of high dose steroids is not rapidly effective in improving vision. Whether surgery also has a role in providing biopsy material is more debatable. This latter objective is fraught with difficulty since there is considerable evidence that changes within the pituitary may be patchy, and that a lymphocytic infiltrate is a frequent concomitant of other pathologies [34], so that the only truly accurate biopsy involves total removal of the pituitary mass [8]. This will frequently amount to total hypophysectomy which means sacrificing potential recovery of pituitary function.

PATHOLOGY

The gross appearance of the pituitary may range in size from atrophic to enlarged, and it frequently has an unusually firm, tough consistency. Light microscopy shows lymphocyte and plasma cell infiltrate in the anterior pituitary which occasionally forms lymphoid follicles and may be accompanied by neutrophils, eosinophils and macrophages [35] (see Figure 11.3). Not only is the severity of the adenohypophyseal destruction variable but also it can be quite patchy with islands and groups of preserved adenohypophyseal cells surrounded by inflammatory infiltrate or fibrous tissue [20]. There is a variable amount of oedema and fibrosis. Granulomas and giant cells are not typical features and suggest an alternative pathology. A necrotizing infundibulohypophysitis has also been described recently by Ahmed *et al.* [36] who felt this was a distinct clinicopathological entity, partly because they were unaware of diabetes insipidus being described within the clinical spectrum of lymphocytic hypophysitis. The presentation was in fact not dissimilar from that seen in the above non-peripartum cases, with MRI evidence of a sellar mass lesion and an abnormally thickened pituitary stalk. Histologically all the above features were evident but there was also extensive necrosis. It is presently unclear whether such cases represent an extreme end of the spectrum of lymphocytic hypophysitis or constitute a separate entity.

Cases have been described [8,34,37] in which otherwise typical lymphocytic hypophysitis has occurred in association with a pituitary tumour. It is now becoming well recognized that a 'secondary hypophysitis' may be a histological accompaniment to a well-defined pathological process in the sellar region, typically a craniopharyngioma or a pituitary adenoma [34]. Pituitary adenomas, particularly prolactinomas and corticotroph adenomas, can secrete IL-6 which may act with other cytokines to produce a local lymphocyte infiltrate and complement activation [38]. It is unclear whether a secondary hypophysitis may nevertheless have similar clinicopathological consequences with respect to loss of hormone production from the pituitary cells.

Thodou reported pituitary immunoreactivity studies in 11 of 16 patients, with the amount of tissue restricting examination to GH and/or prolactin in three of these [20]. The commonest abnormality was a lack of ACTH staining (five out

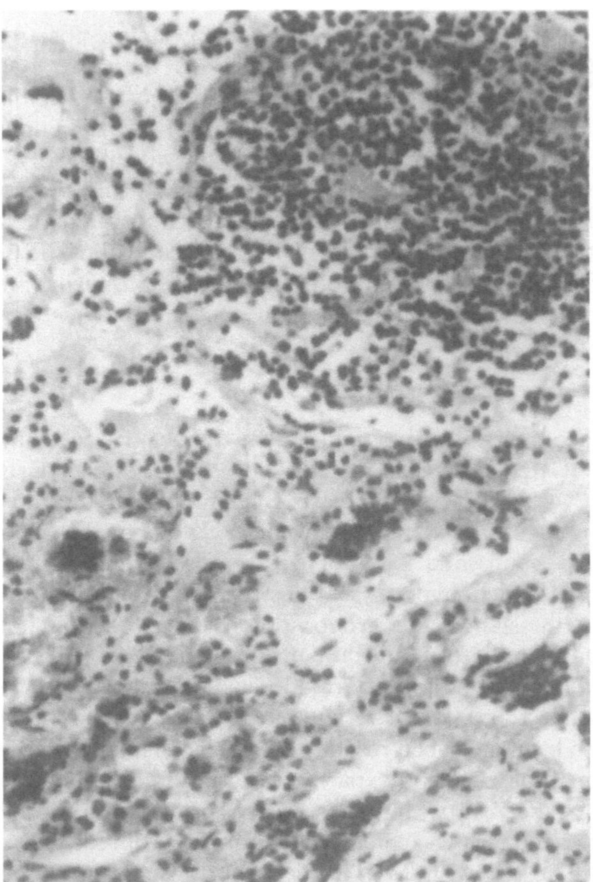

Figure 11.3 Typical light microscopic appearances of autoimmune hypophysitis showing lymphocytic infiltration of anterior pituitary tissue [clinical details reported in Reference 35]. The patient was a 61-year-old woman who presented with headaches and symptoms of hypothyrodism. Total T_4 was reduced at 20 nmol/L but TSH only minimally raised at 9 mU/L; thyroid peroxidase autoantibodies were positive. Detailed pituitary function testing revealed TSH, ACTH, GH and (mild) vasopressin deficiency and prolactin was slightly raised at 690 mU/L. CT demonstrated a pituitary mass with a small suprasellar extension and transsphenoidal biopsy of the tough mass revealed the diagnosis. She remains well on hydrocortisone and thyroxine replacement therapy

of eight tested), not invariably accompanied by documented adrenal insufficiency. There was no immunostaining for β-TSH, β-FSH, β-LH and/or α-subunit in two of the patients but, in the absence of reduced circulating levels of these hormones, this is probably an illustration of the difficulty in obtaining representative samples. All but one case showed immunoreactivity for GH and prolactin. The inflammatory cells were a polyclonal population of T and B cells as indicated by immunohistochemistry. In a few cases, including the non-pregnant woman with diabetes insipidus and autoimmune thyroiditis described by Paja, a predominance of CD4 cells among the infiltrating lymphocytes has been demonstrated [21].

In the case described by Hughes evidence of GH excess was found without clinical features of acromegaly, the patient also having hyperprolactinaemia [23]. At the time of presentation she was 18 months postpartum and had already developed hypoadrenalism, hypothyroidism and hypogonadism as well as a sellar mass. The biopsy material showed typical features of lymphocytic hypophysitis as described above and pituitary cell immunoreactivity for GH, ACTH, prolactin, β-TSH, β-FSH, β-LH and α-subunit. Interestingly there was also prominent extracellular immunostaining for GH and prolactin, tempting speculation that somatotroph and lactotroph cell lysis due to lymphocytic destruction might be resulting in supraphysiological levels of these hormones (analogous to transient hyperthyroidism during postpartum thyroiditis (see Figure 11.2)). Prominent extracellular staining for any of the above hormones has not been commented on in other cases of lymphocytic hypophysitis.

Electron microscopy reveals an inflammatory cell infiltrate, sometimes completely destroying adenohypophyseal architecture, consisting of plasma cells, lymphocytes, macrophages and occasional eosinophils and neutrophils. Activated lymphocytes can be seen interdigitating with pituitary cells in varying stages of cell injury and death.

IMMUNOLOGY

Lymphocytic hypophysitis is considered to be an autoimmune disease, possibly involving a contribution from both humoral and cellular arms of the immune system. There are technical difficulties concerning the detection of tissue antibodies directed against components of the pituitary gland so that humoral immunity cannot be easily assessed, even supposing it has a pathogenetic role alongside the cell-mediated immune process.

Pituitary antibodies

Methods for detecting pituitary antibodies remain controversial. Such antibodies have been sought by immunofluorescence using a variety of substrates. Normal human pituitary causes non-specific binding of immunoglobulins to Fc receptors on corticotrophs [39] but fetal pituitary is devoid of Fc receptors and should therefore provide a more specific substrate [40]. Other substrates have been used, including rat, mouse, monkey and baboon pituitaries, the problems with these being the presence of heterophilic pituitary antibodies in animal sera giving false positive results and the low species cross-reactivity of pituitary autoantibodies. Use of an immunoblotting technique is now being evaluated, but the success of this lies in identifying the appropriate autoantigen, which presently remains elusive [41,42].

Pituitary antibodies have been detected in normal postpartum women, 18% showing a transitory rise at day 5–7 postpartum [43], and also in patients with autoimmune polyglandular endrocrinopathy. Cell surface antibodies reacting with both intact GH prolactin-secreting rat GH_3 and ACTH-secreting mouse AtT-20 cells were detected in 44% of patients with the empty sella syndrome [44]. Furthermore families of patients with hypopituitarism of various aetiologies have been shown to have antibodies to both rat pituitary cytoplasm and cell surface antigens [45].

Investigators have found variable results in patients with hypophysitis, with only a minority of reports (three out of 16) detecting pituitary antibodies, although Mayfield reported a case with antibodies against all anterior pituitary cell types [46]. Few of these patients have been assessed for antibody status at more than one time point. However one recent report [33] documented antibody level in a 50-year-old patient with a clinical course evolving over an eighteen month period from panhypopituitarism associated with a sellar mass to spontaneous full recovery with resolution of the mass. Antibodies against rat pituitary cytosol were positive throughout the period of hypopituitarism, becoming negative with recovery of pituitary function. However antibodies reacting with intact GH_3 and AtT-20 cells were positive and remained so even when pituitary function had normalized. This patient had thyroiditis, as did the woman reported by Bevan in whom pituitary antibodies were not detected (using a fetal pituitary-based assay) during sequential monitoring covering the development of hypocortisolaemia immediately postpartum through its evolution over 14 months to subsequent spontaneous recovery [9].

In an animal study by Yoon, passive transfer of pituitary antibodies failed to induce lymphocytic hypophysitis [47]. In the same study, hamsters which developed inflammatory lesions of lymphocytic hypophysitis (as a specific response to injection with glycosylated membrane-associated E1 and E2 rubella virus proteins) did not develop pituitary antibodies. The implication is that the presence of these antibodies is an epiphenomenon rather than indicating any direct involvement in target cell destruction, but the methodological problems referred to above must also be borne in mind. The usefulness of detecting circulating pituitary antibodies as a means of clarifying the diagnosis therefore still remains unproven, as is their role in pathogenesis.

Immunogenetics

Few patients with lymphocytic hypophysitis have undergone HLA typing and there have been no consistently associated class I or II specificities [2,5,7,27,46]. However three cases have been described with a shared class III-encoded complement allotype [9,14]. An attempt to identify HLA class II antigens on pituitary cells taken from biopsy of patients with lymphocytic hypophysitis was unsuccessful [48].

Associated conditions

The high prevalence of postpartum thyroiditis (Chapter 5), occurring in 4–7% of patients postpartum [49], inevitably results in it being relatively frequently associated with lymphocytic adenohypophysitis. There is also an association with autoimmune disorders associated with either organ-specific antibodies, such as Hashimoto's hypothyroidism or adrenalitis (Chapter 9), or with non-organ specific antibodies (see above).

PATHOGENESIS

Various factors add to the impression that lymphocytic hypophysitis is an autoimmune disorder, not least its frequent association with other autoimmune disorders, notably thyroiditis. It has a propensity to affect individuals peri-partum, a time of intense immunological change. The accompanying pituitary antibodies that may be detected and the increment in CD4/CD8 ratio in peripheral blood as well as predominance of the CD4 subpopulation in lymphocytic infiltrate [21] all reinforce the idea that autoimmunity is implicated.

Several experimental animal models of lymphocytic hypophysitis have been produced. Levine produced lymphocytic hypophysitis by injecting human pituitary tissue with Freund's adjuvant into rat footpads, the pituitary reaction being more florid in pregnant or lactating rats [50]. Klein *et al.* injected homologous pituitary tissue plus adjuvant into rabbits, producing adenohypophyseal inflammation in the majority [51]. They did not detect significant circulating pituitary antibody levels but showed evidence of pituitary lymphocytes being activated by pituitary extract. Cellular immunity therefore appears to play a role in experimentally induced autoimmune pituitary disease.

In more recent animal studies Yoon *et al.* were able to induce lymphocytic hypophysitis, in hamsters by giving multiple injections of glycosylated membrane-associated E1 and E2 rubella virus proteins. Neonatal thymectomy prevented this, indicating that the disease induction was due to an antigen-specific T cell mediated autoimmune mechanism [47].

IDIOPATHIC HYPOPITUITARISM IN ADULTS

There are anecdotal reports of possible autoimmune atrophy of the pituitary. Amongst these is the description by Nishiyama *et al.* of a case of hypopituitarism presenting in a 50-year-old woman with a history of postpartum failure of lactation 24 years previously (following a normal pregnancy), subsequent amenorrhoea and then symptoms of hypoadrenalism [52]. She had panhypopituitarism and positive pituitary antibodies. Neuroimaging revealed an empty sella. Patel *et al.* [2] quote the documentation by Brandes *et al.* of a woman who developed a sellar mass and partial hypopituitarism after her second pregnancy. By the time of her third pregnancy neuroimaging revealed an empty sella.

In patients with the primary empty sella syndrome, Komatsu *et al.* found antibodies to both AtT-20 and GH_3 cells in 44%, with antibodies to the former alone in 75% [44]. This was a considerably higher incidence than that in patients with other pituitary disorder such as adenomas of various types. By contrast, studies of patients with idiopathic hypopituitarism using the immunoblotting technique, taking the hormonal products of the pituitary cells as antigen, have so far been disappointing [53]. By analogy with other endocrinopathies the autoantigen in the case of the pituitary might also be an intracellular enzyme, perhaps specific to the corticotroph, such as a pro-opiomelanocortin processing enzyme.

INFUNDIBULONEUROHYPOPHYSITIS AND DIABETES INSIPIDUS

Central diabetes insipidus is most often caused by surgical trauma to the pituitary stalk, craniopharyngiomas, very large pituitary tumours or, more rarely arises secondary to head injury, granulomatous disease or infections. There are very rare autosomal dominant familial forms described but a third of cases remain idiopathic. A proportion of such cases of diabetes insipidus were shown to have circulating antibodies to the magnocellular neurons which synthesize vasopressin [54] and this has led to the suspicion that some cases of idiopathic cranial diabetes might represent an autoimmune disorder.

A recent study by Imura *et al.* assessed pituitary MRI appearances of 17 patients with established cranial diabetes insipidus without an identified underlying cause [4]. All patients lacked the hyperintense signal normally generated by the neurohypophysis and half of the patients also showed a thickened pituitary stalk and/or neurohypophysis on MRI (Figure 11.4). Biopsy of two such patients revealed inflammatory infiltrate composed mainly of lymphocytes and plasma cells, with scattered eosinophils, neutrophils and histiocytes. Specific staining techniques suggested the lymphocytes were mostly T cells and strenuous efforts were made to exclude granulomatous conditions including Wegener's granulomatosis, histiocytosis and so on. These authors considered this lymphocytic infundibuloneurohypophysitis to be a separate entity from lymphocytic adenohypophysitis, and, although they did demonstrate normal anterior pituitary function (with the exception of occasional borderline growth hormone deficiency) in their group of patients, they did not report any adenohypophyseal histology.

Furthermore they suggested that those patients in whom MRI scan did not show a thickened stalk were at a later stage in the evolution of the same

Figure 11.4 (opposite) High resolution (a) sagittal and (b) coronal gadolinium-enhanced, T_1-weighted magnetic resonance images (MRI) from a 42-year-old man who presented with cranial diabetes insipidus (unpublished case). The pituitary stalk is greatly thickened (arrows) but the anterior pituitary is of normal shape and size. A pituitary biopsy has not been performed and the MRI appearances have remained unchanged during four years observation. The radiology is identical to that reported in biopsy proven cases [4]. This patient also has GH and gonadotrophin deficiency, together with low titres of antinuclear, DNA and Ro autoantibodies

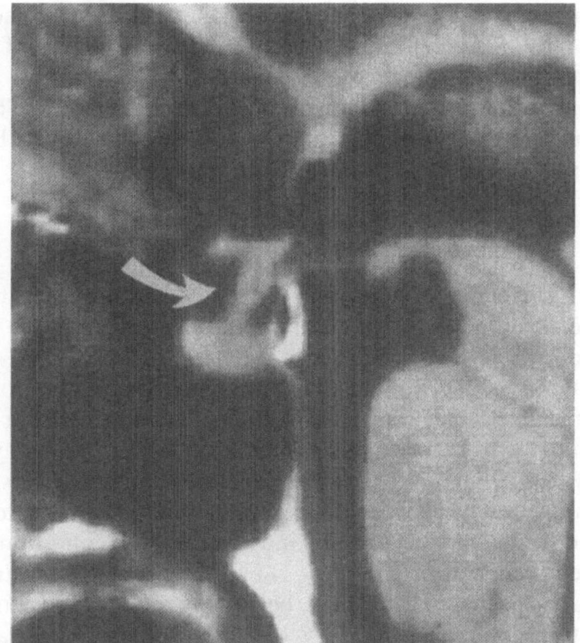

a

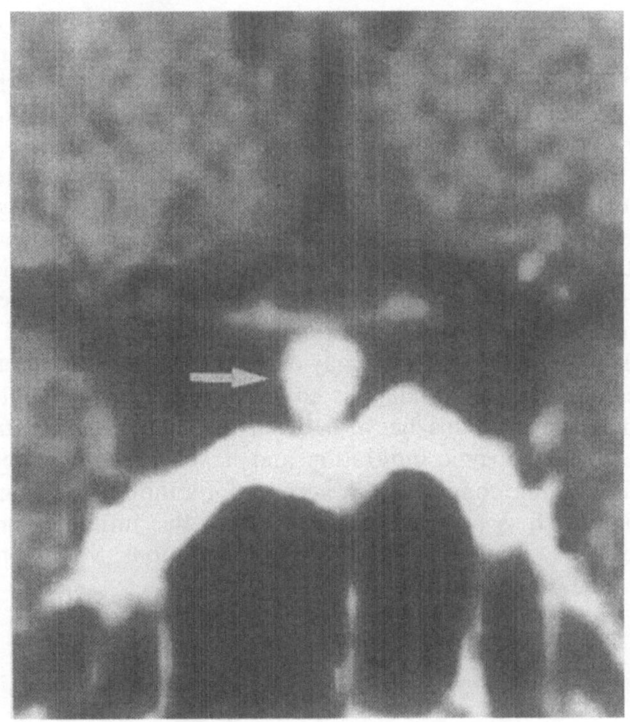

b

inflammatory process where swelling had now subsided and the histology would be expected to show more fibrosis. Within Thodou's review of 16 cases of lymphocytic hypophysitis one patient with hyperprolactinaemia and diabetes insipidus had only a stalk lesion of unspecified type detected on CT scan [20]. It appears that in this case adenohypophyseal and stalk biopsy both showed inflammatory infiltrate with lymphocytes.

SUMMARY

At its broadest there may be a single entity of autoimmune hypophysitis, involving adenohypophysitis, infundibulum and neurohypophysis to a variable degree. At one end of the spectrum is a major subgroup of pregnant or postpartum patients with lymphocytic adenohypophysitis, the posterior pituitary being unaffected. These patients may have a significant sellar mass lesion, particularly when they present during pregnancy itself, or there may be no sellar enlargement. Where there is associated adenohypophyseal dysfunction the pattern of hormone loss is characteristic, preferentially involving loss of ACTH production. The natural history may be indolent and the condition may be self-limiting. Where confirmatory histology is available it shows an infiltrate with polyclonal B and T cells which may be patchy in distribution, leading to difficulty in interpretation of pituitary biopsy specimens. The latter is compounded by the knowledge that other well-defined pituitary pathologies may generate an apparently identical inflammatory response, possibly induced by IL-6 or other cytokines. In their present state of refinement pituitary antibody tests do not add much useful certainty to the diagnostic process, although if an appropriate autoantigen can be identified immunoblotting techniques may override some of the earlier methodological difficulties.

Cases of hypophysitis occurring in men and in women outside of recent pregnancy not only occur in a different immunological milieu, but also involve a pituitary that is unaffected by changes of pregnancy. Their pathogenesis may be different, although still autoimmune, and it is probably no surprise that the clinicopathological spectrum may be different with the process more frequently also including the infundibulum, resulting in diabetes insipidus. At least some cases of adult empty sella syndrome may represent the end stage of a process of lymphocytic hypophysitis, analagous to primary atrophic hypothyroidism. Idiopathic diabetes insipidus has now been associated with pituitary stalk swelling due to lymphocytic infiltration and it has been suggested that this presumed autoimmune condition may account for a third of cases of idiopathic diabetes insipidus. It is not clear to what extent this infundibuloneurohypophysitis is part of a continuum with the above conditions. Much remains to be learnt about these rare disorders.

References

1 Goudie RB, Pinkerton PH. Anterior hypophysitis and Hashimoto's disease in a young woman. J Pathol Bacteriol. 1962;83:584–5.
2. Patel MC, Guneratne N, Haq N, West TET, Weetman AP, Clayton RN. Peripartum hypopituitarism and lymphocytic hypophysitis. Q J Med. 1995;88:571–80.
3 Anonymous. Case records of the Massachusetts General Hospital. Weekly clinicopathological exercises. Case 25. New Engl J Med. 1995;333:441–7.
4. Imura H, Nakao K, Shimatsu A et al. Lymphocytic infundibuloneurohypophysitis as a cause of central diabetes insipidus. New Engl J Med. 1993;329:683–9.
5. Cosman F, Post KD, Holub DA, Wardlaw SL. Lymphocytic hypophysitis. Report of three new cases and review of the literature. Medicine. 1989;68:240–56.
6. Quencer RM. Lymphocytic adenohypophysitis: autoimmune disorder of the pituitary gland. Am J Neuroradiol. 1980;1:343–5.
7. Guay AT, Agnello V, Tronic BC, Gresham DG, Freidberg SR. Lymphocytic hypophysitis in a man. J Clin Endocrinol Metab. 1987;64:631–4.
8. Jenkins PJ, Chew SL, Lowe DG et al. Lymphocytic hypophysitis: unusual features of a rare condition. Clin Endocrinol. 1995;42:529–34.
9 Bevan JS, Othman S, Lazarus JH, Parkes AB, Hall R. Reversible adrenocorticotropin deficiency due to probable autoimmune hypophysitis in a woman with postpartum thyroiditis. J Clin Endocrinol Metab. 1992;74:548–52.
10. Gal R, Schwartz A, Gukovsky-Oren S, Peleg D, Goldman J, Kessler E. Lymphoid hypophysitis associated with sudden maternal death: report of a case and review of the literature. Obstet Gynecol Surv. 1986;41:619–21.
11. Scheithauer BW, Sano T, Kovacs KT, Young WF, Ryan N, Randall RV. The pituitary gland in pregnancy: a clinicopathological and immunohistochemical study of 69 cases. Mayo Clin Proc. 1990;65:461–74.
12. Gonzalez JG, Elizondo G, Saldivar E, Nanez H, Todd LE, Vallarreal JZ. Pituitary gland growth during normal pregnancy: an in vivo study using magnetic resonance imaging. Am J Med. 1988;85:217–20.
13. Nishioka H, Ito H, Miki T, Akada K. A case of lymphocytic hypophysitis with massive fibrosis and the role of surgical intervention. Surg Neurol. 1994;42:74–8.
14. Pestell RG, Best JD, Alford FP. Lymphocytic hypophysitis. The clinical spectrum of the disorder and evidence for an autoimmune pathogenesis. Clin Endocrinol. 1990;33:457–66.
15. Nussbaum CE, Okawara SH, Jacobs LS. Lymphocytic hypophysitis with involvement of the cavernous sinus and hypothalamus. Neurosurgery. 1991;28:440–4.
16. Supler ML, Mickle JP. Lymphocytic hypophysitis. Report of a case in a man with cavernous sinus involvement. Surg Neurol. 1992;37:472–6.
17. Lee JH, Laws ER, Guthrie BL, Dina TS, Nochomovitz LE. Lymphocytic hypophysitis: occurrence in two men. Neurosurgery. 1994;34:159–63.
18. Escobar-Morreale H, Serrano-Gotarredona J, Varela C. Isolated adrenocorticotropic hormone deficiency due to probable lymphocytic hypophysitis in a man. J Endocrinol Invest 1994;17:127–31.
19. Abe T, Matsumoto K, Sanno N. Osamura Y. Lymphocytic hypophysitis. Case report. Neurosurgery. 1995;36:1016–9.
20. Thodou E, Asa SL, Kontogeorgos G, Kovacs K, Horvath E, Ezzat S. Clinical case seminar: lymphocytic hypophysitis: clinicopathological findings. J Clin Endocrinol Metab. 1995;80: 2302–11.
21. Paja M, Estrada A, Ojeda A, Ramon y Cajal S, Garcia-Uria J, Lucas T. Lymphocytic hypophysitis causing hypopituitarism and diabetes insipidus, and associated with autoimmune thyroiditis, in a non-pregnant woman. Postgrad Med J. 1994;70:220–4.
22. Portocarrero CJ, Robinson AG, Taylor AL, Klein I. Lymphoid hypophysitis – an unusual case of hyperprolactinaemia and enlarged sella turcica. J Am Med Assoc. 1981;246:1811–2.
23. Hughes JM, Ellsworth CA, Harris BS. Clinical case seminar: a 33-year-old woman with a pituitary mass and panhypopituitarism. J Clin Endocrinol Metab. 1995;80:1521–5.
24. Levine SN, Benzel EC, Fowler MR, Shroyer JV III, Mirfakhraee M. Lymphocytic adenohypophysitis: clinical, radiological, and magnetic resonance imaging characterization Neurosurgery. 1988;22:937–41.

25. Ahmadi J, Meyers GS, Segall HD, Sharma OP, Hinton DR. Lymphocytic adenohypophysitis: contrast-enhanced MR imaging in five cases. Radiology. 1995;195:30–4.
26. Naik RG, Ammini A, Shah P, Sarkar C, Mehta VS, Berry M. Lymphocytic hypophysitis. Case report. J Neurosurg. 1994;80:925–7.
27. Asa SL, Bilbao JM, Kovacs K, Josse RG, Kreines K. Lymphocytic hypophysitis of pregnancy resulting in hypopituitarism: a distinct clinicopathological entity. Ann Intern Med. 1981;95:166–71.
28. Powrie JK, Powell M, Ayers AB, Lowy C, Sonksen PH. Lymphocytic adenohypophysitis: magnetic resonance imaging features of two new cases and a review of the literature. Clin Endocrinol. 1995;42:315–22.
29. Beressi N, Cohen R, Beressi J et al. Pseudotumoural lymphocytic hypophysitis successfully treated by corticosteroid alone: first case report. Neurosurgery. 1994;35:505–8.
30. Castle D, De Villiers JC, Melvill R. Lymphocytic adenohypophysitis. Report of a case with demonstration of spontaneous tumour regression and a review of the literature. Br J Neurosurg. 1988;2:401–6.
31. Bitton RN, Slavin M, Decker RE, Zito J, Schneider BS. The course of lymphocytic hypophysitis. Surg Neurol. 1991;36:40–3.
32. McGrail KM, Beyerl BD, Black PM, Klibanski A, Zervas NT. Lymphocytic adenohypophysitis of pregnancy with complete recovery. Neurosurgery. 1987;20:791–3.
33. Ozawa Y, Shishiba Y. Recovery from lymphocytic hypophysitis associated with painless thyroiditis: clinical implications of circulating antipituitary antibodies. Acta Endocrinol. 1993;128:493–8.
34. Sautner D, Saeger W, Ludecke DK, Jansen V, Puchner MJ. Hypophysitis in surgical and autoptical specimens. Acta Neuropathol. 1995;90:637–44.
35. Bevan JS, Burke CW, Esiri MM, Adams CBT. Misinterpretation of prolactin levels leading to management errors in patients with sellar enlargement. Am J Med. 1987;82:29–32.
36. Ahmed SR, Aiello DP, Page R, Hopper K, Towfighi J, Santen RJ. Necrotizing infundibulo-hypophysitis: a unique syndrome of diabetes insipidus and hypopituitarism. J Clin Endocrinol Metab. 1993;76:1499–504.
37. McConnon JK, Smyth HS, Horvath E. A case of sparsely granulated growth hormone cell adenoma associated with lymphocytic hypophysitis. J Endocrinol Invest. 1991;14:691–6.
38. Jones TH. Interleukin-6 an endocrine cytokine. Clin Endocrinol. 1994;40:703–13.
39. Pouplard A, Bottazzo G, Doniach D, Roitt M. Binding of human immunoglobulins to pituitary ACTH cells. Nature. 1976;261:142–4.
40. Scherbaum WA, Schrell U, Gluck M, Fahlbusch R, Pfeiffer EF. Autoantibodies to pituitary corticotropin-producing cells: possible marker for unfavourable outcome after pituitary microsurgery for Cushing's disease. Lancet. 1987;1:1394–8.
41. Sauter NP, Toni R, McLaughlin CD, Dyess EM, Kritzman J, Lechan RM. Isolated ACTH deficiency associated with an autoantibody to a corticotroph antigen that is not ACTH or other proopiomelanocortin-derived peptides. J Clin Endocrinol Metab. 1990;70:1391–7.
42. Crock P, Salvi M, Miller A, Wall J, Guyda H. Detection of anti-pituitary autoantibodies by immunoblotting. J Immunol Methods. 1993;162:31–40.
43. Engelberth O, Jezkova Z. Autoantibodies in Sheehan's syndrome. Lancet. 1965;1:1075.
44. Komatsu M, Kondo T, Yamauchi et al. Antipituitary antibodies in patients with the primary empty sella syndrome. J Clin Endocrinol Metab. 1988;67:633–8.
45. Kajita K, Yasuda K, Yamakita N et al. Anti-pituitary antibodies in patients with hypopituitarism and their families: longitudinal observation. Endocrinol Japon. 1991;38:121–9.
46. Mayfield RK, Levine JH, Gordon L, Powers J, Galbraith RM, Rawe SE. Lymphoid adenohypophysitis presenting as a pituitary tumour. Am J Med. 1980;69:619–23.
47. Yoon JW, Choi DS, Liang HC et al. Induction of an organ-specific autoimmune disease, lymphocytic hypophysitis, in hamsters by recombinant rubella virus glycoprotein and prevention of disease by neonatal thymectomy. J Virol. 1992;66:1210–4.
48. McCutcheon IE, Oldfield EH. Lymphocytic adenohypophysitis presenting as infertility. J Neurosurg. 1991;74:821–6.
49. Jansson R, Dahlberg PA, Karlsson FA. Postpartum thyroiditis. In: Lazarus JH, Hall R, eds. Hypothyroidism and Goitre. Baillière's Clin Endocrinol Metab. 1988;2:619–35.
50. Levine S. Allergic adenohypophysitis: new experimental disease of the pituitary gland. Science. 1967;158:1190–1.
51. Klein I, Kraus KE, Martines AJ, Weber S. Evidence for cellular mediated immunity in an animal model of autoimmune pituitary disease. Endocr Res Comm. 1982;9:145–53.

52. Nishiyama S, Takano T, Hidaka Y, Takada K, Iwatani Y, Amino N. A case of postpartum hypopituitarism associated with empty sella; possible relation to postpartum autoimmune hypophysitis. Endocrine J. 1993;40:431–8.
53. Mau M, Phillips TM, Ratner RE. Presence of anti-pituitary hormone antibodies in patients with empty sella syndrome and pituitary tumours. Clin Endocrinol. 1993;38:495–500.
54. Scherbaum WA, Bottazzo GF. Autoantibodies to vasopressin cells in idiopathic diabetes insipidus: evidence for an autoimmune variant. Lancet. 1983;i:897–901.

12
Autoimmune gastritis and pernicious anaemia

P. BURMAN, J.-Y. MA and F. A. KARLSSON

HISTORICAL BACKGROUND

In 1849 in the London Medical Gazette Dr Thomas Addison drew attention to a remarkable form of anaemia of idiopathic origin which in his view had not received the interest it deserved, although its existence had occasionally been pointed out by others. He described the clinical picture in three men with insidious anaemia who at postmortem examination all displayed "a diseased condition of the suprarenal capsules" [1]. Pathogenic relevance of the anaemia was suspected, but this was questioned by Dr Austin Flint, who himself had had experience of patients with insidious anaemia and who considered the possibility of a degenerative disease of the gastric tubular glands. At a clinical lecture at the Long Island College hospital in 1860, he referred to an article by Dr Handfield Jones, who some years earlier had published his findings on light microscopic examinations of a hundred stomachs. In 12 cases considerable degeneration of the gastric tubuli was noted. Dr Flint stated: "It is not difficult to see how fatal anaemia must follow an amount of degenerative disease reducing the amount of gastric juice so far that the assimilation of food is rendered wholly inadequate to the wants of the body. I shall be ready to claim the merit of this idea when the difficult and laborious researches of someone have shown it to be correct" [2]. Seventeen years later Fenwick observed atrophic glands and failure of the scrapings of the gastric mucosa to digest egg white in autopsy studies [3], and during the following decades, after analysis of the amount of 'free acid' in gastric juice from patients with insidious anaemia, several investigators reported achylia to be a constant finding [4].

The name pernicious anaemia was adopted in England in 1874 from a

A.P. Weetman (ed.), Endocrine Autoimmunity and Associated Conditions. 243–267.

description by Biermer in 1872 of patients with severe forms of anaemia [5]. Pernicious means destructive or fatal and relates to the pessimistic prognosis of the disease at that time. Before the introduction of specific therapy, this anaemia was characterized by a slow downhill course with remissions and relapses. A relapse was often precipitated by a change in diet, with increased consumption of dairy products such as butter and cream and a distaste for meat [4]. Three organ systems were affected to a varying extent – the blood, the digestive tract, and the nervous system. At presentation the patients generally complained of a sore tongue, weakness and symmetrical paraesthesias of the hands and feet. In about 30% more severe degenerative changes of the lateral and dorsal columns of the spinal cord and/or of the cerebral cortex developed and led to ataxia, a spastic gait, atony of the bladder and incontinence, and even mental confusion [6]. The anaemia was long considered to be of haemolytic origin. Hurst [7] hypothesized that an abnormal gut flora, favoured by the anacidic environment, had developed, with the production of haemolytic (and neurotoxic) toxins, and advocated administration of diluted hydrochloric acid to the patients.

During the early 1900s many different diets were recommended to anaemic patients, such as fresh vegetables, large amounts of proteins and, especially, blood products and even fresh bone marrow. Whipple *et al.* systematically investigated the effects of various foods on blood formation after acute haemorrhage in dogs, and found that liver was particularly favourable [8]. This inspired Minot and Murphy to treat 45 patients with pernicious anaemia with a special diet consisting of about 200 g of cooked calf's or beef liver per day, which led to a rapid and distinct response by the red blood cell count and clinical improvement [9]. An even better effect was observed when extracts of liver, diluted in water, were given orally and parenterally [10,11]. Minot, Murphy and Whipple were awarded the Nobel prize for this discovery in 1934. A student of Minot's, William Castle, focused attention on the loss of an 'intrinsic factor' of the gastric mucosa in patients with gastric atrophy and pernicious anaemia. He found that the patients benefited from administration of normal gastric juice in combination with beef muscle (referred to as extrinsic factor) and that the anaemia could be reversed just as well as if liver had been administered. The intrinsic factor of gastric juice was found to be separate from hydrochloric acid and pepsin and to be heat labile [12,13].

Vitamin B_{12} was isolated from liver in 1948 [14,15] and was found to be identical to the hematopoietic factor of liver extracts. The molecule was characterized by X-ray diffraction studies in 1956 by Dorothy Hodgkin [16], an achievement for which she received a Nobel prize 8 years later. Low levels of vitamin B_{12} were subsequently observed in sera from patients with pernicious anaemia [17]. Castle's intrinsic factor was later found to be a glycoprotein with a molecular mass of about 45 kDa [18]. In the early 1950s there were several reports on decreased absorption of radiolabelled vitamin B_{12} ($B_{12}{}^{60}Co$) in patients with pernicious anaemia. Schilling found that normal gastric juice given simultaneously with oral vitamin $B_{12}{}^{60}Co$ enhanced the urinary recovery of vitamin $B_{12}{}^{60}Co$ and designed the test which has been given his name [19].

The first evidence that pernicious anaemia is an autoimmune disease was produced by Schwartz, who in 1958 found that an inhibitor of intrinsic factor was present in the sera of patients with the disorder [20]. This finding was confirmed by Taylor in 1959 [21]. The observation was a result of attempts to solve the problem of acquired resistance to treatment with intrinsic factor given orally. In 1960, the inhibiting factor was found to be an immunoglobulin and to be present in the serum in 36 out of 91 patients [22]. *In vitro* methods for detection of the antibody soon followed [23,24]. A second type of autoantibody reactive to parietal cells was discovered shortly after [25,26] and an immunofluorescence method, staining the cytoplasm of parietal cells, was developed [27,28]. Parietal cell autoantibodies (PCA) were demonstrated in 75–86% of the examined patients with pernicious anaemia sera [29–31]. Gastric autoantibodies of both IgG and IgA subclasses also have been found in the gastric juice [32–35]. Strickland reported that 15 out of 20 patients with parietal cell antibodies in the serum also had the antibody in the gastric juice. While the IgG subclass predominated in serum, the IgA subclass was more common in the gastric juice [35].

THE GASTRIC MUCOSA AND THE PARIETAL CELL

The gastric mucosa contains three types of glands: the oxyntic glands, the pyloric glands and the cardiac glands. The oxyntic glands are mainly located in the corpus and fundus (Figure 12.1) and contain chief or zymogen cells, parietal cells, endocrine cells, mucous neck cells, and more undifferentiated stem cells responsible for cell renewal. The gastric acid-producing parietal cell has an ability to secrete H^+ against a two million-fold concentration gradient from the mucosa to the lumen of the stomach [36]. This is mediated by a unique enzyme termed the proton pump, i.e. H^+,K^+-ATPase. Besides hydrochloric acid, the gastric juice contains mucus, pepsinogen and intrinsic factor. The surface cells secrete bicarbonate and a protective mucus layer. Pepsinogen (type A), which is converted to pepsin in an acidic environment, is secreted by the chief cells and the mucous neck cells [37]. A type of pepsinogen termed C is synthesized in the cardia, antrum, and proximal duodenum. In most species, including man, intrinsic factor (IF) is synthesized by the parietal cell [38]. Recent data, however, also indicate a contribution from other foregut derived cells [39]. In rats chief cells are the source of IF [40], and in dogs it is also produced by the secretory ducts of the pancreas and the salivary glands [41].

The pyloric glands are situated in the antrum and contain endocrine cells, namely the G and D cells. The G cells synthesize gastrin, which stimulates gastric acid secretion. Gastrin also promotes growth of the gastric mucosa, and atrophy of the oxyntic mucosa after antrectomy is well documented [42]. The somatostatin-containing D cells possibly function as chemoreceptors and mediate a paracrine inhibitory effect of the adjacent G cells on gastrin secretion when the pH falls too low [43]. The cardiac glands are in the cardiac region of the stomach and secrete mucus. At least five endocrine cell types have been

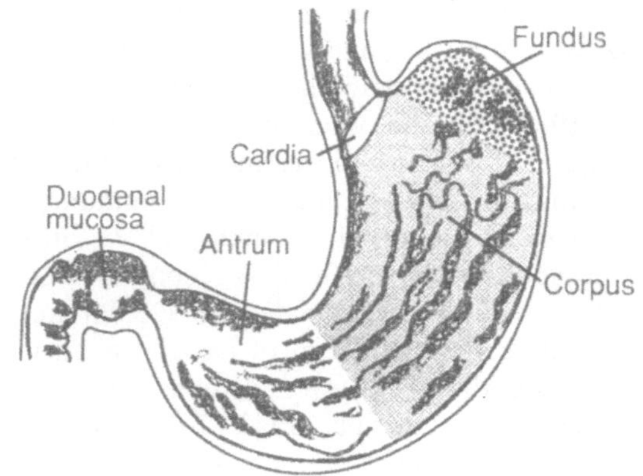

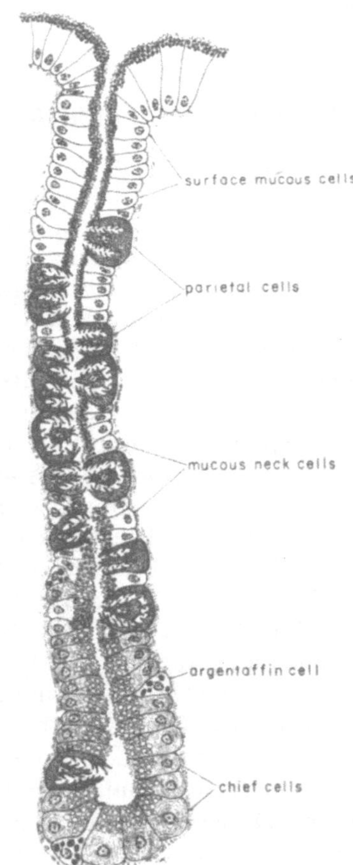

GASTRIC GLAND

found in the human oxyntic mucosa, namely ECL cells (enterochromaffin-like cells), A-like cells, D cells, D1 or P cells and the 5-hydroxytryptamine-containing enterochromaffin cells (EC cells) [44].

H^+,K^+-ATPase

H^+,K^+-ATPase (EC 3.6.1.36) is a membrane-associated enzyme which acidifies the stomach lumen through hydrolysis of ATP. In the resting state this enzyme is predominantly located in numerous tubulovesicles in the apical cytoplasm of the cells. It has been proposed that on stimulation, these tubulovesicles translocate and fuse with narrow canals, referred to as secretory canaliculi, which are invaginations of the apical surface membrane, to form secretory channels [45–47] (Figure 12.2). Concomitantly, according to this concept, an increase in the ion permeability of the canalicular membrane takes place, allowing potassium

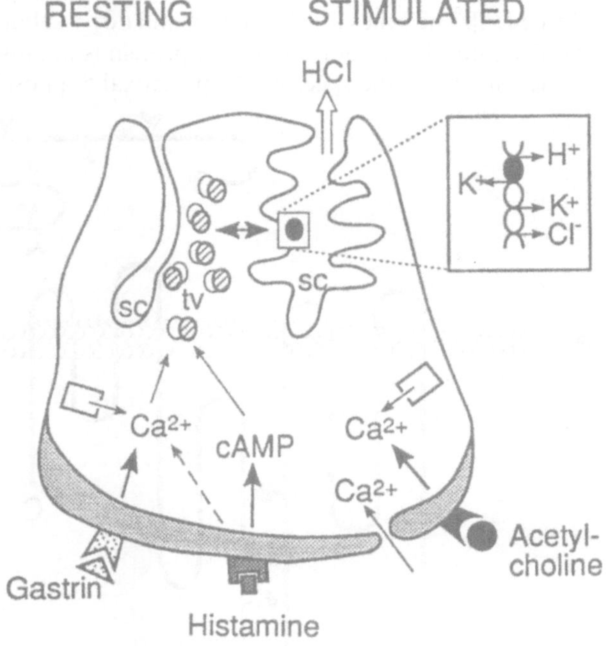

Figure 12.2 A schematic diagram of the parietal cell in a resting and stimulated state. Activation of the gastrin, histamine or acetylcholine receptors leads to stimulation of gastric acid secretion, whereby H^+,K^+-ATPase, which is present in tubulovesicular(tv)-like structures, is translocated to the secretory canaliculi (sc)

Figure 12.1 (opposite) The stomach and its anatomical regions (upper). Gastric acid is produced from the oxyntic glands (lower), which are present in the corpus of the stomach

and chloride ions to diffuse into the canaliculi from the cytosol [47–49]. The acid pump then transports H^+ out of the cell into the lumen in exchange for K^+ ions. As this is an energy-consuming process, more than one third of the cell volume is occupied by mitochondria, a higher proportion than in any other epithelial cell [36].

H^+,K^+-ATPase, together with Na^+,K^+-ATPase and Ca^{2+}-ATPase, belongs to the cation transport ATPase family. They all have a related catalytic subunit (α subunit) and a β subunit (Figure 12. 3). The α subunit of H^+,K^+-ATPase is the major part of the enzyme. Its molecular mass on SDS-PAGE is 94 kDa. It is a single polypeptide chain with 3 N-linked glycosylation sites and eight trans-membrane domains. About 80% of this subunit protrudes into the cytosol, 15% is located within the membrane, and 5% protrudes into the canalicular lumen [49]. The nucleotide sequences of the cDNA and the deduced amino acid sequences (1033–1035 residues, molecular mass 114 kDa) of the H^+,K^+-ATPase α subunit have been cloned from the rat [52], pig [53], rabbit [54], dog [55], mouse [56], and frog [56]. The genes for the human and dog α subunit contain 22 exons [50,51,55]. The phosphorylation site of the protein is at amino acid Asp-385, 386 or 387, depending on the species. The pyridoxal 5′-phosphate-binding

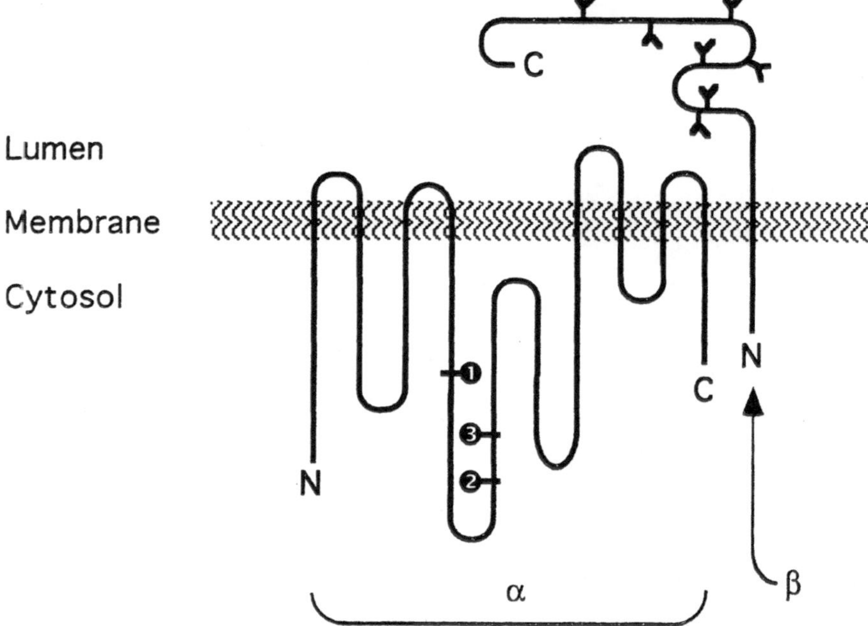

Figure 12.3 A schematic model of the folding of the α and β subunits of H^+,K^+-ATPase. The human α subunit is thought to pass eight times through the secretory membrane [50,51]. A potential catalytic site consists of a phosphorylation site (1, Asp-387), a pyridoxal 5′-phosphate binding site (2, Lys-498) and FITC binding site (3, Lys-519). The β subunit is glycosylated on at least four, probably seven positions on the extracellular portion of the protein

site and a fluorescein isothiocyanate (FITC) binding site are conserved at Lys-497 or 498 and Lys-518 or 519, respectively. The overall sequence homology between the α subunit of H^+,K^+-ATPase and that of Na^+,K^+-ATPase is about 60%.

The β subunit of is a glycoprotein with one transmembrane domain. It was discovered in 1990, 17 years after the identification of the α subunit of this enzyme [57–62]. It is difficult to detect by the Coomassie blue protein stain on SDS-PAGE and appears as a glycoprotein of 60–80 kDa in H^+,K^+-ATPase-containing membranes from several species on lectin blotting. The protein was found to be co-immunoprecipitated with the α subunit of H^+,K^+-ATPase. After deglycosylation with glycosidase, it has a protein core of 32–35 kDa, which is similar to the protein core of the Na^+,K^+-ATPase β subunit. Sequencing analysis of V8 protease-generated peptide fragments showed at least 30% homology with the β subunit of Na^+,K^+-ATPase. Like the α subunit, the nucleotide sequences of the cDNA of the β subunit have been determined in several species: the rat [60,61], pig [62], rabbit [63], human [64], mouse [65], dog [55], and birds [66]. The deduced amino acid sequences, comprising 290 amino acids in the pig and dog, 291 amino acids in the rabbit and man, 294 amino acids in the rat and mouse, and 299 amino acids in avian species with a molecular mass of 33 kDa, show 29–35% and 37–53% homology with those of the Na^+,K^+-ATPase β1 subunit and β2 subunit, respectively. There are six cysteine residues within the extracellular domain which appear to be highly conserved in these species. Seven N-linked glycosylation sites (except in the pig, which has one glycosylation site less, and in avian species, which have one more) are located in the extracellular regions of the protein. The genes encoding this subunit containing seven exons have been cloned and sequenced in the rat [67,68] and mouse [65,69]. The genes of the mouse and man have been mapped to chromosome 8 [61] and chromosome 13q34 [70], respectively. The function of the β subunit of H^+,K^+-ATPase is not known. However, as has been proposed for the Na^+,K^+-ATPase β subunit, it might be essential for cation transport, ATPase activity, or correct insertion of H^+,K^+-ATPase into the membrane [59, 71].

Intrinsic factor

IF is a globular glycoprotein which is synthesized and secreted by parietal cells in man, monkey, cat, ox, rabbit and guinea pig, and by chief cells in the rat and mouse [72]. The function of IF is to promote absorption of vitamin B_{12} at specific sites in the distal small intestine. In the absence of IF less than 2% of ingested cobalamin is absorbed [73]. The cDNAs of rat [74] and human [75] IF have been cloned. The corresponding proteins contain 421 and 417 amino acids, respectively, with a calculated molecular mass of 46 kDa. Rat IF has four N-linked glycosylation sites, and human IF has six. The identity between human and rat IF is 80%. The human IF gene with 10 exons has been localized to chromosome 11 [75].

AUTOIMMUNE GASTRITIS

Characteristics and progression to pernicious anaemia

Atrophic gastritis has been classified into two entities, types A and B, depending on the involvement of the antral mucosa and the presence or absence of gastric autoantibodies [76]. The antral-predominant type B is related to *Helicobacter pylori* infection, and is more common than type A. Autoantibodies are generally absent, although there have been two reports on low-titre anti-gastrin-cell antibodies in a minority of patients [77,78].

Type A chronic atrophic gastritis (i.e. autoimmune gastritis) is characterized by the presence of serum PCA, infiltration of mononuclear cells in the gastric mucosa, and loss of parietal cells and chief cells from the oxyntic glands. The antrum is usually spared or only mildly affected [76]. Hypergastrinemia is present in most but not all cases [79,80], possibly depending on the integrity of the antral mucosa [81,82]. Loss of antral acidification with loss of inhibition of gastrin release has been implicated as a mechanism of hypergastrinemia. Low serum concentrations of pepsinogen A reflect tissue damage and loss of chief cells. In screening for atrophic autoimmune level gastritis, low serum level of pepsinogen A has a high predictive value [83,84]. The combination of a high serum gastrin with a low serum pepsinogen A has been reported to have a specificity of 100% [83].

PCAs are found in the serum in 70–95% of patients with pernicious anaemia but less frequently (30–60%) in atrophic gastritis without pernicious anaemia. The titre is higher in women than in men and is inversely related to the duration of the disease and the residual cell mass, indicating that the autoimmune response is antigen driven [85]. Autoantibodies to IF, which have been reported in 40–75% of patients with pernicious anaemia, are rare in simple atrophic gastritis (i.e. without pernicious anaemia) [86,87]. Contrary to PCA, there is a positive relation between the presence of the IF autoantibody and the duration of the disease [88,89]. The mononuclear infiltrate in the gastric mucosa may be focal in early stages of disease and is then dominated by macrophages and T lymphocytes. The adjacent epithelial cells show an aberrant expression of HLA-DR [90].

Pernicious anaemia results from loss of IF, which is essential for vitamin B_{12} absorption in the ileum. Over a period of 10 years about 20% of investigated patients with autoimmune gastritis were found to develop symptoms of vitamin B_{12} malabsorption [91–93]. A higher incidence was noted in patients who in addition to serum PCA had IF autoantibodies in the serum and/or in the gastric juice, possibly blocking the binding of remaining IF to vitamin B_{12} [91,94]. However, these estimates were based on the presence of anaemia in combination with low serum cobalamin levels. Findings in several studies have now supported the presence of intracellular B_{12} deficiency despite low to normal serum concentrations of the vitamin, and there are also reports of CNS malfunctions in B_{12}-deficient patients despite a normal haemoglobin concentration [95–99]. Thus, the occurrence of clinically relevant cobalamin malabsorption seems previously to have been underestimated.

Presentation and evaluation of vitamin B_{12} deficiency

The classical manifestation of cobalamin deficiency is megaloblastic anaemia with or without neuropathy. The neuropathy is dominated by paraesthesia and ataxia associated with hyperreflexia with or without spasticity, symmetrical loss of proprioception and the sense of vibration affecting the lower limbs first, and distal loss of cutaneous sensation [73]. The anaemia is due to a defect in the synthesis of DNA, which can also affect other rapidly dividing cells, resulting in glossitis, hypospermia and sometimes diarrhoea [100]. The pathogenesis of the neuropathy is still a matter of controversy, but it is presently thought to be related to interference with methylation reactions in the CNS, where vitamin B_{12} is an important co-enzyme [101].

However, patients who benefit from cobalamin therapy may have minimal or no haematological changes and may present with more subtle neurological and psychological manifestations. In 70 patients with pernicious anaemia, defined as either a low serum vitamin B_{12} level in combination with a reduced uptake of cobalamin according to the Schilling test, or the presence of serum IF antibodies, or the absence of IF in the gastric juice, Carmel found no anaemia and no macrocytosis in 19% and 33%, respectively [95]. Lindenbaum *et al.* [96] observed no anaemia in 28% of 141 patients with neuropsychiatric disorders attributable to cobalamin deficiency, including memory loss, spastic gait, and ataxia, most often combined with paraesthesia. In 13.5% both the haematocrit and mean cell volume (MCV) were normal. In certain cases a normal MCV could be explained by a co-existing iron deficiency, which is common in patients with atrophic gastritis. Atypical manifestations, mimicking these in multiple sclerosis, have been reported and may constitute a diagnostic dilemma [102–104]. Psychiatric symptoms of various types, e.g. memory loss, depression, delirium, slow mentation and acute psychosis, have been attributed to B_{12} deficiency, and there is evidence that such symptoms can be alleviated by replacement therapy [105]. An increased frequency of atrophic gastritis and subnormal vitamin B_{12} levels has also been found among patients with dementia [106,107]. It is not known to what extent, if any, the occurrence and degree of vitamin B_{12} deficiency among such patients contributes to their dementia.

The diagnosis of vitamin B_{12} deficiency has been based on measurements of serum cobalamin levels, bone marrow or peripheral blood abnormalities, and tests of cobalamin absorption such as the Schilling test. However, each of these tests has its shortcomings and at present there is no golden standard for assessing the vitamin B_{12} status. As a result of inherent methodological problems in the current assays, as well as variations in cobalamin binding proteins, serum cobalamin concentrations may not accurately reflect the tissue availability of this vitamin [108]. It has been suggested that perhaps as many as one-half of all patients with low serum levels of vitamin B_{12} do not have demonstrable B_{12} deficiency [109]. The positive predictive value of a low serum cobalamin concentration, defined as < 133 pmol/L, has been found to be as low as 22.2% in an in- and outpatient population suspected of having vitamin B_{12}

deficiency [110]. This indicates the need for complementary diagnostic tools before initiating lifetime parenteral therapy. The serum levels of methylmalonic acid (MMA) and/or homocysteine (HCYS), metabolites that accumulate in the presence of cellular cobalamin deficiency, and their response to vitamin B_{12} injections, have been suggested to be sensitive indices of significant cobalamin deficiency [96,98,99,108]. A high prevalence (14.5%) of elevated MMA and HCYS has been found in subjects of ages above 65 years [111]. However, as the serum levels of both MMA and HCYS increase in patients with renal failure and as the serum level of HCYS is also increased in patients with folate or pyridoxine deficiency, the result of an individual test has to be interpreted with some caution.

Identification of groups at risk of developing the disease

Severe atrophic gastritis has been reported to occur in 2–6% of the populations of Finland and Estonia, and is mainly seen in elderly subjects [112]. The overall prevalence of pernicious anaemia has been estimated to be 1–2/1000, women being affected about twice as often as men. Pernicious anaemia is primarily a disease of old age with an average onset at 65 years, and the prevalence at older ages is 1% or higher in northern European countries [73,113,114]. There are racial differences; in the USA the prevalence among subjects older than 60 years was recently reported to be 1.9% and highest in black or white women, but rare in persons of Latin American, Asian or other origin [97]. Among first-degree relatives of patients with pernicious anaemia, the proportion of subjects with severe atrophic gastritis was found to be significantly higher (13%) than in controls (1%) matched for age and sex. In addition, the mean age of probands with less severe gastric mucosal damage was lower than that of controls with corresponding mucosal lesions. An inherited propensity for the disease, with early onset and rapid progression from mild to severe forms, was suggested [115].

The frequency of gastric autoantibodies, atrophic gastritis and pernicious anaemia, is clearly increased in other organ-specific autoimmune endocrine diseases and related disorders [114,116] (Table 12.1). Autoimmune gastric disease is particularly often found in patients with autoimmune thyroiditis, and in patients with insulin-dependent diabetes mellitus. In the latter group B_{12} deficiency may also be found in younger individuals and the symptoms may be mistaken for diabetes-related neuropathy. Another risk group for development pernicious anaemia at a young age is women with postpartum thyroiditis. Such women show a high frequency of PCA in the serum and may develop a flare-up of the gastric autoimmune disease after delivery [90].

PARIETAL CELL AUTOANTIGENS AND AUTOANTIBODIES

In early studies the parietal cell autoantigen was localized to a microsome fraction of homogenized gastric mucosa [129], and Hoedemaeker and Ito [130]

Table 12.1 Prevalence (%) of pernicious anaemia (PA), autoimmune gastritis (AIG), parietal cell autoantibodies (PCA) and intrinsic factor autoantibodies (IFA) in various autoimmune organ-specific disorders

Disease	*PA*	*AIG*	*PCA*	*IFA*	*Reference*
Hyperthyroidism					
($n = 410$)	1.7				[117]
($n = 300$)	2.3		22	4.7	[118]
($n = 1623$)	1.7			2.6	[119]
<40 yrs ($n = 291$)	0			0.3	
>40 yrs ($n = 1332$)	2.1			2.9	
Hashimoto's thyroiditis					
($n = 394$)			32		[29]
($n = 120$)	4.2			5	[119]
Postpartum thyroiditis					
($n = 54$)	4	7	33		[90]
Primary hypothyroidism					
($n = 73$)	12.3	46			[120]
($n = 297$)	11.4			6.7	[119]
Addison's disease					
($n = 118$)	5.1				[121]
($n = 321$)	3.7				[116]
($n = 97$)	1	5.2	24		[122]
Vitiligo					
($n = 65$)		15	17		[123]
Hypoparathyroidism					
($n = 74$)	9.5				[124]
IDDM					
20–80 yrs ($n = 200$)	4.0		28	4	[125]
<30 yrs ($n = 771$)		4.5	9		[126]
0–14 yrs ($n = 389$)			3		[127]
Reference population					
15–65 yrs ($n = 629$)			5.0		[119]
21–65 yrs ($n = 3492$)			4.8		[128]
21–30 yrs			2.2		
61–65 yrs			6.3		
0–15 yrs ($n = 321$)			0.3		[127]

demonstrated specific binding of PCA to the secretory canaliculi of the parietal cells. PCA reactive to the cytoplasm of the parietal cells were found also to react with the cell surface of such living cells [131]. Evidence for a complement-dependent cytotoxic effect *in vitro* of the autoantibodies was provided by an Australian group [132]. In a radioreceptor assay, sera from six of 20 patients with pernicious anaemia blocked the binding of gastrin to rat gastric mucosal cells [133], and it was proposed that the gastrin receptor might be the parietal cell autoantigen. In immunoblotting studies with separated proteins from gastric mucosal membrane fractions of the dog, mouse and rat, sera from patients with pernicious anaemia recognized a 65–70 kDa protein, claimed not to be a glycoprotein, and identified as the presumptive parietal cell autoantigen [134]. However, the researchers later found the gastrin receptor to be a 78 kDa protein [135], refuting their previous hypothesis. Absence of gastrin receptor blocking antibodies was subsequently demonstrated by our research group [136] and others [137].

Autoantibodies to the H^+,K^+-ATPase α and β subunits

The discovery of H^+,K^+-ATPase as the major parietal cell autoantigen was reported in 1988 [138]. PCA were found to immunoblot a 92 kDa protein of gastric and parietal cell membrane preparations separated by electrophoresis in SDS–polyacrylamide gels. In addition, patient immunoglobulins were found to adsorb in parallel parietal cell antigens and H^+,K^+-ATPase from a solubilized gastric membrane fraction [138]. In the SDS–polyacrylamide gels a broad blurred band of 65–75 kDa was seen in some experiments with non-reduced material, and the protein of this band did not stain with Coomassie blue (Figure 12.4). Subsequently, Goldkorn *et al.* showed that sera containing PCAs precipitated a 60–90 kDa protein from solubilized gastric membrane fractions [139]. The identity of this protein as the β subunit of H^+,K^+-ATPase was clarified in 1990 by Toh *et al.* [62]. The antigenicity of the β subunit critically depends on the presence of a full complement of N-linked carbohydrates. Unglycosylated recombinant protein [140], partial deglycosylation of the native protein, and COS cells bearing high mannose N-glycan recombinant proteins all failed to bind the antibody [141]. This suggests that the B cell autoepitopes are located on the luminal side of the β subunit.

The B cell autoepitopes of the α subunit have been investigated after generation of recombinant fusion proteins from cDNA fragments encoding different portions of the domain (Figure 12.5). Epitopes have been localized to residues 606–964 and also to the amino-terminal 79 amino acids of the porcine α subunit [142], to residues 360–525 on the cytosolic side of the human α subunit [143] and further to residues 506–961 incorporating the catalytic cytoplasmic domain and the ATP-binding sites, respectively, of the rat protein [141], indicating heterogeneity of the antibody repertoire.

The reported presence of autoantibodies to the α and the β domains has varied in different series of patients. Wang *et al.* found that each of nine patient sera immunoblotted the α subunit, whereas no other protein was recognized [142], Goldkorn *et al.* found that 24 of 34 PCA positive sera reacted only with the β subunit on immunoblotting [139]. However, under appropriate, but mutually exclusive conditions it was found that all PCA-containing sera immunoblotted both subunits [141].

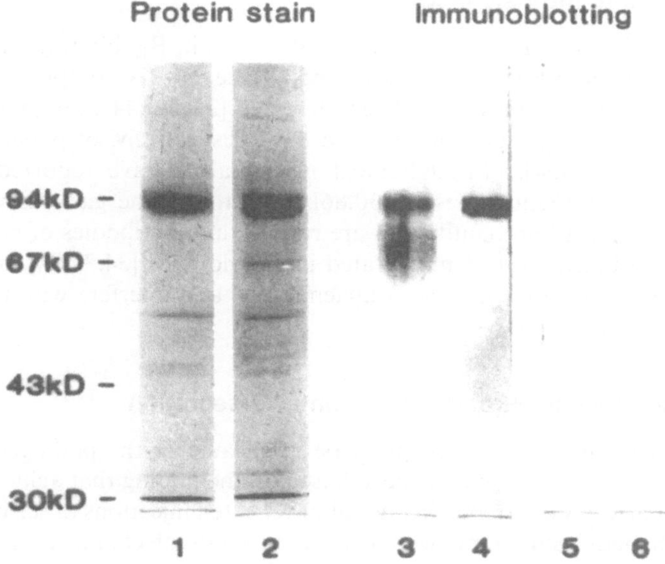

Figure 12.4 Identification of the α subunit as the parietal cell autoantigen. SDS polyacrylamide gel electrophoresis of a non-reduced (1,3,5) and a reduced and alkylated (2,4,6) vesicular membrane preparation. In immunoblotting a serum positive for parietal cell autoantibody (3,4) and a control serum (5,6) were used. Note the identical mobility of the major protein of the vesicular membranes, H^+,K^+-ATPase, and the immunoblotting signal at the 92 kDa position. The wide, blurred band of higher mobility was not explained at the time. Later studies revealed the presence of the β subunit in H^+,K^+-ATPase. (Reproduced from *Journal of Clinical Investigation* 1988;81:475–9 by copyright permission of The Rockefeller University Press)

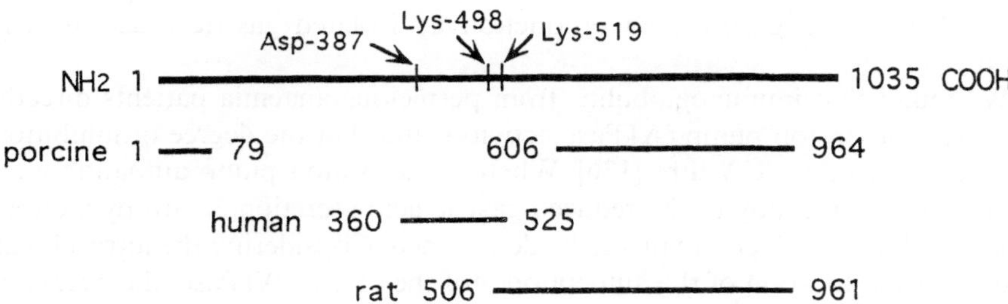

Figure 12.5 Map of epitopes on the H^+,K^+-ATPase α subunit. Arrows point to the amino acid residues with the potential phosphorylation site (Asp-387), pyridoxal 5′-phosphate binding site (Lys-498) and FITC binding site (Lys-519). The epitopes of the porcine (142), human (143) and rat (141) are indicated

Autoantibodies to intrinsic factor

Two types of IF autoantibodies, reactive to the vitamin B_{12} binding site of IF (type I antibody or blocking antibody) and to the IF-B_{12} complex (type II antibody or binding antibody) have been identified [23,24,144,145]. Type I and II antibodies have been found in 70% and 34%, respectively, of patients with pernicious anaemia [31], although most investigators have reported lower frequencies of IF autoantibodies [27,30,86]. In autoimmune gastritis without pernicious anaemia, IF autoantibodies are rare. IF autoantibodies of both IgA and IgG isotypes have been demonstrated in gastric juice [34,35,94] and may hasten the development of pernicious anaemia [94] and interfere with tests for cobalamin absorption.

Effects of parietal cell autoantibodies on acid secretion

It has been suggested that PCAs might be implicated in the pathogenesis of atrophic gastritis. This concept has been based on the finding that achlorhydria and glandular atrophy developed in dogs after repeated injections of serum from rabbits which had been immunized with a microsomal canine parietal cell fraction. The rabbit anti-canine serum specifically stained the cytoplasm of the parietal cells [146]. In a set of experiments designed by Loveridge *et al.* [147], immunoglobulins from patients with pernicious anaemia were shown to inhibit spontaneous and gastrin-stimulated gastric acid secretion in an experimental animal. Similarly, passive transfer of immunoglobulins containing PCAs from patients with pernicious anaemia to rodents resulted in hypochlorhydria and a significant reduction of the parietal cell mass and mucosal thickness [148]. Another group reported the presence of a blocking immunoglobulin in about 50% of sera from patients with pernicious anaemia, which specifically inhibited gastrin-stimulated gastric acid production by isolated gastric mucosal cells [149].

We found that immunoglobulins from pernicious anaemia patients directly inhibited the proton pump (ATPase activity), and that the degree of inhibition was related to the PCA titre [136]. Whether the proton pump autoantibodies contribute significantly to the reduced gastric acid secretion *in vivo* by a direct binding/blocking effect remains to be determined. Considering the intracellular and/or apical location of the autoepitopes of the H^+,K^+-ATPase, the access of circulating autoantibodies to the proton pump seems limited. However, aberrant expression of target molecules has been demonstrated in other autoimmune diseases such as primary biliary cirrhosis and insulin-dependent diabetes mellitus. In primary biliary cirrhosis the dihydrolipoamide acetyltransferase component of the mitochondrial pyruvate dehydrogenase complex, the antigen most closely associated with this cirrhotic disease, was found to be located on the membrane of cultured human intrahepatic biliary epithelial cells, in contrast to a cytoplasmic location in cells from normal livers [150]. Recently it was demonstrated that a portion of tyrosine phosphatase ICA 512, a key autoantigen in autoimmune diabetes localized to neurosecretory granules, appears transiently at the cell surface during insulin secretion [151]. In patients with early autoimmune gastritis, selective localization of immunoglobulins, in particular IgG, to parietal cells has been observed, suggesting *in vivo* access of PCAs to the antigen [90]. The potential contribution of the autoantibodies in the acidic gastric secretions to the achlorhydria has not been assessed.

AUTOIMMUNE GASTRITIS IN EXPERIMENTAL MODELS

In early studies, achlorhydria, degeneration of oxyntic glands, and development of circulating PCA were observed in various species after immunization with homologous and autologous gastric juice or mucosal extracts [152–154]. In recent years, experimental murine models have been introduced which have enabled important immunological events in the induction of autoimmune gastritis to be defined.

The murine models – characteristics

Several endocrine organ-specific autoimmune diseases including gastritis can be induced in some strains of mice by thymectomy performed 2–4 days after birth [155], by neonatal administration of cyclosporin A [156], and by total lymphoid irradiation with high fractionated doses in adult mice [157]. Forty to 60% of BALB/c mice thymectomized on day 2–4 developed autoimmune gastritis accompanied by decreased vitamin B_{12} absorption and macrocytic anaemia within 12 weeks [158]. Like the human disease, murine gastritis is characterized by loss of parietal and chief cells, mononuclear cell infiltrates in the gastric mucosa and circulating antibodies to the proton pump [159,160]. In general it is the α subunit of H^+,K^+-ATPase that is targeted; a proportion of the animals also develop antibodies to the β subunit, and in rare cases also to IF [159–161]. Unlike in the human disease, the gastric mucosa is thicker than normal as a result of hyperplasia of the mucous cells. In early stages of the disease (week 4) the gastric mucosal mononuclear infiltrate has been found to consist mainly of macrophages and $CD4^+$ T cells. At week 8 after birth, coinciding with the peaking of serum antibodies to H^+,K^+-ATPase, B cells appear, while $CD8^+$ T cells increase marginally during the first 12 weeks of life [162].

T cell reactivity and transfer of disease

The murine gastric disease appears to be cell-mediated, since spleen cells, but not serum, from the thymectomized animals cause autoimmune gastritis when transferred to nude BALB/c mice [163]. The mechanisms involved in the breakdown of self-tolerance are not known. Neonatal thymectomy has been found to result in disappearance of a $CD4^+$ T cell subset (CD5) from peripheral lymphoid organs [164]. Spleen cells from BALB/c nu/+ mice freed of this particular T cell subset were able to induce endocrine organ-specific autoimmune diseases, including autoimmune gastritis, when transferred to BALB/c nude mice [165]. In the murine model with total lymphoid irradiation, this treatment was found to eliminate the majority of the mature thymocytes and peripheral T cells for one month. Inoculation of spleen cells, thymocytes or bone marrow suspensions from syngeneic naive mice within 2 weeks prevented the development of autoimmunity. It was found that $CD4^+$, but not $CD8^+$ T cells mediated this prevention [157]. $CD4^+$ T cells also appeared to induce autoimmune disease when transferred from disease-bearing to syngeneic naive mice.

The autoantigens recognized by T cells have been investigated in neonatally thymectomized BALB/c mice. A $CD4^+$ T cell line responding to murine, human and porcine parietal cells was established from regional lymph nodes of the stomach from a mouse with autoimmune gastritis [166]. Adoptive transfer of this cell line to nude mice resulted in gastritis, albeit without circulating autoantibodies to parietal cells. The T cells recognized two peptides, identical in all but one amino acid, from the α subunit of porcine (amino acids 891–905) and of human (amino acids 892–906) H^+,K^+-ATPase, respectively. No reactivity towards the murine β subunit was found. In affected animals a delayed-type hypersensitivity reaction toward parietal cell-enriched, but not chief cell-enriched fractions of gastric cells, has been observed [163]. In both the human and the murine disease, however, chief cells also disappear from the glands. Recently, T cells reactive to H^+,K^+-ATPase-enriched preparations of parietal cell microsomes (enzyme purified by lectin affinity chromatography) were found in lymph nodes in the immediate proximity of the stomach, but little or no response was seen when mesenteric or peripheral lymph nodes were examined [167].

ATTEMPTS TO PREVENT OR ARREST THE DEVELOPMENT OF THE DISEASE

During the 1950s and 1960s trials with corticosteroids [168–174] and azathioprine [175] were conducted in patients with pernicious anaemia with promising results. Regeneration of gastric parietal cells was observed by means of repeat gastric biopsies. Significant improvement of vitamin B_{12} absorption and an increase in IF secretion were evident in a majority of the patients. Reductions in circulating autoantibodies to IF were also described. The amelioration produced by corticosteroids was not, however, mediated by suppression of autoantibodies to IF, since reappearance of IF in the gastric juice preceded any decline in the autoantibody level [170,174]. The doses administered were usually high and relapse occurred shortly after withdrawal of the steroids.

In BALB/c mice thymectomized on day 3, intrathymic injection of syngeneic parietal cells within 24 h of birth resulted in almost complete prevention of autoimmune gastritis [176]. The preventive effect was parietal cell-specific, since the occurrence of oophoritis, which usually developed in about 25% of the female mice (Chapter 10), was not affected. Intraperitoneal injection of parietal cells had no effect, suggesting that the parietal cell autoantigens had to be specifically recognized by autoreactive cells in the thymus.

This approach was taken further by Alderuccio *et al.* [177], who showed that transgenic expression of the β subunit of H^+,K^+-ATPase under the control of a major histocompatibility complex class II I-E promotor specifically prevented autoimmune gastric disease, but that the incidence of oophoritis was identical to that in non-transgenic littermates (Figure 12.6). In addition, autoimmune gastritis could be transferred by thymocytes from adult BALB/c mice to nude mice, as previously described [178], but could not be transferred by thymocytes from the transgenic mice, suggesting that tolerance to pathogenic autoreactive T cells was induced within the thymus. Interestingly, in neonatal mice the protein

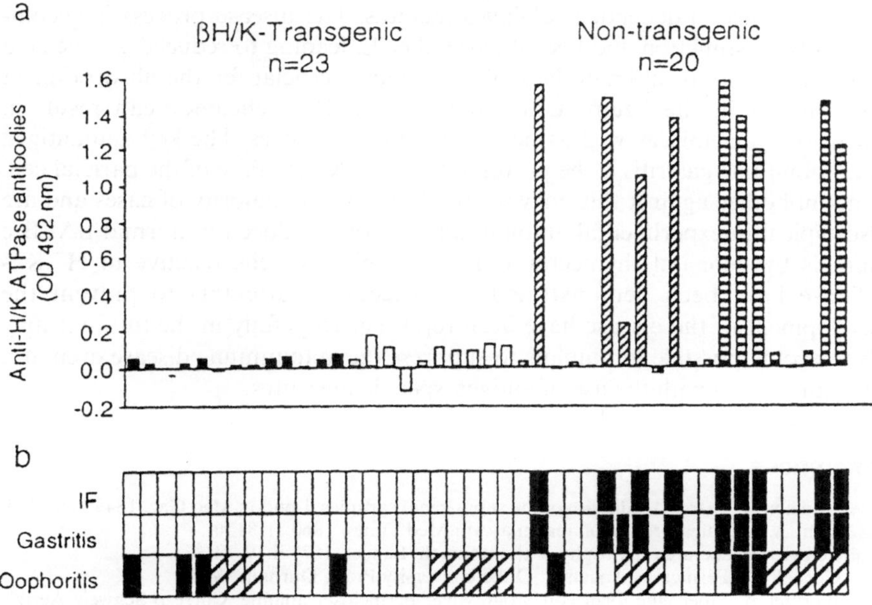

Figure 12.6 H^+,K^+-ATPase autoantibodies, gastritis, and oophoritis in neonatally thymectomized mice. (a) Mice from line 25 were thymectomized on day 3 and the transgenic status was determined at weaning. At 3 months, sera were collected from all mice and approximately half the βH/K-transgenic and non-transgenic mice were killed for histological examination. Sera were collected from the remaining mice at 5 months of age. Anti-H^+,K^+-ATPase antibodies were detected by ELISA. Filled bars: βH/K-transgenic mice at 3 months; open bars: βH/K-transgenic mice at 5 months; diagonally striped bars: non-transgenic mice at 3 months; horizontally striped bars: non-transgenic mice at 5 months. (b) Immunofluorescence (IF) for detection of anti-parietal cell autoantibodies and histological examination of stomachs and ovaries of mice from (a). Mice are represented in the same order as in (a) and are shown directly below the corresponding ELISA readings. The presence of parietal cell autoantibodies, gastritis or oophoritis is indicated by a filled box. Striped boxes indicate male mice excluded from analysis of oophoritis. (Reproduced from *Journal of Experimental Medicine* 1993;178:419–26 by copyright permission of The Rockefeller University Press)

levels of the two subunits of the gastric proton pump in the gastric mucosa have been found to be very low up to day 15. Adult levels were reached by day 30 [179], suggesting that the gastric antigen does not accumulate at a concentration sufficient to induce thymic tolerance during fetal life. In another mouse strain (C3H/HeN) administration of IL-2 for 7 days after day-3 thymectomy inhibited the development of anti-gastric autoantibodies [180].

CONCLUSION

Autoimmune gastritis is a common disorder affecting females more often than males. Individuals with autoimmune endocrine diseases are at increased risk of developing this type of gastritis, especially patients with autoimmune thyroid disease or insulin-dependent diabetes mellitus. The disease process is accompanied by dysfunction and loss of parietal cells, leading to reduced gastric acid production and an ultimate lack of IF, a factor crucial for the absorption of vitamin B_{12} in the ileum. Untreated vitamin B_{12} deficiency can result in pernicious anaemia as well as neurological disturbances. The key autoantigen in autoimmune gastritis is the proton pump, H^+,K^+-ATPase of the parietal cell. Autoantibodies against this enzyme are found in the majority of cases and are also typical in experimental autoimmune gastritis, induced in normal BALB/c animals by neonatal thymectomy. In such mice, T cells reactive to H^+,K^+-ATPase have been demonstrated and successful attempts to prevent the development of the disease have been reported. Hopefully in the future it may also become possible in humans to suppress the autoimmune disease even at a subclinical level with the use of antigen-specific measures.

References

1. Addison T. Anaemia – disease of the supra-renal capsules. London Med Gaz. 1849;43:517–8.
2. Flint A. A clinical lecture of anaemia. Am Med Times. 1860;1:181–6.
3. Fenwick S. Lecture on atrophy of the stomach. Lancet. 1877;ii:39–41.
4. Cornell BS. Pernicious Anaemia. Duke University Press, Durham 1927.
5. Biermer A. Uber eine form von progressiver perniciöser anämie. Corresp Schweiz Aertze. 1872;2:15–17.
6. Wintrobe MM. Nutritional factors in the production and function of erythrocytes. In: Wintrobe MM, Lee GR, Boggs DR, eds. Clinical Hematology. Philadelphia: Lea and Febiger; 1981:136–70.
7. Hurst AF. Achlorhydria: its relation to pernicious anaemia and other diseases. Lancet. 1923; i:111–5.
8. Whipple GH, Hooper CW, Robscheit FS. Blood regeneration following simple anaemia. Am J Physiol. 1920:53:151–67.
9. Minot GR, Murphy WP. Treatment of pernicious anaemia by a special diet. J Am Med Assoc. 1926;87:470–6.
10. Minot GR, Cohn EJ, Murphy WP, Lawson HA. Treatment of pernicious anaemia with liver extract: effects upon the production of immature and mature red blood cells. Am J Med Sci. 1928;175:599–621.
11. Minot GR. The development of liver therapy in pernicious anaemia. A Nobel lecture. Lancet. 1935;i:361–4.
12. Castle WB. Observations on the etiologic relationship of achylia gastrica to pernicious anaemia. I. The effect of the administration to patients with pernicious anaemia of the

contents of the normal human stomach recovered after the ingestion of beef muscle. Am J Med Sci. 1929;178:748–64.

13. Castle WB, Townsend WC. Observations on the etiologic relationship of achylia gastrica to pernicious anaemia. II. Effect of the administration to patients with pernicious anaemia of beef muscle after incubation with normal human gastric juice. Am J Med Sci. 1929;178:764–77.
14. Smith EL. Purification of anti-pernicious anaemia factors from liver. Nature. 1948;161:638–9.
15. Rickes EL, Brink NG, Koniuszy FR, Wood TR, Folkers K. Crystalline vitamin B_{12}. Science. 1948;107:396–7.
16. Hodgkin DC, Kamper J, Mackay M, Pickworth J, Trueblood KN. Structure of vitamin B_{12}. Nature. 1956;178:64–6.
17. Ross GIM. Vitamin B_{12} assay in body fluids. Nature. 1950;166:270–1.
18. Allen RH, Mehlman CS. Isolation of gastric vitamin B_{12}-binding proteins using affinity chromatography. I. Purification and properties of human intrinsic factor. J Biol Chem. 1973; 248:3660–9.
19. Schilling RF. Intrinsic factor studies. II. The effect of gastric juice on the urinary excretion of radioactivity after the oral administration of radioactive vitamin B_{12}. J Lab Clin Med. 1953; 42:860–6.
20. Schwartz M. Intrinsic-factor-inhibiting substance in serum of orally treated patients with pernicious anaemia. Lancet. 1958;ii:61–2.
21. Taylor KB. Inhibition of intrinsic factor by pernicious sera. Lancet. 1959; ii:106–8.
22. Schwartz M. Intrinsic factor antibody in serum from patients with pernicious anaemia. Lancet. 1960;ii:1263–7.
23. Jeffries GH, Hoskins HW, Sleisenger MH. Antibody to intrinsic factor in serum from patients with pernicious anaemia. J Clin Invest. 1962;41:1106–15.
24. Ardeman S, Chanarin I. Method for assay of human gastric intrinsic factor and for detection and titration of antibodies against intrinsic factor. Lancet. 1963;ii:1350–4.
25. Irvine WJ, Davies SH, Delamore IW, Williams AW. Immunological relationship between pernicious anaemia and thyroid disease. Br Med J. 1962;2:254–6.
26. Markson JL, Moore JM. Autoimmunity in pernicious anaemia and iron deficiency anaemia. Lancet. 1962;ii:1240–3.
27. Taylor KB, Roitt IM, Doniach D, Couchman KG, Shapland C. Autoimmune phenomena in pernicious anaemia: gastric antibodies. Br Med J. 1962;2:1347–52.
28. Irvine WJ. Gastric antibodies studied by fluorescence microscopy. Quart J Exp Physiol. 1963; 48:427–38.
29. Doniach D, Roitt IM. An evaluation of gastric and thyroid auto-immunity in relation to hematologic disorders. Semin Hematol. 1964;1:313–43.
30. Irvine WJ. Immunologic aspects of pernicious anaemia. N Engl J Med. 1965;273:432–9.
31. Samloff MI, Kleinman MS, Turner MD, Sobel MV, Jeffries GH. Blocking and binding antibodies to intrinsic factor and parietal cell antibody in pernicious anaemia. Gastroenterology. 1968;55:575–83.
32. Fisher JM, Rees C, Taylor KB. Antibodies in gastric juice. Science. 1965; 150:1467–9.
33. Jeffries GH, Sleisenger MH. Studies of parietal cell antibody in pernicious anaemia. J Clin Invest. 1965;44:2021–8.
34. Rose MS, Chanarin I. Dissociation of intrinsic factor from its antibody: application to study of pernicious anaemia gastric juice specimens. Br Med J. 1969;1:468–70.
35. Strickland RG, Baur S, Ashworth LAE, Taylor KB. A correlative study of immunological phenomena in pernicious anaemia. Clin Exp Immunol. 1971;8:25–36.
36. Helander H. Physiology and pharmacology of the parietal cell. Baillières Clin Gastroenterol. 1988;2:539–54.
37. Meuwissen SG, Mullink H, Bosma A et al. Immunocytochemical localization of pepsinogen I and II in the human stomach. In: Pepsinogens in man: Clinical and Genetic Advances. New York: Alan R Liss, Inc.; 1985:185–97.
38. Smolka A, Donaldson RM. Monoclonal antibodies to human intrinsic factor. Gastroenterology. 1990;98:607–14.
39. Alpers DH, Becich MJ, Tang L-H, Gordon MM, Simpson KW. Intrinsic factor. In: Bhatt HR, James VHT, Besser GM, Bottazzo HF, Keen H, eds. Advances in Thomas Addison's Diseases. Bristol: Journal of Endocrinology Ltd; 1994;2:287–92.

40. Hoedemaeker PJ, Abels J, Wachters JJ, Arends A, Nieweg HO. Further investigations about the site of production of Castle's intrinsic factor. Lab Invest. 1966;15:1163–73.
41. Simpson KW, Alpers DH, De Wille J, Swanson P, Farmer S, Sherding RG. Cellular localization and hormonal regulation of pancreatic intrinsic factor secretion in dogs. Am J Physiol. 1993;265:G178–88.
42. Johnson LR. Regulation of gastrointestinal growth. In: Johnson LR, ed. Physiology of the Gastrointestinal Tract. New York: Raven Press; 1987:131–42.
43. Brand SJ, Stone D. Reciprocal regulation of antral gastrin and somatostatin gene expression by omeprazole-induced achlorhydria. J Clin Invest. 1988;82:1059–66.
44. Simonsson M, Eriksson S, Håkansson R et al. Endocrine cells in human oxyntic mucosa. A histochemical study. Scand J Gastroenterol. 1988;23:1089–99.
45. Forte TM, Machen RE, Forte JG. Ultrastructural changes in oxyntic cells associated with secretory function: a membrane recycling hypothesis. Gastroenterology. 1977;73:941–55.
46. Smolka A, Helander HF, Sachs G. Monoclonal antibodies against the gastric (H^+,K^+)-ATPase. Am J Physiol. 1984;245:G589–96.
47. Urushidani T, Forte J. Stimulation-associated redistribution of H^+,K^+-ATPase activity in isolated gastric glands. Am J Physiol. 1987;252;G458–65.
48. Sachs G, Chang HH, Rabon E, Schackman R, Lewin M, Saccomani G. A non electrogenic H^+ pump in plasma membrane of hog stomach. J Biol Chem. 1976;251:7690–8.
49. Sachs G, Hersey SJ. The gastric parietal cell. Its clinical relevance in the management of acid-related diseases. Oxford: Oxford Clinical Communications: AB Astra, 1990.
50. Maeda M, Oshiman K-I, Tamura S, Futai M. Human gastric (H^+,K^+)-ATPase gene. J Biol Chem. 1990;265:9027–32.
51. Newman PR, Greeb J, Keeton TP, Reyes AA, Shull GE. Structure of the human gastric H,K-ATPase gene and comparison of the 5′-flanking sequences of the human and rat genes. DNA Cell Biol. 1990;9:749–62.
52. Shull GE, Linrel JB. Molecular cloning of the rat stomach (H^+-K^+)-ATPase. J Biol Chem. 1986;261:16788–91.
53. Maeda M, Ishiaki J, Futai M. cDNA cloning and sequence determination of pig gastric (H^+,K^+)-ATPase. Biochem Biophys Res Commun.1988;157:203–9.
54. Bamberg K, Mercier F, Reuben MA, Kobayashi Y, Munson KB, Sachs G. cDNA cloning and membrane topology of the rabbit gastric H^+/K^+-ATPase α-subunit. Biochim Biophys Acta. 1992;1131:69–77.
55. Song II, Mortell MP, Gantz I, Brown DR, Yamada T. Molecular cloning and structural analysis of canine gastric H^+,K^+-ATPase. Biochem Biophys Res Commun. 1993;196:1240–7.
56. Mathews PM, Claeys D, Jaisser F et al. Primary structure and functional expression of the mouse and frog α-subunit of the gastric H^+-K^+-ATPase. Am J Physiol. 1995;268:C1207–14.
57. Callaghan JM, Toh B-H, Pettitt JM, Humphris DC, Gleeson PA. Poly-N-acetyllactosamine-specific tomato lectin interacts with gastric parietal cells. Identification of a tomato-lectin binding 60–90 × 10^3 Mr membrane glycoprotein of tubulovesicles. J Cell Sci. 1990;95:563–76.
58. Hall K, Perez G, Anderson D et al. Location of the carbohydrates present in the HK-ATPase vesicles isolated from hog gastric mucosa. Biochemistry. 1990;29:701–6.
59. Okamoto CT, Karpilow JM, Smolka A, Forte JG. Isolation and characterization of gastric microsomal glycoproteins. Evidence for a glycosylated β-subunit of the H^+,K^+-ATPase. Biochim Biophys Acta. 1990;1037:362–72.
60. Shull GE. cDNA cloning of the β-subunit of the rat gastric H,K-ATPase. J Biol Chem. 1990; 265:12123–6.
61. Canfield VA, Dkamoto CT, Chow DC et al. Cloning of the H,K-ATPase β-subunit. Tissue-specific expression, chromosomal assignment, and relationship to Na,K-ATPase β-subunit. J Biol Chem. 1990;265:19878–84.
62. Toh B-H, Gleeson PA, Simpson RJ et al. The 60- to 90-kDa parietal cell autoantigen associated with autoimmune gastritis is a β subunit of the gastric H^+/K^+-ATPase (proton pump). Proc Natl Acad Sci USA. 1990;87:6418–22.
63. Reuben MA, Lasater LS, Sachs G. Characterization of a β subunit of the gastric H^+/K^+-transporting ATPase. Proc Natl Acad Sci USA. 1990;87: 6767–71.
64. Ma JY, Song YH, Sjöstrand SE, Rask L, Mårdh S. cDNA cloning of the β-subunit of the human gastric H,K-ATPase. Biochem Biophys Res Commun. 1991;180:39–45.
65. Morley GP, Callaghan JM, Rose JB, Toh BH, Gleeson PA, Driel IRV. The mouse gastric H,K-ATPase β subunit. J Biol Chem. 1992;267:1165–74.

66. Yu H, Ishii T, Pearson WR, Takeyasu K. Primary structure of avian H^+/K^+-ATPase β-subunit. Biochim Biophys Acta. 1994;1190:189–92.
67. Newman PR, Shull GE. Rat gastric H,K-ATPase β-subunit gene: intron/exon organization, identification of multiple transcription initiation sites, and analysis of the 5′-flanking region. Genomics. 1991;11:252–62.
68. Maeda M, Oshiman KI, Tamura S, Kaya S, Mahmood S. The rat H^+/K^+-ATPase β subunit gene and recognition of its control region by gastric DNA binding protein. J Biol Chem. 1991;266:21584–8.
69. Canfield VA, Levenson R. Structural organization and transcription of the mouse gastric H^+,K^+-ATPase β subunit gene. Proc Natl Acad Sci USA. 1991;88:8247–51.
70. Song II, Brown DR, Yamada T, Trent JM. Mapping of the gene encoding the β-subunit of H^+,K^+-ATPase to human chromosome 13q34 by fluorescence in situ hybridization. Genomics. 1992;14:1114–5.
71. Chow DC, Browning CM, Forte JG. Gastric H^+-K^+-ATPase activity is inhibited by reduction of disulfide bonds in β-subunit. Am J Physiol. 1992;32:C39–C46.
72. Donaldson RM. Intrinsic factor and transport of cobalamin. In: Johnson LR, ed. Physiology of the Gastrointestinal Tract. Second Edition, New York: Raven Press; 1987:959–73.
73. Antony AC. Megaloblastic anaemias. In: Hoffman R, Benz EJ Jr, Shattil SJ, Furie B, Cohen HJ, eds. Hematology. Basic Principles and Practice. New York: Churchill Livingstone; 1991: 392–421.
74. Dieckgraefe BK, Seetharam B, Banaszak L, Leykam JF, Alpers DH. Isolation and structural characterization of a cDNA clone encoding rat gastric intrinsic factor. Proc Natl Acad Sci USA. 1988;85:46–50.
75. Hewitt JE, Gordon MM, Taggart RT, Mohandas TK, Alpers DH. Human gastric intrinsic factor: characterization of cDNA and genomic clones and localization to human chromosome 11. Genomics. 1991;10:432–40.
76. Strickland RG, Mackay IR. A Reappraisal of the nature and significance of chronic atrophic gastritis. Dig Dis. 1973;18:426–39.
77. Vandelli C, Bottazzo GF, Doniach D, Franceschi F. Autoantibodies to gastrin-producing cells in antral (Type B) chronic gastritis. N Engl J Med. 1979;300:1406–10.
78. Uibo R, Krohn K. Demonstration of gastrin cell autoantibodies in antral gastritis with avidin-biotin complex antibody technique. Clin Exp Immunol. 1984;58:341–7.
79. Ganguli PC, Cullen DR, Irvine WJ. Radioimmunoassay of plasma gastrin in pernicious anaemia. Lancet. 1971;ii:155–8.
80. McGuigan JE, Trudeau WL. Serum gastrin concentrations in pernicious anaemia. N Engl J Med. 1970;282:358–61.
81. Stockbrugger R, Larsson L-I, Lundquist G, Angervall L. Antral gastrin cells and serum gastrin in achlorhydria. Scand J Gastroenterol. 1977;12:209–13.
82. Strickland RG, Bhathal PS, Korman MG, Hansky J. Serum gastrin and the antral mucosa in atrophic gastritis. Br Med J. 1971;4:451–3.
83. Varis K, Samloff IM, Ihamaki T, Siurala M. An appraisal of tests for severe atrophic gastritis in relatives of patients with pernicious anaemia. Dig Dis Sci. 1979;24:187–91.
84. Borch K, Axelsson CK, Halgreen H, Damkjaer Nielsen M, Ledin T, Szesci PP. The ratio of pepsinogen A to pepsinogen C: a sensitive test for atrophic gastritis. Scand J Gastroenterol. 1989;24:870–6.
85. Burman P, Karlsson FA, Lööf L, Szesci PB, Borch K. H^+,K^+-ATPase antibodies in autoimmune gastritis: observations on the development of pernicious anaemia. Scand J Gastroenterol. 1991;26:207–14.
86. Cheli R, Perasso A, Giacosa A. Chronic gastritis. Immunological mechanisms. In: Cheli R, Perasso A, Giacosa A, eds. Gastritis – A Critical Review. Berlin: Springer-Verlag; 1987:98–109.
87. Kaye MD. Immunological aspects of gastritis and pernicious anaemia. Baillières Clin Gastroenterol. 1987;1:487–506.
88. Ungar B, Whittingham S, Francis CM. Pernicious anaemia: incidence and significance of circulating antibodies to intrinsic factor and to parietal cells. Aust Ann Med. 1967;16:226–9.
89. Davidson RJL, Atrah HI, Sewell HF. Longitudinal study of circulating gastric antibodies in pernicious anaemia. J Clin Pathol. 1989;42:1092–5.
90. Burman P, Kämpe O, Kraaz W et al. A study of autoimmune gastritis in the postpartum period and at a 5-year follow-up. Gastroenterology. 1992;103:934–42.

91. Irvine WJ, Mawhinney H, Cullen DR. Natural history of autoimmune achlorhydric atrophic gastritis. Lancet. 1974;ii:482–5.
92. Wood IJ, Ralston M, Ungar B, Cowling DC. Vitamin B_{12} deficiency in chronic gastritis. Gut. 1964;5:27–37.
93. Siurala M, Varis K, Wiljasalo M. Studies of patients with atrophic gastritis: a 10–15-year follow-up. Scand J Gastroenterol. 1966;1:40–8.
94. Rose MS, Chanarin I, Doniach D, Brostoff J, Ardeman S. Intrinsic-factor antibodies in absence of pernicious anaemia. Lancet. 1970;ii:9–12.
95. Carmel R. Pernicious anaemia. The expected findings of very low serum cobolamin levels, anaemia, and macrocytosis are often lacking. Arch Intern Med. 1988;148:1712–4.
96. Lindenbaum J, Healton EB, Savage DG et al. Neuropsychiatric disorders caused by cobolamin deficiency in the absence of anaemia or macrocytosis. N Engl J Med. 1988;318: 1720–8.
97. Carmel R. Prevalence of undiagnosed pernicious anaemia in the elderly. Arch Intern Med. 1996;156:1097–100.
98. Joosten E, Pelemans W, Devos P et al. Cobalamin absorption and serum homocysteine and methylmalonic acid in elderly subjects with low serum cobalamin. Eur J Haematol. 1993;51: 25–30.
99. Naurath HJ, Joosten E, Riezler R, Stabler SP, Allen RH, Lindenbaum J. Effects of vitamin B_{12}, folate, and vitamin B6 supplements in elderly people with normal serum vitamin concentrations. Lancet. 1995;346:85–9.
100. Colon-Otero G, Wheby MS. Disorders of cobalamin and folate metabolism. In: Thorup OA Jr, ed. Fundamentals of Clinical Hematology, 5th edn. Philadelphia: WB Saunders; 1987: 185–211.
101. Weir DG, Scott JM. The biochemical basis of the neuropathy in cobalamin deficiency. Baillières Clin Hematol. 1995;8:479–97.
102 Reynolds EH, Linnell JC. Vitamin B_{12} deficiency, demyelination, and multiple sclerosis. Lancet. 1987;ii:920.
103. Ransohoff RM, Jacobsen DW, Green R. Vitamin B_{12} deficiency and multiple sclerosis. Lancet. 1990;335:125–6 (letter).
104. Kandler RH, Davies-Jones GAB. Internuclear ophthalmoplegia in pernicious anaemia. Br Med J. 1988;297:1583.
105. Hector MH, Burton JR. What are the psychiatric manifestations of vitamin B_{12} deficiency? J Am Geriatr Soc. 1988;36:1105–12.
106. Regland B. Low B_{12} levels related to high activity of platelet MAO in patients with dementia disorders. Acta Psychiatr Scand. 1988;78:451–7.
107. Kristensen MO, Gulmann NC, Christensen JE, Ostergaard K, Rasumssen K. Serum cobalamin and methylmalonic acid in Alzheimer dementia. Acta Neurologica Scand. 1993; 87:475–81.
108. Nexø E, Hansen M, Rasmussen K, Lindgren A, Gräsbeck R. How to diagnose cobalamin deficiency. Scand J Clin Lab Invest. 1994;54 (Suppl 219):61–76.
109. Green R. Metabolite assays in cobolamin and folate deficiency. Baillières Clin Hematol. 1995;8:533–66.
110. Matchar DB, McCrory DC, Millington DS, Feussner JR. Performance of the serum cobalamin assay for diagnosis of cobalamin deficiency. Am J Med Sci. 1994;308:276–83.
111. Pennypacker LC, Allen RH, Kelly JP et al. High prevalence of cobalamin deficiency in elderly outpatients. J Am Geriatr Soc. 1992;40:1197–204.
112. Villako K, Siurala M. The behaviour of gastritis and related conditions in different populations. Ann Clin Res. 1981;13:114–8.
113. Borch K, Liedberg G. Prevalence and incidence of pernicious anaemia. Scand J Gastroenterol.1984;19:154–6.
114. Chanarin I. Pernicious anaemia as an autoimmune disease. Br J Haematol (Suppl). 1972;238: 101–7.
115. Varis K, Ihamäki T, Härkönen M, Samloff IM, Siurala M. Gastric morphology, function and immunology in first-degree relatives of probands with pernicious anaemia and controls. Scand J Gastroenterol. 1979;14:129–39.
116. Irvine WJ. Autoimmunity in endocrine disease. Rec Progr Horm Res. 1980;36:509–56.
117. Furszyfer J, McConahey WM, Kurland LT, Maldonado JE. On the increased association of Graves' disease with pernicious anaemia. Mayo Clin Proc. 1971;46:37–9.

118. Schiller KFR, Spray GH, Wangel AG, Wright R. Clinical and precursory forms of pernicious anaemia in hyperthyroidism. Q J Med. 1968;147:451–62.
119. Irvine WJ. The association of atrophic gastritis with autoimmune thyroid disease. Clinics in Endocrinol Metab. 1975;4:351–77.
120. Tudhope GR, Wilson GM. Deficiency of vitamin B_{12} in hypothyroidism. Lancet. 1962;i:703–6.
121. Blizzard RM, Chee D, Davis W. The incidence of adrenal and other antibodies in the sera of patients with idiopathic insufficiency (Addison's disease). Clin Exp Immunol. 1967;2:19–30.
122. Winqvist O, Söderbergh A, Norheim I et al. Adrenal autoantibodies, adrenal function and organ-specific autoimmunity in patients with Addison's disease receiving replacement therapy. In: Comprehensive Summaries of Uppsala Dissertations from the Faculty of Medicine; 1994:505.
123. Zauli D, Tosti A, Biasco G et al. Prevalence of autoimmune atrophic gastritis in vitiligo. Digestion. 1986;34:169–72.
124. Blizzard RM, Chee D, Davis W. The incidence of parathyroid and other antibodies in sera of patients with idiopathic hypoparathyroidism. Clin Exp Immunol. 1966;1:119–28.
125. Ungar B, Stocks AE, Martin FIR, Whittingham S, Mackay IR. Intrinsic-factor antibody, parietal-cell antibody, and latent pernicious anaemia in diabetes mellitus. Lancet. 1968;ii: 415–18.
126. Riley WJ, Toskes PP, Maclaren NK, Silverstein JH. Predictive value of gastric parietal cell autoantibodies as a marker for gastric and hematologic abnormalities associated with insulin-dependent diabetes. Diabetes. 1982;31:1051–5.
127. Landin-Olsson M, Karlsson A, Dahlquist G et al. Islet cell and other organ-specific autoantibodies in all children developing Type I (insulin-dependent) diabetes mellitus in Sweden during one year and in matched control children. Diabetologica. 1989;32:387–95.
128. Hooper B, Whittingham S, Mathews JD, Mackay IR, Curnow DH. Autoimmunity in a rural community. Clin Exp Immunol. 1972;12:79–87.
129. Bauer S, Roitt IM, Doniach D. Characterization of the human gastric parietal cell autoantigen. Immunology. 1965;8:62–8.
130. Hoedemaeker PJ, Ito S. Ultrastructural localization of gastric parietal cell antigen with peroxidase-coupled antibody. Lab Invest. 1970;22:184–8.
131. Masala C, Smurra G, Di Prima MA, Amandolea MA, Celestino D, Salsano F. Gastric parietal cell antibodies: demonstration by immunofluorescence of their reactivity with the surface of the gastric parietal cells. Clin Exp Immunol. 1980;41:271–80.
132. De Aizpurua HJ, Cosgrave LJ, Ungar B, Toh B-H. Autoantibodies cytotoxic to gastric parietal cells in serum of patients with pernicious anaemia. N Engl J Med. 1983;309:625–9.
133. De Aizpurua HJ, Ungar B, Toh B-H. Autoantibody to the gastrin receptor in pernicious anaemia. N Engl J Med. 1985;313:479–83.
134. Dow CA, de Aizpurua HJ, Pedersen JS, Ungar B, Toh B-H. 65-70 kD protein identified by immunoblotting as the presumptive gastric microsomal autoantigen in pernicious anaemia. Clin Exp Immunol. 1985;62:732–7.
135. Mu F-T, Balwin G, Weinstock J, Stockman D, Toh B-H. Monoclonal antibody to the gastrin receptor on parietal cells recognizes a 78-kDa protein. Proc Natl Acad Sci USA. 1987;84: 2698–702.
136. Burman P, Mårdh S, Norberg L, Karlsson FA. Parietal cell antibodies in pernicious anaemia inhibit $H,^{+}K^{+}$-adenosine triphosphatase, the proton pump of the stomach. Gastroenterology. 1989;96:1434–8.
137. Smith JTL, Garner A, Hampson SE, Pounder RE. Absence of gastrin inhibitory factor in the IgG fraction of serum from patients with pernicious anaemia. Gut. 1990;31:871–4.
138. Karlsson FA, Burman P, Lööf L, Mårdh S. The major parietal cell antigen in autoimmune gastritis with pernicious anaemia is the acid-producing H^{+},K^{+}-ATPase of the stomach. J Clin Invest. 1988;81:475–9.
139. Goldkorn I, Gleeson PA, Toh B-H. Gastric parietal cell antigens of 60–90, 92, and 100–120 kDa associated with autoimmune gastritis and pernicious anaemia. J Biol Chem. 1989;264: 18768–74.
140. Ma JY, Borch K, Mårdh S. Human gastric H,K-adenosine triphosphate β-subunit is a major autoantigen in atrophic gastritis. Expression of the recombinant human glycoprotein in insect cells. Scand J Gastroenterol. 1994;29:790–4.

141. Callaghan JM, Khan MA, Alderuccio F, Van Driel IR, Gleeson PA, Toh B-H. α and β subunits of the gastric H^+,K^+-ATPase are concordantly targeted by parietal cell antibodies associated with autoimmune gastritis. Autoimmunity. 1993;16:289–95.
142. Wang XH, Miyazaki Y, Shinomura Y et al. Characterization of human autoantibodies reactive to gastric parietal cells. Biochem Biophys Res Commun. 1993;15:207–14.
143. Song YH, Ma JY, Mårdh S et al. Localization of a pernicious anaemia autoantibody epitope on the α-subunit of human H,K-adenosine triphosphatase. Scand J Gastroenterol. 1994;29: 122–7.
144. Abels J, Bouma W, Janz A, Wolring MG, Bakker MG, Nieweg HO. Experiments on the intrinsic factor antibody in serum of patients with pernicious anaemia. J Lab Clin Med. 1963; 61:893–906.
145. Roitt IM, Doniach D. Intrinsic factor autoantibodies. Lancet. 1964;ii:469–70.
146. Walder AI. Experimental achlorhydria: techniques of production with parietal cell antibody. Surgery. 1968;64:175–84.
147. Loveridge N, Bitensky L, Chayen J et al. Inhibition of parietal cell function by human gammaglobulin containing gastric parietal cell antibodies. Clin Exp Immunol. 1980;41: 264–70.
148. Tanaka N, Glass GBJ. Effect of prolonged administration of parietal cell antibodies from patients with atrophic gastritis and pernicious anaemia on the parietal cell mass and hydrochloric acid output in rats. Gastroenterology. 1970;58:482–94.
149. De Aizpurua HJ, Ungar B, Toh B-H. Serum from patients with pernicious anaemia blocks gastrin stimulation of acid secretion by parietal cells. Clin Exp Immunol. 1985;61:315–22.
150. Joplin R, Lindsay JG, Johnson GD, Strain A, Neuberger J. Membrane dihydrolipoamide acetyltransferase (E2) on human biliary epithelial cells in primary biliary cirrhosis. Lancet. 1992;339:93–4.
151. Solimena M, Dirkx Jr R, Hermel J-M et al. ICA 512, an autoantigen of type I diabetes, is an intrinsic membrane protein of neurosecretory granules. EMBO J. 1996;15:2102–14.
152. Hennes AR, Sevelius H, Lewellyn T, Joel W, Woods AH, Wolf S. Atrophic gastritis in dogs. Production by intradermal injection of gastric juice in Freund's adjuvant. Arch Path (Chic). 1962;73:281–7.
153. Andrada JA, Rose NR, Andrada EC. Experimental autoimmune gastritis in the rhesus monkey. Clin Exp Immunol. 1969;4:293–310.
154. Krohn KJE, Finlayson NDC. Interrelations of humoral and cellular immune responses in experimental canine gastritis. Clin Exp Immunol. 1973;14:237–45.
155. Kojima A, Prehn RT. Genetic susceptibility of postthymectomy autoimmune diseases in mice. Immunogenetics. 1981;14:15–27.
156. Sakaguchi S, Sakaguchi N. Organ-specific disease induced in mice by elimination of T cell subsets. V. Neonatal administration of cyclosporin A causes autoimmune disease. J Immunol. 1989;142:471–80.
157. Sakaguchi N, Miay K, Sakaguchi S. Ionizing radiation and autoimmunity. Induction of autoimmune disease by high dose fractionated total lymphoid irradiation and its prevention by inoculating normal T cells. J Immunol. 1994;152:2586–95.
158. Kojima A, Taguchi O, Nishizuka Y. Experimental production of possible autoimmune gastritis followed by macrocytic anaemia in athymic nude mice. Lab Invest. 1980;42:387–95.
159. Mori Y, Fukuma K, Adachi Y et al. Parietal cell autoantigens involved in thymectomy-induced murine autoimmune gastritis. Studies using monoclonal antibodies. Gastroenterology. 1989;97:364–75.
160. Jones CM, Callaghan JM, Gleeson PA, Mori Y, Masuda T, Toh B-H. The parietal cell autoantibodies recognized in neonatal thymectomy-induced murine gastritis are the α and β subunits of the gastric proton pump. Gastroenterology. 1991;101:287–94.
161. Kontani K, Taguchi O, Takahashi T. Involvement of the H^+,K^+-ATPase α subunit as a major antigenic protein in autoimmune gastritis induced by neonatal thymectomy in mice. Clin Exp Immunol. 1992;89:63–7.
162. Martinelli T M, van Driel IR, Alderuccio F, Gleeson PA, Toh BH. Analysis of mononuclear cell infiltrate and cytokine production in murine autoimmune gastritis. Gastroenterology. 1996;110:1791–802.
163. Fukuma K, Sakaguchi S, Kuribayashi K et al. Immunologic and clinical studies on murine experimental autoimmune gastritis induced by neonatal thymectomy. Gastroenterology. 1988;94:274–83.

164. Sakaguchi S, Takahashi T, Nishizuka Y. Study on cellular events in post-thymectomy autoimmune oophoritis in mice. I. Requirement of Lyt-1 effector cells for oocytes damage after adoptive transfer. J Exp Med. 1982;156:1565–76.
165. Sakaguchi S, Fukuma K, Kuribayashi K, Masuda T. Organ-specific autoimmune diseases induced in mice by elimination of a T cell subset. J Exp Med. 1985;161:72–87.
166. Nishio A, Hosono M, Watanabe Y, Sakai M, Okuma M, Masuda T. A conserved epitope on H^+,K^+-adenosine triphosphatase of parietal cells discerned by a murine gastritogenic T-cell clone. Gastroenterology. 1994;107:1408–14.
167. Suri-Payer E, Kehn PJ, Cheever AW, Shevach EM. Pathogenesis of post-thymectomy autoimmune gastritis. Identification of anti-H/K adenosine triphosphatase-reactive T cells. J Immunol. 1996;157:1799–805.
168. Doig A, Girdwood RH, Duthie JJR, Knox JDE. Response of megaloblastic anaemia to prednisolone. Lancet. 1957;ii:966–72.
169. Frost JW, Goldwein MI. Observations on vitamin B_{12} absorption in primary pernicious anaemia during administration of adrenocortical steroids. N Engl J Med. 1958;258:1096–8.
170. Ardeman S, Chanarin I. Steroids and addisonian pernicious anaemia. N Engl J Med. 1965; 273:1352–3.
171. Jeffries GJ, Todd JE, Sleisenger MH. The effect of prednisolone on gastric mucosal histology, gastric secretion, and vitamin B_{12} absorption in patients with pernicious anaemia. J Clin Invest. 1966;45:803–12.
172. Rødbro P, Dige-Petersen H, Schwartz M, Dalgaard OZ. Effects of steroids on gastric mucosal structure and function in pernicious anaemia during prednisolone therapy. Acta Med Scand. 1967;181:445–52.
173. Wall AJ, Whittingham S, Mackay IR, Ungar B. Prednisolone and gastric atrophy. Clin Exp Immunol. 1968;3:359–66.
174. Baggett RT, Welsh JD. Observations on the effects of glucocorticoid administration in pernicious anaemia. Am J Dig Dis. 1970;15:871–81.
175. Jorge AD, Sanchez D. The effect of azathioprine on gastric mucosal histology and acid secretion in chronic gastritis. Gut. 1973;14:104–6.
176. Murakami K, Maruyama H, Nishio A et al. Effects of intrathymic injection of organ-specific autoantigens, parietal cells, at the neonatal stage on autoreactive effector and suppressor T cell precursors. Eur J Immunol. 1993;23:809–14.
177. Alderuccio F, Toh BH, Tan SS, Gleeson PA, van Driel IR. An autoimmune disease with multiple molecular targets abrogated by the transgenic expression of a single autoantigen in the thymus. J Exp Med. 1993;178:419–26.
178. Sakaguchi S, Sakaguchi N. Thymus and autoimmunity: capacity of the normal thymus to produce self-reactive T cells and the conditions required for their induction of autoimmune disease. J Exp Med. 1990;172:537–45.
179. Morley GP, Callaghan JM, Rose JB, Toh BH, Gleeson PA, van Driel IR. The mouse gastric H,K-ATPase beta subunit. Gene structure and co-ordinate expression with the alpha subunit during ontogeny. J Biol Chem. 1992;267:1165–74.
180. Classen JB, Shevach EM. Post-thymectomy organ-specific autoimmunity: enhancement by cyclosporin A and inhibition by IL-2. Autoimmunity. 1993;15:55–9.

13 Vitiligo

D. J. GAWKRODGER

DEFINITION AND PREVALENCE

Vitiligo is an acquired idiopathic hypomelanotic disorder characterized by circumscribed depigmented macules. There is frequently a family history of the condition or of autoimmune endocrine disease. Vitiligo can lead to social embarrassment, psychological disturbance, and cosmetic disability.

Large population surveys have shown a prevalence of 0.4% in Denmark and 0.46% in Calcutta, India [1,2], although in certain subpopulations, the prevalence may be higher.

PATHOLOGY

Involved skin shows loss of functional melanocytes and of melanin in the epidermis (Figure 13.1). Electron microscopic and immunohistochemical studies using a variety of monoclonal and polyclonal antibodies confirm loss of melanocytes [3,4]. The epidermis of the areas around the margins of vitiligo shows degenerating melanocytes and abnormalities of keratinocytes [3]. Inflammatory vitiligo is characterized clinically be a raised erythematous border and, on histology, by a lymphohistiocytic infiltrate which may be found in non-inflamed marginal areas [5].

GENETICS

Familial cases of vitiligo are common, a family history being found in between 6 and 38% of cases [6]. An autosomal dominant pattern of inheritance with incomplete penetrance has been suggested [7]. Majumder and colleagues [8]

A.P. Weetman (ed.), Endocrine Autoimmunity and Associated Conditions. 269–284.

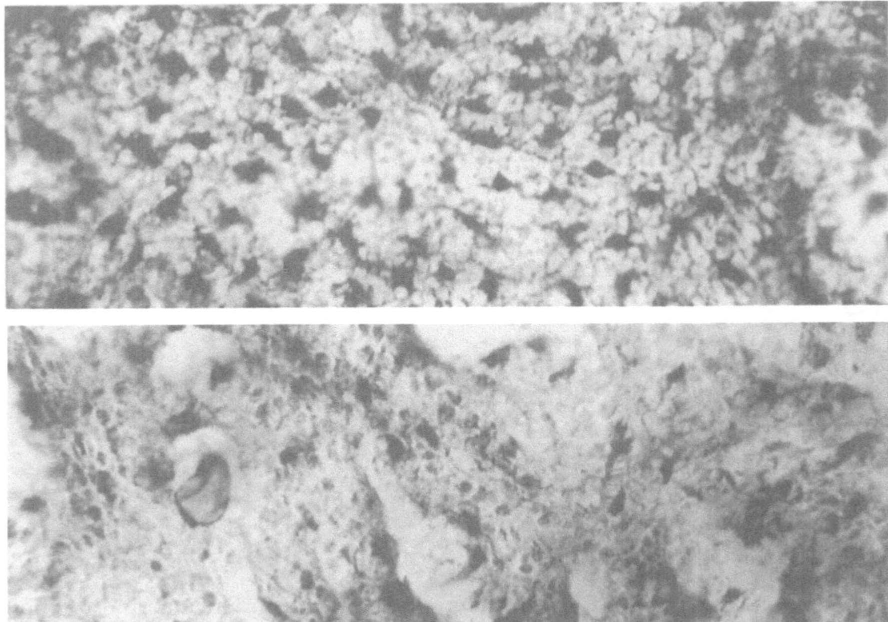

Figure 13.1 (a) Melanocytes in a sheet of normal epidermis, revealed by DOPA staining; (b) DOPA-positive melanocytes in an epidermal sheet from a patient with vitiligo, showing a much reduced cell density (courtesy of Professor S.S. Bleehen)

postulated a genetic model with recessive alleles at a set of four unlinked diallelic loci. In a study of 160 Caucasian kindreds in the USA, vitiligo affected a first-degree relative in 20% of cases [9]. The relative risk was calculated as 7 for patients, 12 for siblings, 36 for children and between 1 and 16 for second-degree relatives [9]. In this study, there was no significant association of vitiligo with thyroid disease.

A recent study of 131 patients with non-segmental vitiligo showed a family history in 22% [10]. Familial cases were associated with HLA-B46 whereas non-familial cases were associated with HLA-A31 and –Cw4. Different ethnic groups have different HLA phenotypic associations with vitiligo [1]. In 50 Omani patients with vitiligo, HLA-Bw6 was found in 66% of cases (compared to 49% of controls), and HLA-DR7 in 40% (compared to 9% of controls) [12]. All those who had a family history had consanguinous parents: all of these vitiligo patients were positive for HLA-Bw4 compared to a 48% prevalence in consanguinous patients with no family history. In 102 vitiligo patients from north Germany, significantly increased prevalences of HLA DRw12, HLA A2 and, in adults, HLA Bw60 were found [13].

A further study from the Netherlands showed a negative association of vitiligo with HLA-DR3, a positive association with HLA-DR4, and an increased frequency of heterozygous C4 and C2 deficiency [14]. In vitiligo patients, the frequency of one C4B*Q0 allele was three times higher than controls, and that of two other C4B**Q0 alleles was five times higher. Several autoimmune disorders are associated with homozygous or heterozygous deficiencies of C4 and C2 [15].

These findings suggest that, although a 'vitiligo gene' has not yet been discovered, certain C4B alleles and HLA associations may be risk factors in vitiligo.

ASSOCIATED DISORDERS

Vitiligo is frequently associated with autoimmune disease, for example with thyroid disease [16], pernicious anaemia [17], diabetes mellitus [3], Addison's disease [18], myasthenia gravis [19], alopecia areata [20], morphoea and lichen sclerosus [20,21], and autoimmune hypoparathyroidism [1].

In a case-matched study of 35 vitiligo patients from Denmark, six had hyperthyroidism and two had hypothyroidism compared with none of the 35 controls [22]. Nine patients had positive thyroid autoantibodies compared with two controls. An enlarged thyroid gland was found in six vitiligo patients and five controls. This study suggests that all vitiligo patients should be screened for thyroid disease. Confirmation is given by a German study of 321 vitiligo patients, in which the authors showed a 7.8% prevalence of thyroid disease, although an increase in other autoimmune disorders in this instance was not evident [23].

The occurrence of two or more endocrinopathies in a single patient generally indicates the autoimmune polyendocrine syndrome type 2 (APS), and this syndrome includes vitiligo (see Chapter 9). In a study of 224 patients with Addison's disease and APS type 2, 5% had vitiligo [24]. Vitiligo is also seen with the much more rare APS type 1. This usually has its onset in childhood and is often manifest as chronic mucocutaneous candidiasis and hypoparathyroidism followed, after 5–10 years, by Addison's disease. In two reported series of 71 and 45 patients with this condition, 8% and 13% respectively had vitiligo [24,25]. Vitiligo was present in two of 14 patients with type B insulin resistance, a syndrome characterized by autoantibodies against insulin receptors, insulin-resistant diabetes, acanthosis nigricans and autoimmune disorders including systemic lupus erythematosus and haemolytic anaemia [26].

Halo naevi (Figure 13.2) may be associated with and not frequently predate the onset of vitiligo [27]. Premature greying of the hair (canities), uveitis and ocular abnormalities may also be found in patients with vitiligo [28,29]. There is a suggestion that deafness may be more common [19]. The combination of vitiligo with uveitis, neurological involvement and canities is known as Vogt-Koyanagi syndrome [30]. Areas of depigmentation are sometimes found in patients with malignant melanoma [31].

An unusual but possibly important clinical observation is that the depigmented skin of vitiligo shows a reduced capacity for the induction and elicitation of the allergic contact dermatitis response, a form of type IV hypersensitivity [32].

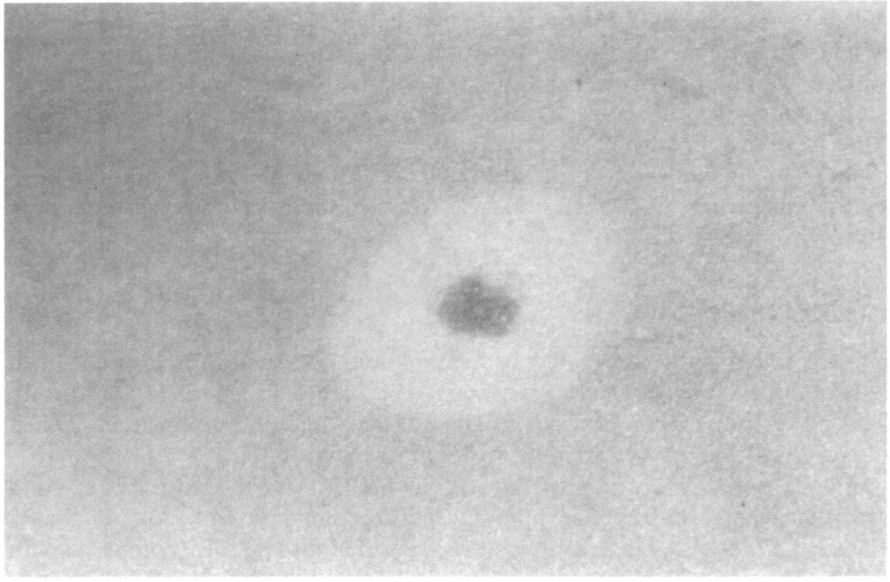

Figure 13.2 A halo naevus: an area of depigmentation is seen surrounding an involuting melanccytic naevus

THEORIES OF AETIOLOGY

The cause of the melanocyte destruction in vitiligo is not known and it is possible that there may be many more than one mechanism and that vitiligo is more than one disease [33,34]. Four theories have been proposed: autoimmune, self-destructive, neuronal and composite (the latter bringing together elements from the other three). In addition, it is recognized that loss of pigment, often identical to that seen with 'idiopathic' vitiligo, may be induced by exposure to certain chemicals.

The autoimmune theory is based on the clinical association of autoimmune diseases, the frequent finding of autoantibodies in the serum of patients with vitiligo, and the finding of antibodies to melanocytes in some patients with vitiligo (see below). The neuronal theory is supported by clinical observations, discussed below, as well as occasional case reports of sparing by vitiligo of denervated skin [35]. In addition, neuropeptide and neuronal marker abnormalities have been found in vitiligo skin [36]. The self-destructive theory suggests that melanocytes destroy themselves due to a defect in the natural protective mechanism that removes toxic melanin precursors [27].

The neuronal theory

Clinical evidence supporting this includes a segmental distribution in some patients, the symmetrical distribution of the common type, sparing below the level of neurological damage in certain patients who have suffered severe spinal cord injury, spontaneous repigmentation occasionally seen in patients with diabetic neuropathy, and an association with psychological stress. Other indirect evidence for the involvement of nerves includes the requirement for innervation for skin transplants to repigment an area, the known control over skin colour exerted by nerves in fish and reptiles, and the demonstration of abnormal levels of neuropeptides in the lesional skin of vitiligo patients.

Using immunohistochemistry of lesional and perilesional vitiligo skin sections it has been possible to identify abnormalities in skin neuropeptides [36]. Five of 10 patients with non-segmental symmetrical type vitiligo, including three with active disease, had increased activity against neuropeptide Y antibody in marginal areas (Figure 13.3), and three with active disease had positive findings in areas of lesional skin. Reactivity against vasoactive intestinal polypeptide was minimally increased, but substance P and calcitonin gene-related peptide were no different from control skin. Electron microscopy has also demonstrated regenerative and degenerative changes in dermal nerves in lesional and perilesional vitiligo skin [37].

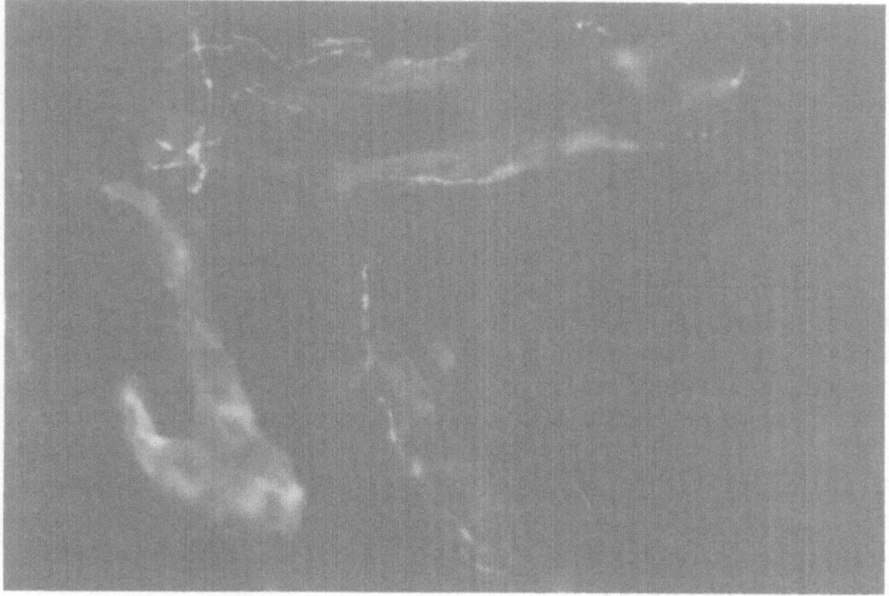

Figure 13.3 Neuropeptide Y around blood vessels is increased in perilesional and lesional vitiligo skin (immunohistochemical stain: courtesy of the editor of the British Journal of Dermatology [36])

Further evidence for a neural component to vitiligo comes from the finding that met-enkephalin and β-endorphin oscillations are no longer circadian in patients with the condition [38].

The self-destructive theory

This hypothesis is based on experimental studies and on clinical observations of patients exposed to certain chemical compounds who develop a pattern of depigmentation which is indistinguishable from vitiligo. It has been suggested that, in vitiligo, melanocytes destroy themselves due to a defect of a natural protective mechanism that removes toxic melanin precursors [27]. Mercapto-amines and other compounds that have a selective lethal effect on functioning melanocytes can cause cutaneous depigmentation [39]. The resulting leuko-derma, as seen clinically in occupational vitiligo (see below), is indistinguishable from idiopathic vitiligo.

Recently, attention has been focussed on catecholamine metabolism in vitiligo. Noradrenaline levels are increased in the plasma and epidermis of vitiligo patients [40] and, in lesional vitiligo skin, catechol-*o*-methyl transferase (COMT) is increased [41]. COMT is the enzyme that methylates catecholamines, thereby inactivating these potentially cytotoxic compounds, and a rise in this enzyme may indicate an elevated amount of catecholamines in vitiligo skin. Studies on the regulation of catecholamines led to the discovery that the cofactor, (6R)-5,6,7,8-tetrahydrobiopterin, is fundamentally involved in the regulation of melanin biosynthesis [42]. This cofactor is rate-limiting for the production of L-tyrosine from L-phenylalanine by phenylalanine hydroxylase, and for the formation of L-DOPA from L-tyrosine.

Schallreuter and colleagues [42] have demonstrated that biopterins accumulate in the involved and uninvolved epidermis of patients with vitiligo, and suggest that this build-up is due to *de novo* synthesis and defective recycling. A consequence of this is an accumulation of hydrogen peroxide and the non-enzymatic by-product 7-tetrahydrobiopterin, a potent inhibitor of phenylalanine hydroxylase in keratinocytes and melanocytes. In addition, levels of catalase are very low in vitiligo epidermis [43]. Defective catecholamine biosynthesis in vitiligo epidermis may lead to the formation of hydrogen peroxide which cannot be cleared because of low catalase levels, resulting in cytotoxic concentrations of hydrogen peroxide and destruction of the melanocyte. This has led to the suggested treatment of vitiligo with a pseudocatalase [44].

The autoimmune theory

The main supportive evidence for this hypothesis is the clinical association with disorders considered to be autoimmune in origin and the finding of circulating organ-specific antibodies more commonly than in the general population. Specific immune responses have also been detected.

Autoantibodies

Circulating anti-melanocyte antibodies have been demonstrated in patients with vitiligo [45], demonstrating an alteration in specific immunity to melanocytes [46]. A correlation has been described between the incidence and level of pigment cell antibodies and disease activity in vitiligo [47]. Antimelanocyte antibodies were found in the serum of 57% of 56 patients with vitiligo and in 6% of 47 controls [48]. Those patients with active disease were more likely to have antibodies than those whose disease was inactive. The antibodies were most commonly directed against antigens with molecular weights of 40–45 kDa, 75 kDa and 90 kDa and were found in 74%, 57% and 35% of vitiligo subjects respectively. Vitiligo patients also have autoantibodies to keratinocytes, but cytotoxicity has not been shown *in vitro* and these antibodies could arise secondarily to cellular damage [49]. In fact, keratinocytes from vitiligo skin, especially marginal areas, may show ultrastructural changes such as disturbed expression of cytokeratins, although the exact significance of these is unclear [50].

In a model using human skin grafted onto nude mice, it has been shown that autoantibodies from the sera of vitiligo patients can destroy melanocytes *in vivo* [51]. There is recent evidence that tyrosinase may be the target for autoantibodies in vitiligo [52]. Sera from 20 of 26 patients with vitiligo and type 2 APS had antibodies specific for a 69 kDa protein in HTB-70 human melanoma cells, which proved to be tyrosinase. This finding has yet to be confirmed.

T cell immunity

There is also evidence for the involvement of cell-mediated immunity. A dermal T cell infiltrate has been described in skin biopsies from areas of vitiligo [53]. An accumulation of $CD3^+$, $CD4^+$ and $CD8^+$ T lymphocytes has been described in the epidermis and upper dermis in vitiligo [54] and many of the infiltrating lymphocytes express the IL-2 receptor [55]. Cytotoxicity responses from natural killer and lymphokine-active killer cells in patients with vitiligo are no different from those in controls [56], and these cells are probably not responsible for the melanocyte destruction.

Langerhans cells

The Langerhans cells in the depigmented areas of vitiligo are thought to be functionally impaired [57]. The number of Langerhans cells within the depigmented areas of vitiligo is normal although a modest increase has been found in perilesional (marginal) areas [58]. In depigmented vitiligo skin there is impairment of migration of $CD\text{-}1^+$ Langerhans cells from the epidermis, following the injection of interferon-γ, in comparison to pigmented skin [57]. This defective migration may explain the reduced capacity for vitiligo skin to show an allergic contact dermatitis response as the Langerhans cells have to migrate from the epidermis to the regional lymph nodes for this response to occur.

Adhesion molecules and class II antigens

Recent studies have shown expression of intercellular adhesion molecule-1 (ICAM-1) by keratinocytes and melanocytes (in 13 of 21 cases) in areas of vitiligo [59,60]. In one study, the expression of ICAM-1 by melanocytes at the edge of vitiligo lesions was found to be increased six-fold, and was present in 19 of 20 biopsies from perilesional skin, compared to six of seven biopsies from non-lesional skin and five of eight samples from control skin [60]. Similar abnormal expression of HLA-DR and ICAM-1 is shown by the pancreatic islet cells in type I diabetes mellitus [61] and by the thyroid follicular cells in autoimmune thyroid disease [62], as discussed in Chapters 3 and 8.

The adhesion receptor E-cadherin is important for the adhesion of melanocytes to keratinocytes [63], but has not as yet been specifically studied in vitiligo.

Cytokines, matrices and melanocyte migration

Leukotriene C_4 and transforming growth factor-α enhance melanocyte migration *in vitro* [64]. Melanocytes migrate preferentially over a matrix containing type IV collagen, and their migration is blocked by antibodies to α_2- and α_3- but not α_5-integrin [65]. Proteins in the extracellular matrix also have an effect on the activity of tyrosinase in cultured melanocytes [66].

These observations in vitiligo strongly support the concept of the involvement of immune mechanisms specifically directed against the melanocyte in the aetiopathogenesis of the disease. There are now animal models of vitiligo, in the mouse and in the Smyth chicken [67,68], which may allow further study of autoimmunity in vitiligo.

CHEMICALLY-INDUCED VITILIGO

Depigmentation due to a chemical was first reported in 1939 when tannery workers in Chicago were found to have loss of pigment of the skin on their forearms and the dorsal aspects of their hands [69]. The operators thought that rubber gloves were to blame. It was discovered that monobenzylether of hydroquinone, added to the rubber to make it more durable, was responsible.

The substituted phenols are destructive to functional melanocytes. Many of these compounds cause permanent depigmentation of the skin similar to that seen in idiopathic vitiligo. The chemicals most commonly responsible are para-tertiary butyl phenol, para-tertiary butyl catechol, monobenzyl ether of hydroquinone, hydroquinone and related compounds. The depigmentary effect of the phenolic compounds is thought to be by a toxic mechanism on the melanocyte. It is proposed that the chemical requirement for depigmentation is the hydroxyl group in the 4 position with a nonpolar side group in the 1 position. Alkyl phenols are chemically similar to tyrosine and may be oxidized by tyrosinase to give rise to a free radical derivative which is highly toxic to the melanocyte.

p-Tertiary butylphenol was recognized as causing leukoderma in the 1960s

[70] and has caused occupational vitiligo in workers who manufacture *p*-tertiary butylphenol formaldehyde resin, in shoe manufacturers, and after contact with cleaning fluid: *p*-tertiary butylcatechol is a similar agent [71]. It has been used as an antioxidant in oils and is a contaminant in coal tar distillation.

CLINICAL PRESENTATION

Vitiligo is characterized by loss of pigment from the skin and hair, and is often manifested as macular areas of white skin.

Onset and progression

Vitiligo can begin at any age but in 50% it develops before the age of 20 years. It is usually slowly progressive although there may be quite long intervals when the disease is static and other times when it progresses in fits and starts. Occasionally vitiligo shows rapid progression. When it starts in a child, vitiligo is more likely to be segmental than in adult cases. A history of severe sunburn or emotional or physical stress preceding the onset of vitiligo is found in 20% of cases [72].

Bilateral/symmetrical type

The hypopigmented macules are often first noticed on the sun-exposed and sunburn-prone sites of the face or dorsal aspects of the hands (Figure 13.4). Hypopigmented macules may be found on areas that are normally hyperpigmented, e.g. the face, axillae, groins, areolae and genitalia. The distribution of the lesions is normally symmetrical but sometimes vitiligo occurs unilaterally or in a segmental or dermatomal distribution.

Unilateral/segmental type

Unilateral and bilateral vitiligo differ in several respects apart from their distribution (Figure 13.5). In unilateral vitiligo there is an earlier age of onset and associated autoimmune diseases are less likely [73]. Vitiligo involving the near entirity of the skin surface may occur but is very rare.

Trichrome vitiligo

In a vitiligo macule, the pigment loss may be partial or complete, or there can be both partial and complete in the same area ('trichrome' vitiligo). The macules have a convex outline and, as they progress, fuse with neighbouring lesions to form complex patterns. Hair in involved patches may remain normally pigmented but ultimately can depigment. Normally pigmented skin adjacent to an area of vitiligo may become hyperpigmented.

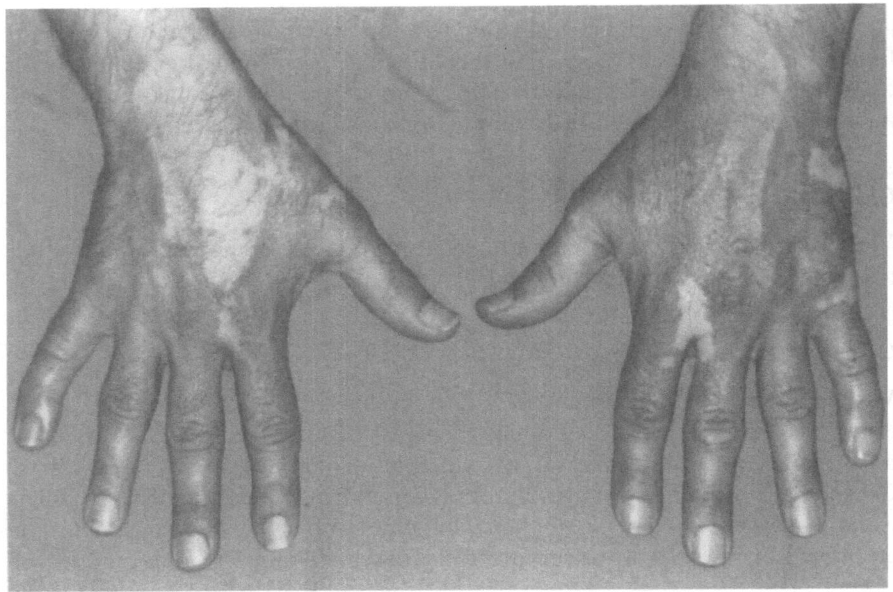

Figure 13.4 Bilateral symmetrical vitiligo on the dorsal aspects of the hands

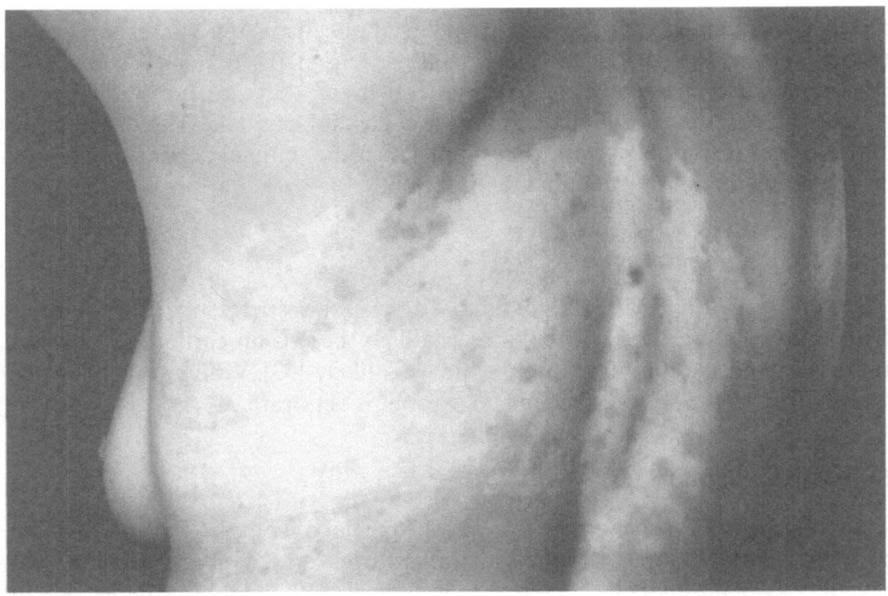

Figure 13.5 Unilateral segmental type vitiligo, affecting one side of the back

Spontaneous repigmentation

Spontaneous repigmentation, which is often perifollicular, is seen in 10–20% of cases, most frequently in sun-exposed sites and more commonly in children. Trauma to the skin in subjects with vitiligo frequently leads to the development of depigmentation in the damaged area, an occurrence known as the Koebner phenomenon.

Occupational vitiligo

In some individuals with occupational vitiligo, the leukoderma is confined to the parts of the body exposed to the chemical, usually the hands and forearms. However, in many reported cases, the depigmentation is more extensive and away from areas of skin in which direct contact would be expected. This has given rise to the suggestion that the depigmentation is due to systemic exposure to the chemical, either by percutaneous absorption, inhalation or ingestion. In support of this is the observation that some workers with occupational leukoderma due to *p*-tertiary butylphenol also have had abnormal liver function tests.

The minimum time for skin depigmentation to develop is 2–4 weeks. Laboratory studies suggest that pigment loss through repeated contact with chemicals may take 6 months to become visible. Of several workers with apparently the same level of exposure to a chemical, only a minority will develop occupational leukoderma. The reason for this is not known.

Idiopathic vitiligo is much more common than occupationally-induced leukoderma, although often the two cannot be differentiated on the basis of the clinical pattern of disease.

DIFFERENTIAL DIAGNOSIS

The diagnosis is rarely in doubt due to the distribution and the age of onset of the condition and the hyperpigmented border. In piebaldism, the lesions are present at birth, usually confined to the head and trunk, and do not normally show a hyperpigmented edge. Lichen sclerosus and morphoea are distinguishable as they are characterized by an alteration in the texture of the hypopigmented skin.

Post-inflammatory depigmentation is seen particularly in darkly pigmented races, but can be differentiated by irregular mottling of hypo- and hyperpigmented areas. Contact leukoderma associated with allergic contact dermatitis to hair colourants is recorded [74]. The hypopigmented patches in pityriasis alba and pityriasis versicolor are slightly scaly, and the hypopigmented macules of tuberculoid leprosy are anaesthetic.

TREATMENT

Topical therapy

At the moment, the treatment of vitiligo is unsatisfactory [33]. The use of topical corticosteroids is often recommended; this is effective in some patients and is worth trying, especially if the area of vitiligo is relatively small. The commonest treatment is the use of camouflage cosmetic creams. These can make a big difference to patients and allow them to go out without the cosmetic embarrassment of white patches, but professional advice about the mixing and method of application is needed. Patients with vitiligo in exposed parts should use a sunscreen in sunny weather.

Photochemotherapy

Psoralen photochemotherapy (psoralen and ultraviolet A: 'PUVA') is often suggested for the treatment of vitiligo. This treatment involves the patient either taking psoralen tablets orally or using the psoralen topically, and being exposed to ultra violet irradiation of the 'A' wavelengths. This treatment is usually given three times a week, and the dose of UV-A is increased in an incremental fashion up to a maximum. The risks of this treatment are those of excess sun exposure and can include, if high doses of UV are used, the development of skin cancers.

The response rates to treatment with photochemotherapy differ in the reported clinical trials. In one study, repigmentation rates of 44% were reported, with 61% of those who responded getting more than 50% repigmentation [75]. Another report details that 61% of patients obtained 25% or more repigmentation [76]. A recent British study [77] found that, although 69% of patients noticed some improvement, which was 'significant' in 28%, the relapse rate was high (66%), meaning that only 10% of those treated had a good response without subsequent relapse. At present it does not seem possible to identify prior to treatment those patients who are going to do well without relapse and those who will not.

Khellin/UV-A

An alternative to psoralens is to use khellin. This does not require a phototoxic response to achieve repigmentation. Khellin may be used systemically or topically and with UV-A irradiation or with natural sunlight. However, it has been suggested that topical khellin is no more effective than natural sunlight alone [78] and there are concerns that khellin may be hepatotoxic.

Pseudocatalase and antioxidants

The observation that vitiligo epidermis has low levels of catalase and defective catecholamine metabolism led to the treatment with a topical pseudocatalase [44]. Vitiligo patients treated with a pseudocatalase cream, who also received ultraviolet B and a topical calcium preparation, were reported to show complete repigmentation of the face and dorsa of the hands in 90% of cases. This study has not yet been repeated. Other investigators have used antioxidants such as vitamin E acetate, methionine, selenio-methionine and ubiquinone 10, with the apparent effect of inhibiting the progression of depigmentation in patients with vitiligo [79]. The full results of this trial have not yet been reported.

Melanocyte autotransplantation

The culture of normal melanocytes (Figure 13.6) from the patient with grafting back onto the vitiligo areas is now possible [80], but this treatment remains experimental at present, as the culture methods are difficult and the grafting requires the help of plastic surgeons. It remains to be determined whether melanocyte destruction will follow as a result of renewed autoimmunity in such patients.

Depigmentation

If the degree of vitiligo is extreme, the use of depigmenting agents may be appropriate but this should usually only be considered after referral to a dermatologist.

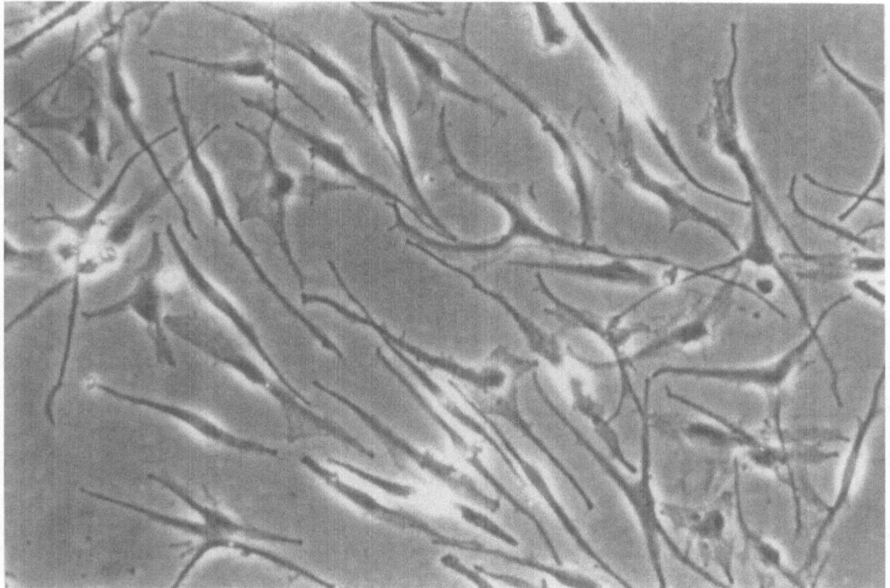

Figure 13.6 Melanocytes from a patient with vitiligo in laboratory culture (courtesy of Miss S.J. Hedley and Dr S. MacNeil)

References

1. Howitz J, Brodthagen H, Schwartz M et al. Prevalence of vitiligo. Arch Dermatol. 1977;113: 47–52.
2. Das SK, Majumder PP, Chakraborty R et al. Studies on vitiligo. I: Epidemiological profile in Calcutta, India. Genet Epidemiol. 1985;2:71–8.
3. Meollmann G, Klein-Angerer S, Scollay DA, Nordlund JJ, Lerner AB. Extracellular granular material and degeneration of keratinocytes in the normally pigmented epidermis of patients with vitiligo. J Invest Dermatol. 1982;79:321–30.
4. Le Poole IC, van den Wijngaard RMJGJ, Westerhof W et al. Presence or absence of melanocytes in vitiligo lesions: an immunohistochemical investigation. J Invest Dermatol. 1993;100:816–22.
5. Bleehen SS. Vitiligo. In: Klaus SN, ed. Pigment Cell, Vol 5. Basel: Karger AG; 1979:54.
6. Ortonne JP, Mosher DB, Fitzpatrick TB. Vitiligo and other hypomelanosis of hair and skin. New York: Plenum Press; 1983:257–8.
7. Butterworth T, Stream LP. Vitiligo. Baltimore: Williams and Wilkins; 1962:4–6.
8. Majumder PP, Das DK, Li CC. A genetic model for vitiligo. Am J Hum Genet. 1988;43:119–25.
9. Majumder PP, Nordlund JJ, Nath SK. Pattern of familial aggregation of vitiligo. Arch Dermatol. 1993;129:994–8.
10. Ando I, Chi HI, Nakagawa H, Otsuka F. Differences in clinical features and HLA antigens between familial and non-familial vitiligo of non-segmental type. Br J Dermatol. 1993;129: 408–10.
11. Orrecchia GL, Perfetti L, Malagoli P et al. Vitiligo is associated with a significant increase in HLA-A30, Cw6 and DQw3 and a decrease in C4AQ0 in Northern Italian patients. Dermatology. 1992;185:123–7.
12. Venkataram MN, White AG, Lenny WA et al. HLA antigens in Omani patients with vitiligo. Clin Exp Dermatol. 1995;20:35–7.
13. Schallreuter KU, Levenig C, Kuhnl P et al. Histocompatibility antigens in vitiligo: Hamburg study on 102 patients from Northern Germany. Dermatology. 1993;187:186–92.
14. Venneker GT, Westerhof W, de Vries IJ et al. Molecular heterogeneity of the fourth component of complement (C4) and its genes in vitiligo. J Invest Dermatol. 1992;99:853–8.
15. Kahl LE, Atkinson JP. Autoimmune aspects of complement deficiency. Clin Aspects Autoimmun. 1988;5:8–20.
16. Cunliffe WJ, Hall DJ, Newell DJ et al. Vitiligo, thyroid disease and autoimmunity. Br J Dermatol. 1968;80:135–9.
17. Parrish JA, Fitzpatrick TB, Shea C et al. Photochemotherapy of vitiligo. Arch Dermatol. 1976;112:1531–4.
18. Dunlop D. Eighty-six cases of Addison's disease. Br Med J. 1963;ii:887–91.
19. Tosti A, Bardazzi F, Tosti G et al. Audiologic abnormalities in cases of vitiligo. J Am Acad Dermatol. 1987;17:230–3.
20. Lerner AB, Halaban R, Klaus SN et al. Transplantation of human melanocytes. J Invest Dermatol. 1987;89:219–24.
21. Macaron C, Winter RJ, Traisman HS et al. Vitiligo and juvenile diabetes mellitus. Arch Dermatol. 1977;113:1515–17.
22. Hegedus L, Heidenheim M, Gervil M et al. High frequency of thyroid dysfunction in patients with vitiligo. Acta Derm Venereol. 1994;74:120–3.
23. Schallreuter KU, Lemke R, Brandt O et al. Vitiligo and other diseases: coexistence or true association? Dermatology. 1994;188:269–75.
24. Neufeld M, Maclaren NK, Blizzard RM. Two types of autoimmune Addison's disease associated with different polyglandular autoimmune syndromes. Medicine (Baltimore). 1981;60:355–62.
25. Ahonen P, Koskimies S, Lokki ML et al. The expression of autoimmune polyglandular disease type I appears associated with several HLA-A antigens but not with HLA-DR. J Clin Endocrinol Metab. 1988;66:1151–7.
26. Tsokos GC, Gorden P, Antonovych T et al. Lupus nephritis and other autoimmune features in patients with diabetes mellitus due to autoantibody to insulin receptors. Ann Intern Med. 1985;102:176–81.
27. Lerner AB. On the etiology of vitiligo and gray hair. Am J Med. 1971;51:141–7.

28. Nordlund JJ, Todes-Taylor N, Albert DM et al. The presence of vitiligo and poliosis in patients with uveitis. J Am Acad Dermatol. 1981;4:528–36.
29. Cowan CL, Halder RM, Grimes PE, Chakrabarti SG, Kenney JA. Ocular disturbances in vitiligo. J Am Acad Dermatol. 1986;15:17–24.
30. Barnes L. Vitiligo and the Vogt–Koyanagi–Harada syndrome. Dermatol Clin. 1988;6:229–39.
31. Frenk E. Depigmentation vitiligineuses chez des patients atteints de melanomes malins. Dermatologica. 1969;1139:84–91.
32. Veharaa M, Mayauchi H, Tanaka S. Diminished contact sensitivity response in vitiliginous skin. Arch Dermatol. 1984;120:195–8.
33. Morelli JG. The cause and treatment of vitiligo. Curr Opin Dermatol. 1995;1:105–8.
34. Ortonne JP, Bose SK. Vitiligo: where do we stand? Pigment Cell Res. 1994;6:61–72.
35. Lerner AB. Vitiligo. J Invest Dermatol. 1959;32:285–310.
36. Al'Abadie MSK, Senior HJ, Bleehen SS, Gawkrodger DJ. Neuropeptide and neuronal marker studies in vitiligo. Br J Dermatol. 1994;131:160–5.
37. Al'Abadie MSK, Warren MA, Bleehen SS, Gawkrodger DJ. Morphologic observations on the dermal nerves in vitiligo: an ultrastructural study. Int J Dermatol. 1995;34:837–40.
38. Mozzanica N, Villa ML, Foppa S et al. Plasma α-melanocyte-stimulating hormone, -endorphin, met-enkephalin and natural killer cell activity in vitiligo. J Am Acad Dermatol. 1992;26:693–700.
39. Bleehen SS, Pathak MA, Hori Y et al. Depigmentation of skin with 4-isopropylcatechol mercaptoamines, and other compounds. J Invest Dermatol. 1968;50:103–17.
40. Schallreuter KU, Wood JM, Ziegler I et al. Defective tetrahydrobiopterin and catecholamine biosynthesis in the depigmentation disorder vitiligo. Biochim Biophys Acta. 1994;1226:181–92.
41. Le Poole C, van der Wijngaard R, Smit NPM et al. Catechol-o-methyltransferase in vitiligo. Arch Dermatol Res. 1994;286:81–6.
42. Schallreuter KU, Wood JM, Pittelkow MR et al. Regulation of melanin biosynthesis in the human epidermis by tetrahydrobiopterin. Science. 1994;2631:21444–6.
43. Schallreuter KU, Wood JM, Berger I. Low catalase levels in the epidermis of patients with vitiligo. J Invest Dermatol. 1991;97:1081–5.
44. Schallreuter KU, Wood JM, Lemke KR, Levenig C. Treatment of vitiligo with a topical application of pseudocatalase and calcium in combination with short-term UVB exposure: a case study on 33 patients. Dermatology. 1995;190:223–9.
45. Naughton GK, Eisenger M, Bystryn JC. Antibodies to normal melanocytes in vitiligo. J Exp Med. 1983;158:246–51.
46. Bystryn JC. Serum antibodies in vitiligo patients. Clin Dermatol. 1989;2:136–45.
47. Harning R, Cui J, Bystryn JC. Relationship between the incidence and level of pigment cell antibodies and disease activity in vitiligo. J Invest Dermatol. 1991;97:1078–80.
48. Cui J, Arita Y, Bystryn JC. Cytolytic antibodies to melanocytes in vitiligo. J Invest Dermatol. 1993;100:812–15.
49. Yu CL, Kao CH, Yu HS. Co-existence and relationship of antikeratinocyte and antimelanocyte antibodies in patients with non-segmental-type vitiligo. J Invest Dermatol. 1993;100:823–8.
50. Abdel Nasser MB, Gollnick H, Orfanos CE. Evidence of primary involvement of keratinocytes in vitiligo. Arch Dermatol Res. 1991;283:47–8.
51. Gilhar A, Zelickson B, Ulman Y, Etzioni A. In vivo destruction of melanocytes by the IgG fraction of serum from patients with vitiligo. J Invest Dermatol. 1995;105:683–6.
52. Song YH, Connor E, Li Y et al. The role of tyrosinase in autoimmune vitiligo. Lancet. 1994;344:1049–52.
53. Grimes PE, Ghoneum M, Stockton T, Payne C, Kelly P, Alfred L. T-cell profiles in vitiligo. J Am Acad Dermatol. 1986;14:196–201.
54. Abdel Nasser MB, Kruger S, Krasagakis K et al. Evidence for involvement of both cell mediated and humoral immunity in generalized vitiligo. J Invest Dermatol. 1991;96:1024.
55. Gross A, Tapis FJ, Mosea W et al. Mononuclear cell subpopulations and infiltrating lymphocytes in erythema dyschromiscum perstans and vitiligo. Histol Histopathol. 1987;2:277–87.
56. Durham-Pierre DG, Walters CS, Halder RM et al. Natural killer cell and lymphokine-associated killer cell activity against melanocytes in vitiligo. J Am Acad Dermatol. 1995;33:26–30.

57. Gilhar A, Aizen E, Ohana N, Etzioni A. Vitiliginous vs pigmented skin response to intradermal administration of interferon gamma. Arch Dermatol. 1993;129:600–4.
58. El Magrabi IAS. Clinical, histological and immunopathological studies on vitiligo. PhD thesis, University of Sheffield, 1990.
59. Norris DA. Cytokine modulation of adhesion molecules in the regulation of immunocytotoxicity of epidermal targets. J Invest Dermatol. 1990;95:111S–20S.
60. Al Badri AMT, Foulis AK, Todd PM et al. Abnormal expression of MHC class II and ICAM-1 by melanocytes in vitiligo. J Pathol. 1993;169:203–6.
61. Campbell IL, Harrison LC. Molecular pathology of type I diabetes. Mol Biol Med. 1990;7: 299–309.
62. Zheng RQH, Abney ER, Grubeck-Loebenstein B et al. Expression of intercellular adhesion molecule-1 and lymphocyte function-associated antigen-3 on human thyroid epithelial cells in Graves' and Hashimoto's diseases. J Autoimmun. 1990;3:727–36.
63. Nakazawa K, Bonnard M, Damour O, Collombel C. Functional role of E-cadherin in melanocyte-keratinocyte adhesion in vitro. Melanoma Res. 1995;5(2):40.
64. Morelli JG, Kincannon J, Yohn JJ et al. Leukotriene C4 and TGF-α are stimulators of human melanocyte migration in vivo. J Invest Dermatol. 1992;98:290–5.
65. Morelli JG, Yohn JJ, Zekman T, Norris DA. Melanocyte movement in vitro: role of matrix proteins and integrin receptors. J Invest Dermatol. 1993;101:605–8.
66. Hedley SJ, Gawkrodger DJ, Weetman AP, MacNeil S. Extracellular matrix proteins stimulate melanocyte tyrosinase. Melanoma Res. 1995;5(2):38–9.
67. Lerner AB, Shiohara T, Boissy RE et al. A mouse model for vitiligo. J Invest Dermatol. 1986; 87:299–304.
68. Gilhar A, Pillar T, Eidelman S, Etzioni A. Vitiligo and idiopathic guttate hypomelanosis. Repigmentation of skin following engraftment onto nude mice. Arch Dermatol. 1989;125: 1363–6.
69. Oliver EA, Schwartz L, Warren LH. Occupational leukoderma. Arch Dermatol Syphilol. 1940;101:163–9.
70. Malten KE, Seutter E, Hara I, Nakajima T. Occupational vitiligo due to paratertiary butyl phenol and homologues. Trans St John's Dermatol Soc. 1971;57:115–31.
71. Gellin GA, Possick PA, Perone VB. Depigmentation from 4-tertiary butyl catechol. J Invest Dermatol. 1970;55:190–7.
72. Nordlund JJ, Lerner AB. Vitiligo: is it important? Arch Dermatol. 1982;118:5–8.
73. Barona MI, Arrunategui A, Falabella R, Alzate A. An epidemiological case–control study in a population with vitiligo. J Am Acad Dermatol. 1995;33:621–5.
74. Taylor JS, Maibach HI, Fisher AA, Bergfeld WF. Contact leukoderma associated with the use of hair colors. Cutis. 1993;52:273–80.
75. Grimes PE. Vitiligo: an overview of therapeutic approaches. Dermatol Clin. 1993;11:325–38.
76. Wildfang IL, Jacobsen FK, Thestrup-Pedersen K. PUVA treatment of vitiligo: a retrospective study of 59 patients. Acta Derm Venereol. 1992;72:305–6.
77. Anstey A, Hawk JLM. PUVA treatment of vitiligo. Br J Dermatol. 1994;131(44):18.
78. Orrecchia G, Perfetti L. Photochemotherapyy with topical khellin and sunlight in vitiligo. Dermatology. 1992;184:120–3.
79. Passi S, Picardo M, De Luca M et al. Treatment of vitiligo with an antioxidant pool. Melanoma Res. 1995;5(2):25.
80. Zachariae H, Zachariae C, Deleuran B, Kristensen P. Autotransplantation in vitiligo: treatment with epidermal grafts and cultured melanocytes. Acta Derm Venereol. 1993;73: 46–8.

Index

A.P. Weetman (ed.), Endocrine Autoimmunity and Associated Conditions. 285–292.

Immunology and Medicine Series

1. A.M. McGregor (ed.). *Immunology of Endocrine Diseases.* 1986 ISBN: 0-85200-963-1
2. L. Ivanyi (ed.). *Immunological Aspects of Oral Diseases.* 1986 ISBN: 0-85200-961-5
3. M.A.H. French (ed.). *Immunoglobulins in Health and Disease.* 1986 ISBN: 0-85200-962-3
4. K. Whaley (ed.). *Complement in Health and Disease.* 1987 ISBN: 0-85200-954-2
5. G.R.D. Catto (ed.). *Clinical Transplantation: Current Practice and Future Prospects.* 1987 ISBN: 0-85200-960-7
6. V.S. Byers and R.W. Baldwin (eds.). *Immunology of Malignant Diseases.* 1987 ISBN: 0-85200-964-X
7. S.T. Holgate (ed.). *Mast Cells, Mediators and Disease.* 1988 ISBN: 0-85200-968-2
8. D.J.M. Wright (ed.). *Immunology of Sexually Transmitted Diseases.* 1988 ISBN: 0-74620-087-0
9. A.D.B. Webster (ed.). *Immunodeficiency and Disease.* 1988 ISBN: 0-85200-688-8
10. C. Stern (ed.). *Immunology of Pregnancy and its Disorders.* 1989 ISBN: 0-7462-0065-X
11. M.S. Klempner, B. Styrt and J. Ho (eds.). *Phagocytes and Disease.* 1989 ISBN: 0-85200-842-2
12. A.J. Zuckerman (ed.). *Recent Developments in Prophylactic Immunization.* 1989 ISBN: 0-7923-8910-7
13. S. Lightman (ed.). *Immunology of Eye Disease.* 1989 ISBN: 0-7923-8908-5
14. T.J. Hamblin (ed.). *Immunotherapy of Disease.* 1990 ISBN: 0-7462-0045-5
15. D.B. Jones and D.H. Wright (eds.). *Lymphoproliferative Diseases.* 1990 ISBN: 0-85200-965-8
16. C.D. Pusey (ed.). *Immunology of Renal Diseases.* 1991 ISBN: 0-7923-8964-6
17. A.G. Bird (ed.). *Immunology of HIV Infection.* 1991 ISBN: 0-7923-8962-X
18. J.T. Whicher and S.W. Evans (eds.). *Biochemistry of Inflammation.* 1992 ISBN: 0-7923-8985-9
19. T.T. MacDonald (ed.). *Immunology of Gastrointestinal Diseases.* 1992 ISBN: 0-7923-8961-1
20. K. Whaley, M. Loos and J.M. Weiler (eds.). *Complement in Health and Disease, 2nd Edn.* 1993 ISBN: 0-7923-8823-2
21. H.C. Thomas and J. Waters (eds.). *Immunology of Liver Disease.* 1994 ISBN: 0-7923-8975-1
22. G.S. Panayi (ed.). *Immunology of Connective Tissue Diseases.* 1994 ISBN: 0-7923-8988-3
23. G. Scadding (ed.). *Immunology of ENT Disorders.* 1994 ISBN: 0-7923-8914-X
24. R. Hohlfeld (ed.). *Immunology of Neuromuscular Disease.* 1994 ISBN: 0-7923-8844-5
25. J.G.P. Sissons, L.K. Borysiewicz and J. Cohen (eds.). *Immunology of Infection.* 1994 ISBN: 0-7923-8968-9
26. J.G.J. van de Winkel and P.M. Hogarth (eds.). *The Immunoglobulin Receptors and their Physiological and Pathological Roles in Immunity.* 1998 ISBN: 0-7923-5021-9
27. A.P. Weetman (ed.). *Endocrine Autoimmunity and Associated Conditions.* 1998 ISBN: 0-7923-5042-1

Kluwer Academic Publishers – Dordrecht / Boston / London